Praise for *Health at E*

"*Health at Every Size* is a must-read for bot[...]
sional dieter, as well as for health care professionals who readily give advice about weight loss, but know little about the actual impact of dieting on metabolism, weight, and health. Bacon challenges the false promises of the weight-loss industry and translates the science underlying the health-at-every-size movement into practical, easily digestible truths. From the politics of fat and food, to the facts about the human body's instinctive response to starvation, this timely resource helps readers understand how to heal their relationship to food and to their bodies, and to commit to good health instead of wasting time and energy dieting."

—MARGO MAINE, PhD, FAED, psychologist, coauthor of several books,
including *The Body Myth: Adult Women and the Pressure to Be Perfect*
and *Body Wars: Making Peace with Women's Bodies*

"Dr. Linda Bacon has done what very few other 'diet book' authors have ever done: She has conducted legitimate academic research to show what happens in the real world with real people who try the HAES approach. And what happens should give us all hope. In the midst of all the hype, the fads, the panic, and the confusion, there emerges a quiet and simple way to make peace with one's body, improve health, and get on with life. It works, it lasts, and it is a way to put all the craziness to rest. Thank you, Dr. Bacon!"

—DEB BURGARD, PhD, psychologist, coauthor of *Great Shape: The First Fitness
Guide for Large Women*, Founder of the BodyPositive.com

"In our body-obsessed culture, *Health at Every Size* is a breath of fresh air. Linda Bacon reminds us of a core truth: Our bodies will naturally gravitate toward health if we could only hear what they're saying above the cacophony of media and advertising."

—ANNA LAPPÉ, coauthor of *Grub: Ideas for an Organic Kitchen* and *Hope's Edge:
The Next Diet for a Small Planet*

"Outstanding! Dr. Bacon offers a compelling and comprehensive understanding of why we are the weight we are and how to maximize our physical and emotional well-being. Based on solid scientific research, Bacon provides us with new concepts that will forever change the way we think about hunger, nourishment, and weight regulation."

—JUDITH MATZ AND ELLEN FRANKEL, psychotherapists, authors of *The Diet
Survivor's Handbook: 60 Lessons in Eating, Acceptance and Self-Care* and *Beyond
a Shadow of a Diet: The Therapist's Guide to Treating Compulsive Eating*

"There are thousands of self-help books directed at plus-sized people, who make up two-thirds of humanity. Nearly every one of these books promises to trim away your body fat, and as a result improve your health and life satisfaction. Every one of these books is a sham. *Health at Every Size* differs from all the rest because it offers a new road to travel, one that will lead you to better health and a better life. This revolutionary book is based on a solid foundation of biomedical research. The book is true to the real science, not the press releases from diet promoters that pass for health news today. Readers will achieve a new understanding of how their bodies really work and how to work with your body and not against it to achieve better balance in life."

—PAUL ERNSBERGER, PHD, researcher/professor,
Case Western Reserve School of Medicine

"Linda Bacon's book is a major contribution to the health-at-every-size movement. Any person contemplating going on a diet to lose weight should read this book first. Every health professional who counsels people about weight control should absolutely read this book, read it again, and make sure [his or her] clients read it. It's a dogma-busting book that provides a sensible alternative to mainstream fairytales of easily attainable weight loss for all, and offers reassurance to all those who have struggled with their weight that the road to a fitter and healthier body is wide enough for everyone."

—GLENN GAESSER, PHD, researcher/professor, Arizona State University, author
of *Big Fat Lies: The Truth About Your Weight and Your Health*

"Linda Bacon deftly exposes the $50 billion lie of the diet industry. In plain language, she describes the indisputable science behind why millions of Americans' failed attempts to lose weight is hardly the result of personal failing, and how if we'd just get out of the way, our bodies already know how to be healthy. Indeed, the nation's collective obsession with the alleged 'obesity epidemic' (another myth Bacon convincingly debunks) is only distracting us from facing the true menace—an industrialized food system driven solely by profit motive. Anyone who has suffered through endless weight-loss programs should read this book and follow Bacon's simple, commonsense guide to better health, improved self-esteem, and the enjoyment of real food as a source of nourishment."

—MICHELE SIMON, JD, MPH, public health attorney, author of *Appetite for Profit: How the Food Industry Undermines Our Health and How to Fight Back*

"At a time when there is tremendous medical and media pressure to be extremely thin, Linda Bacon's new book *Health at Every Size* comes as a breath of fresh air. She insists that, for people of all sizes, the focus needs to be on health, not weight. It needs to be on acceptance and self-respect, not trying to change their bodies to fit 'society's hurtful standards.' The section 'Respect Yourself, Body and Soul' is especially valuable for women caught up in appearance issues. Rather than dieting and waiting to be thin, a clear set-up for failure, Dr. Bacon encourages women to let go of magical thinking and start living life fully now, in their present bodies. Trying to achieve respect and happiness through weight loss 'provides a hollow and tenuous victory, not the core satisfaction that you are really seeking,' she says. 'Cultivate a value system that puts appearance in its place and honors bodies for more than their packaging.' She assures readers that feeling good about themselves is motivating for making healthy changes, unlike punishing or shaming themselves. 'When you feel better about yourself, you make better choices.'"

—FRANCES M. BERG, MS, nutritionist and professor, author of several books, including *Women Afraid to Eat: Breaking Free in Today's Weight-Obsessed World* and *Underage and Overweight: America's Childhood Obesity Crisis—What Every Family Needs to Know*, editor of the Healthy Weight Network

"Free at last! Here's liberation from the tyranny of useless weight-loss regimens and the feelings of failure they provoke. Linda Bacon offers a welcome, practical alternative to obsessing about your weight and shape—eating and exercising according to your body's built-in wisdom. She shows you how to enjoy sound health and unstoppable self-esteem whatever size your body may be. If you're ready to escape from self-loathing and discover the pleasures of self-affirmation, toss out those diet books and dump the bathroom scale. Treat yourself to this sane and friendly guide, scientifically proven to help you make peace with your body, improve your health, and nourish all of who you are."

—LISA SARASOHN, bodywork and yoga therapist, author of *The Woman's Belly Book: Finding Your True Center for More Energy, Confidence, and Pleasure*

"*Health at Every Size* is essential reading for anyone who believes that health or happiness depends on weight. The truth will not only surprise you, but set you free."

—PEGGY ELAM, PHD, psychologist, publisher, Pearlsong Press

"A compassionate yet critical look at how the converging forces of science, economics, and culture drive the weight-loss industry and ultimately undermine the very goal an individual seeks—physical and emotional health. Written by a scientist who has been in the trenches as a dieter struggling through the weight-loss gauntlet. Here's a solution to help you off the dieting treadmill with your sanity intact."

—EVELYN TRIBOLE, MS, RD, nutrition therapist, author of several books, including *Intuitive Eating: A Revolutionary Program That Works* and *Stealth Health: How to Sneak Nutrition Painlessly into Your Diet*

"Dr. Bacon has amazing evidence and shares it with you: Feeding yourself well and trusting your body works better—lots better—than starving yourself and trying to force your weight down. If you are caught in a struggle with your weight, this book shows you the way out."

—ELLYN SATTER, MS, RD, LCSW, BCD, therapist, author of several books, including *Secrets of Feeding a Healthy Family: Orchestrating and Enjoying the Family Meal* and *Your Child's Weight: Helping Without Harming*

"Read this book and it will stop you in your tracks toward weight loss with health as your new goal. Make peace with your body and move on with the rest of your life."

—LINDA OMICHINSKI, RD, founder, Hugs International, author of several books, including *You Count, Calories Don't* and *Staying Off the Diet Rollercoaster*

"Linda Bacon's groundbreaking experiment proved what many of us had discovered in our own lives and work: that learning to honor our bodies and their messages is better for our health than any diet, pill, or operation. Bacon reveals the financial interests fueling body hatred and poor nutrition. She offers many suggestions, facts, and even documents to help people befriend and enjoy their bodies, while also benefiting the health of the earth. Her keen intelligence, strong curiosity, and the powerful, healing commitment of someone who's been there and now helps others, provide a wealth of information and support for readers of any size."

—BARBARA ALTMAN BRUNO, PhD, ACSW, clinical social worker, author of *Worth Your Weight: What You Can Do About a Weight Problem*

"If you have ever been on a diet, you have successfully and thoroughly tested the many, endlessly appearing weight-loss programs. They have failed us. We did what they said. Each and every program fails almost every one of us—they were not capable of delivering on their promise. Dr. Linda Bacon delivers! With solid, clearly explained research, she tells us what works, over a lifetime, is reasonable and doable. *Health at Every Size* is a MUST-READ for each and every person who has ever wanted a different body!"

—BONNIE BERNELL, EdD, psychologist, author of *Bountiful Women: Large Women's Secrets for Living the Life They Desire*

"*Health at Every Size* will change your life! Linda Bacon has painstakingly explained, in understandable language, data from hundreds of sources to help us at long last end the war we've waged against our bodies. Her wise guidance goes beyond enlightening us—it provides a recipe for transforming our lives, our comfort in our own skin, and our health irrelevant of weight. Every person beyond childhood needs a copy of this book!"

—DORIS SMELTZER, MA, psychotherapist, author of *Andrea's Voice: Silenced by Bulimia* and the Gurze Book's "Advice for Parents" blog

"Dr. Bacon's approach to the complex and often self-contradictory questions of body habitus vis-à-vis diet is well thought out, well explained, and offers a revolutionary approach. Her bottom line is that we must not be intimidated by the cultural mores and by those who would take advantage of [us] for monetary gain and, instead, should focus on the positives of the hands we are dealt, i.e., our bodies, and concentrate on maximizing our individual health, both physical and psychological. Her book is informative, instructive, and motivational. I believe it is unique. I can think of many instances in my thirty-five years of practicing orthopedic surgery where this book, the messages of which to some extent I did offer my patients on my own, would have been a wonderful adjunct in the often long and difficult road to joint replacement surgery."

—DAVID HELLER, MD, orthopedic surgeon

"*Health at Every Size* is eye-opening. I was not aware of much of the research indicating that body fat is not the death sentence many of us in the health professions are led to believe. Anyone who wants to lose weight needs to read this book. I will be urging many of my friends and colleagues to do so."

—JACK NORRIS, RD, director, Vegan Outreach

"*Health at Every Size: The Surprising Truth About Your Weight* is a fascinating insight into the complex issues of health and weight. In this book, Linda Bacon has managed to investigate the biological, sociological, cultural, economic, and political aspects of this issue, yet somehow managed to keep it highly readable and interesting. *Health at Every Size* dismantles some of the biggest myths about weight and health, and provides a positive pathway forward for anyone [who] wants to maximize [his or her] health and well being."

—LILY O'HARA, faculty, University of the Sunshine Coast

"A great manifesto of health, based on a deeply humanistic worldview."

—CHRISTIAN BACHMANN, author and Web master, Med Journal Watch

"We are bombarded from every direction about how awful the obesity epidemic is, how much obesity leads to poor health, and how much obesity increases medical care costs. There is enormous bias and discrimination related to obesity, and those who are obese are often considered to lack willpower. After all, the story goes, if they really wanted to do so, they could lose weight. The data are clear, and the obesity epidemic is a fact; but our strategies for dealing with it are not working and may be counterproductive. I believe that Dr. Bacon identifies a much better approach to addressing the obesity epidemic, and these principles are clearly described in *Health at Every Size*. Dr. Bacon encourages size acceptance, and focusing on healthful eating and regular physical activity, with less emphasis on the scale. Her recommendations are sound and should be widely adopted. Let us get off the soap box of ranting about how bad obesity is, and turn our attention to healthful habits."

—STEVEN BLAIR, MD, professor, University of South Carolina

"You weren't born with a user's manual for living happily and in good health. What do you eat? What exercise do you do? How do you think and feel about your body? I'm tempted to say that this book writes the chapters on these crucial questions for the user's manual. What you hold here is even better—a description and proof of how you (and your body) are already the best possible how-to guide available. Linda Bacon's *Health at Every Size* is a humane and necessary resource for everybody."

—MARILYN WANN, activist, author of *Fat!So?: Because You Don't Have to Apologize for Your Size*

"A more sensible approach to thinking about body weight regulation than the current mainstream view and a welcome change from the diet-of-the-month roller coaster. Perfect for repeat dieters looking for a new path and those interested in taking the first step toward size acceptance."

—SONDRA SOLOVAY, JD, author of *Tipping the Scales of Justice: Fighting Weight-Based Discrimination,* director, Fat Legal Advocacy, Rights and Education Project

"In *Health at Every Size,* Linda Bacon offers a fascinating exploration of the science behind weight gain and loss, or more to the point, why we have such a hard time losing weight and keeping it off. The *coup de grace,* though, is her presentation of an approach to giving up the weight struggle and getting on with your life in a healthy, happy way. If you want to end weight worries, buy this book."

—MARSHA HUDNALL, MS, RD, CD, program director, Green Mountain at Fox Run

"Dr. Bacon eloquently provides readers with a clear understanding of the science regarding the body's physiological response to restrictive dieting and excellent tools for building a new relationship with one's self in respect to food, body image, physical activity, and attitude."

—MARCI GETZ, MPH, health educator

"Every person considering a diet should first read Dr. Bacon's book *Health at Every Size.* Dr. Bacon does an excellent job of explaining the science behind the failure of dieting to successfully maintain weight loss. She offers an alternative health model that takes the emphasis off of weight, and results in people enjoying food and physical activity and making peace with their bodies. Well done Dr. Bacon!"

–CONNIE SOBCZAK, director, The Body Positive

"Now, I finally have a concise clear source for my clients who are casualties of the 'war on obesity.' In *Health at Every Size,* Linda Bacon introduces the concept of self-care and body appreciation for every body of every size! This is a profoundly new way to make peace with our bodies and with food. This is the end to the battle of the bulge."

—KELLY BLISS, MED, ACE, psychotherapist, author of *Don't Weight: Eat Healthy and Get Moving Now!* and *Kelly Bliss' Yellow Pages*

"One would think that with as much emphasis in advertising and public health policy on weight loss that a great deal of research has been done as to the benefits of dieting for weight loss. One would think that logically, but one would be wrong. While statistical correlations between weight and health are constantly being calculated, the truth is very little direct study has been done regarding dieting, weight loss, and health. *Health at Every Size* is based upon groundbreaking research by Linda Bacon, PhD, which set out to see if going on a diet really makes one healthier. What Bacon's research discovered is what every fat person who has spent years conducting [his or her] own personal experiments already knew: *Diets Don't Work*. This book should revolutionize America's obsession with weight!"

—PATTIE THOMAS, PHD, coauthor of *Taking Up Space: How Eating Well and Exercising Regularly Changed My Life*

"This book will revolutionize the way people think about what it means to be at a "healthy weight." Linda Bacon is at the forefront of an exciting new field of research that is debunking many of the myths about weight and health: myths that combine to make Americans less healthy, less happy, and often heavier than they would otherwise be. As Dr. Bacon illustrates, the key to a happy, healthy weight is to recognize that one person's own "ideal" weight is quite independent of—and often radically different than—that of other people's. This simple but powerful idea is crucial to understanding what it means to achieve health at every size."

—PAUL CAMPOS, professor of law, University of Colorado, and author of *The Obesity Myth: Why America's Obsession With Weight Is Hazardous To Your Health*

"Dr. Linda Bacon's *Health at Every Size* makes laudable strides toward a long overdue revolution of the diet industry and the war we have waged against our bodies. She eloquently details the science of nourishing oneself and maintaining a healthy body amidst a culture fraught with political and economically driven agendas. With scientific reasoning accessible to a popular audience and abundant data to support her arguments, this book is a must-read not only for people struggling with their weight, but also for those in the health care profession who treat people struggling with their weight. This book is a sobering reality check of the unforeseen consequences of America's obsession with weight, and more importantly, *Health at Every Size* provides a tenable solution."

—JANELL MENSINGER, PHD, director, Office of Research, The Reading Hospital and Medical Center

"*Health at Every Size: The Surprising Truth About Your Weight* is the book we've all been waiting for. Dr. Linda Bacon has translated complicated information about the physiology of weight, food, dieting, and eating into manageable, understandable language. She intersperses her own life experiences into the text, making her book highly personal and readable. The interactive checklists will help individuals put the *Health at Every Size* concepts into practice immediately. I plan to recommend this book to all my clients and colleagues."

—ELLYN HERB, PhD, CEDS, psychologist and eating disorder specialist

"For years, Linda Bacon has been the voice of reason to professionals working with clients who have eating, exercise, and body-image problems. We now have a great way to offer that same assistance to our clients. *Health at Every Size* will definitely be on the 'Top 10 Recommended' list I give to clients."

—LAURA MCKIBBIN, MSW, LISW, clinical social worker

"Packed full of surprising but convincing information about nutrition, food politics, and fat politics, *Health at Every Size* is an eye-opener. Linda Bacon cuts right through the lies, half-truths, biased reports, and questionable science about eating and exercise, and teaches us how to treat our bodies with genuine care and respect."

—KATE HARDING, co-creator, Shapely Prose blog

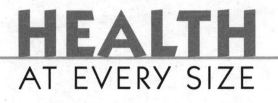

HEALTH
AT EVERY SIZE

HEALTH

AT EVERY SIZE

The Surprising Truth About Your Weight

Linda Bacon, PhD

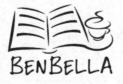

BENBELLA BOOKS, INC.
Dallas, TX

Copyright © 2008 by Linda Bacon, PhD
Additional Materials © 2010 by Linda Bacon, PhD

BenBella Books, Inc.
10440 N. Central Expressway, Suite 800
Dallas, TX 75231
www.benbellabooks.com
Send feedback to feedback@benbellabooks.com

Printed in the United States of America
20 19 18 17 16 15 14 13 12 11

Library of Congress Cataloging-in-Publication Data is available for this title.
ISBN 978-1-935618-25-6

Proofreading by Stacia Seaman, Emily Brown, and Yara Abuata
Cover design by Allison Bard
Text design and composition by PerfecType, Nashville, TN
Index by Shoshana Hurwitz
Printed by Lake Book Manufacturing

Distributed to the trade by Two Rivers Distribution, an Ingram brand
tworiversdistribution.com

Special discounts for bulk sales (minimum of 25 copies) are available.
Please contact bulkorders@benbellabooks.com.

TABLE OF CONTENTS

DEDICATION

For Meg Tara Webster, a role model for a life well lived.

I asked Meg to help me live more fully in the present. She advised that I choose an ordinary action and imbue it with meaning. Each time I did this action, I was to take a few deep breaths and appreciate the present. I chose a challenging action to serve as this cue, something I do many times each day: beginning and ending work on my computer. This process has been invaluable to me as I've written this book, helping me to be productive and appreciative of the work and also supporting me in letting go of my work at appropriate times.

The value of cultivating an appreciation for the present has become even more painfully vivid to me as I watch Meg bravely confront her mortality, providing yet another lesson in how to live life with gratitude, immediacy, authenticity, and heart.

Thank you, Meg, for your contribution to this book and to my world.

MEG TARA WEBSTER
Died 10/8/08

PREFACE

I am tempted to weigh myself, to reassure myself and you, the reader, that I am qualified to write a book about weight regulation and can lead you through your own journey of understanding and making peace with your body. Withstanding the temptation has at times been like the fight of an alcoholic to stay sober, the drive a clear statement of the insidious nature of the cultural attitudes that have lodged inside my psyche.

Only through extraordinary effort and education have I been able to free myself from my obsession with weight. Starting in early adolescence, I stayed abreast of the day-to-day differences on the scale. Convinced that I would be more popular if I weighed less, I started dieting to escape a weight problem that existed only in my head. I would endure weeks on a semi-starvation diet until my desperation for food drove me to eat everything in sight. I thought there was something deeply wrong with me because I could not control my unrelenting drive to eat.

Despite my preoccupation with losing weight and my repeated attempts to shed pounds, however, the scale continued to document my failure. My weight inched up. My self-esteem plummeted.

Both my parents are well practiced in the art of weight loss. During many dinners, I watched my mom exhibit extraordinary self-control, barely eating or nursing her shrimp cocktail, while the rest of us dined on course after course of sumptuous, heavy restaurant foods. The next day a large bag of potato chips would mysteriously disappear from the pantry. My dad was also adept. He would order his turkey sandwich dry and then carefully remove a piece of bread, only to experience an attack of the munchies later at home, where he would wolf down ice cream and cookies.

But I don't blame them for my own dieting history. If I didn't get it from them, I doubt I would have escaped the culture outside our home.

My pain regarding my weight reached an intolerable level by the time I was in college. I became convinced that if only I could lose weight, I could change my life. And so my life deteriorated as I obsessed about food and activity to the detriment of my studies and social relationships. I weighed myself daily and let the scale determine my mood.

My junior year of college, when I studied for a year in India, was a turning point. My surface reason for going was a fascination with India's spiritual traditions and the hope for discovering some sense of inner peace. But I was even more motivated by the idea of escaping my family, friends, and social insecurities so that I could diet in earnest. I naïvely pictured myself meditating and rising above earthly needs, especially food.

For short periods, I did find solace. Even better (or so I believed at the time), I accomplished my goal: returning to the United States thin. It only took a few months, however, for my weight to zoom back to its previous level—and then higher.

My pain preoccupied me so completely that I felt little choice in deciding on a course of study when I returned to college. To save myself, I became determined to understand everything I could about weight regulation.

At first, I studied the cultural issues, which taught me the "why" behind my body image issues. I came to understand that the shame I felt about my body was part of the North American female experience, reflective of a cultural pathology regarding a woman's appearance. Since that time, cultural pressure on women has bumped up several notches, with accompanying pressure on men, many of whom now share women's eating and body image dissatisfaction.

I then earned a master's degree in psychotherapy, with a specialty in eating disorders and body image, and worked as a psychotherapist.

I learned more about myself: how I often turned to food for solace, how it had served as a crutch to protect me from pain, and how it had become a close companion I counted on. My body fat served as a convenient excuse for avoiding intimacy and new challenges. It was also a punching bag to blame when anything went wrong. I learned that I didn't have an eating problem, but I clearly had a problem taking care of myself.

As this wasn't a problem of psychology alone, I went back to school. This time I earned a master's degree in exercise science, specializing in metabolism. I became aware that exercise had turned into a "workout" for me, a means for weight control, and that I had lost the joy I remembered from playing sports and being generally active as a youth.

At the same time, I learned that exercise programs are not the definitive panacea for weight control. Both research and personal observation document many heavy people excelling in sports or just exercising regularly—and not losing weight. I learned to differentiate weight from health: Body weight might be a marker for an imprudent lifestyle in some people, but its role in determining health, particularly when compared to regular activity, is grossly exaggerated.

I subsequently continued to broaden my education and went on to complete a doctoral program in physiology with a focus on nutrition and weight regulation. There, too, I learned dramatically new ideas: that dieting wasn't healthy, nor did it achieve long-term weight loss; and that modern food processing often diminishes the quality of foods, thus disrupting our health and encouraging weight gain. I was shocked to note that dramatic scientific advances frequently failed to reach the general public or influence public health policy and recommendations.

Every discipline I studied revealed the same disconnect: The science of weight regulation directly contradicts cultural assumptions as well as those promoted by the "experts." It is not surprising that so many Americans are unsuccessful in their weight-loss attempts and confused about how to achieve their goals.

My experiences and academic training led me to an entirely different paradigm in weight regulation, where I finally found relief from my painful preoccupation with food and losing weight. I not only recovered from my obsession, but I even managed to develop a healthy and pleasurable relationship with my body and with food. The scale no longer holds the power to weigh my self-esteem.

Food is simple now. I appreciate the sensuality and pleasure of eating. When I am full, I typically lose interest in food. After a few magical bites of chocolate, I am satisfied and the drive dissipates. When I finish eating, I rarely think about food until I am hungry again. I don't feel guilty afterward.

And I take pleasure in my body. I move because it feels good. I enjoy being touched. I dress in clothes that I like and don't consider whether or not they hide my fat.

As wonderful as food is, it is only one of many pleasures in my life. I am no longer waiting to lose weight before I live my life fully. Having freed up all the energy and time that I spent on dieting or obsessing about my weight or food and having let go of my shame about these, I have greater depth and fulfillment in my life, including deeper intimacy with others.

I don't think about my weight, and it stays fairly consistent. Oddly, after this new eating pattern became firmly rooted, I actually lost about thirty pounds—but the difference was, I wasn't trying.*

I am fortunate to have survived my food and weight obsession, but I am still haunted by the pain of others. I was luckier than many people. I was too young to be offered amphetamines, and I recovered before the even more insidious diet drugs were routinely prescribed. Though I received some social condemnation for my size, I was never fat enough to suffer the more intense pain and ridicule routinely experienced by heavier girls and women. I didn't get my jaw wired, my stomach stapled or banded, my intestines shortened, nor did I get injections of pregnant mare's urine. (Believe it or not, this was a very popular diet aid from the mid-seventies until recently.)

---

*You've heard this before. Every book about weight starts with the weight loss testimonial. It gets your hopes up and sells books. And when it doesn't work the same way for you, that's always your fault—you must have done something wrong, if you didn't get the same results. So let me be clear: My weight-loss results aren't typical, and I don't mean to use my experience to promote any weight loss technique. I'll be talking about this more later in the book.

I empathize with the many others engaged in their own personal battle with food and weight. This preoccupation sucks the fun out of life. It saddens me that shame and anxiety regarding the scale and mirror overshadow most people's enjoyment of food, their comfort in their bodies, and their full development as individuals.

Many of us have a disturbing preoccupation with food and an intense fear of being fat. Instead of eating for enjoyment and fuel, we regard food as our enemy, as a test of our resolve and willpower— and even of our moral superiority. Instead of moving for the sheer joy of feeling our bodies and our power, we view exercise as a work-out, our penance for eating or weighing too much. Instead of putting our energy into thinking about how we can improve the world, we obsess about how we can change our bodies.

The degree of ignorance and deception that is practiced by health care providers and the weight-loss industry angers me. The health care community and U.S. public policy have fed our fears. Dietitians, under the auspices of the Department of Health and Human Services and the National Institutes of Health, provide us with calorie restriction diets and a food pyramid to direct our choices. Exercise physiologists, with guidance from the Centers for Disease Control and Prevention, give us prescriptions for target heart rates and calorie burning goals. Even psychologists and psychotherapists exhort us to use their behavior-modification techniques to moderate our eating habits. The former top health authority in the United States, Surgeon General Richard Carmona, labels obesity as the "terror within," naming it to be "every bit as threatening to us as is the terrorist threat we face today."

Because every authority and institution urges us to fight fat, weight control is no longer merely a public health issue, but a moral imperative. From every pulpit of weight control we hear a singular message: Follow my plan, you'll lose weight, improve your health, become a better person, and have a happier life.

Dieting has become such a major force in our cultural landscape that most people view weight control as the normal, right thing to do. While exercising may not be as common, we are all certainly aware that we should exercise and feel the guilt of not doing enough.

Americans desperately want to lose weight—no doubt about that. Our failure to do so is certainly not for lack of trying. Collectively, we spend about $59 billion per year on weight-loss programs and products. We invest an enormous amount of time and energy on our weight-loss goals.

Despite these efforts, we just keep getting fatter and fatter. Until the very recent leveling off, we had several decades of unprecedented weight gain. As the national waistline grew, so did the bottom line of the weight-loss industry.

Although I also fell into the trap of believing what the "experts" told me, I now know how misinformed they are and how damaging their message is. *Health at Every Size* is my attempt to correct America's "weight problem." The answer has nothing to do with dieting or self-denial and everything to do with eating and self-affirmation.

Naming the roots of weight gain is not complicated: Weight gain occurs whenever the food energy we take in exceeds the energy our bodies spend. This maxim is basic biological fact, an application of the well-established first law of thermodynamics.

The conventional approach to weight loss exploits the obvious, directing us to eat less and/or exercise more. As logical as it may seem in theory, it has become increasingly clear that it just does not work. Something is undermining our ability to control our weight.

Recent breakthroughs in scientific research provide the explanation. We now know that weight gain is in part a biologically induced result of the dietary habits that are currently encouraged and common among Americans. Dieting activates "thrifty genes" that induce weight gain, both by increasing your hunger drive and decreasing your metabolism, and triggers other weight-gain mechanisms, many of which are beyond your conscious control. Also, some food choices that have become increasingly common bypass your internal weight-regulation system: Since their calories don't register, eating them can result in an insatiable appetite, even when sufficient (or more than sufficient) calories are consumed.

Dieting is not only ineffective at producing long-term weight loss and satisfaction, but actually promotes the opposite. "Common wisdom" has led us down the wrong path.

Researchers have actually located the control centers in our brain that regulate our weight and identified many of the pathways through which they exert control. We can name the hormones released by fat cells to inform a control center whenever body fat is lost. We can also trace the neurotransmitters released after fat loss that increase our appetite and decrease our metabolism, ultimately leading to weight regain.

This information substantiates what millions of Americans know from personal experience: Diets are a setup for failure—even the more "sensible" diet plans commonly encouraged by health care practitioners. It really isn't your fault that you can't keep lost weight off; your body is simply doing its best to protect and support you!

The news that your body undermines your efforts at weight control is actually good, because it also indicates that your body is enormously successful at manipulating your weight. You can harness that power to your advantage. Your body is ready to help you achieve a healthy weight, if you simply allow it to do its job. You can reclaim sensitivity to its signals, and you can also adopt lifestyle habits, such as changing the types of food you eat and your activity habits, that will improve your health and support you in achieving and maintaining the weight that is right for you.

In other words, the best way to win the war against fat is to give up the fight. Turn over control to your body and you will settle at a healthy weight. And regardless of whether you do lose weight, your health and well-being will markedly improve. You will find that biology is much more powerful than willpower.

Health at Every Size: The Surprising Truth About Your Weight describes the new scientific discoveries and provides you with practical, research-based advice to reconceptualize and permanently overcome your weight problem. It is intended to educate you, support you in achieving and maintaining the weight that is right for you, and help redirect you to adopt healthy habits for the sake of health, enjoyment, and vitality.

I hope that *Health at Every Size* will touch you deeply. While I expect it will make you angry about your wasted years of guilt-laden eating, failed diets, and self-blame, may it also give you hope and inspire you into action and good health.

INTRODUCTION

You want to lose weight. You look in the mirror and you see "fat and ugly." You've heard the obesity fears trumpeted repeatedly in newspapers, magazines, and on the television news: 65 percent of Americans are overweight or obese . . . growing numbers of overweight kids . . . we don't know how to eat . . . we're not exercising enough . . . we're the first generation that's going to die younger than our parents . . . blah, blah, blah. So you buy one diet book after another, desperate for the one that will finally save you. But they never do, at least not in any lasting way.

Face it, the "D" word is dead. A new diet isn't going to get you what you want. You've been there, done that, and there's no point in trying again. Even exercise programs don't deliver.

So you picked up this book, *Health at Every Size: The Surprising Truth About Your Weight*, hoping it will finally provide the cure. This book can cure your weight woes, but the answer may be different from what you've imagined.

Health at Every Size is *not* a weight-loss book. It's not a diet book. It's not an exercise program. *Health at Every Size* is a book about healthy living, one designed to support you as you shift your focus from hating yourself and fighting your body to learning to appreciate yourself, your body, and your life. It's a book designed to help you break free of the weight-loss mentality and embrace the health-and-happiness mentality. Because really, what's beneath your weight-loss quest? Isn't your ultimate goal to feel better about yourself, to feel love, acceptance, vitality, or good health?

That's the Health at Every Size promise. You *can* feel better about yourself. You *can* feel loved, accepted, and vital—and you can improve your health—*regardless* of whether you lose weight.

Health at Every Size is not speculation or unproven theory. It's based on a scientifically tested program. The program was evaluated through a government-funded academic study, its data published in well-respected scientific journals.[1, 2, 3] It showed that the program *can* give you what you want. Even the United States Department of Agriculture (USDA) touts the Health at Every Size program as the "new hope" for people struggling with their weight.[4]

"Oh, no, no, no," you may be thinking. "To feel better about myself, I've got to lose weight!" That's what the women in our research study initially thought. When my colleagues and I recruited participants for the study, we ran open-ended ads for large women who were struggling with their weight and interested in feeling better about themselves and improving their health. Every respondent assumed they were applying to participate in a weight-loss program. After all, they figured, how can large women feel better about themselves and improve their health without losing weight?

The disappointment was palpable during the orientation session when the women randomly assigned to the Health at Every Size program learned they would not be part of the weight-loss group (the control group). If they could have walked out then, I think they would have. Fortunately, they all decided to stay through the initial meeting.

During that meeting, I asked the women to reflect on their history of trying to lose weight. We shared stories of diet and exercise routines; stress management techniques; years spent working with nutritionists, physicians, psychotherapists, hypnotherapists, personal trainers, clergy, and psychic healers. We laughed and cried as we remembered the money and energy we wasted on fat magnets, slimming slippers, thigh creams, ear staples, and even headbands purported to help dream the fat away.

We bonded over the underlying pain and desperation that led us to try everything and anything, from the mundane to the outrageous, and repeatedly go back for more. It became clear that, in contrast to the negative stereotype of the lazy and undisciplined fat person, everyone in this group had exhibited tremendous determination, strength of character, and willpower in their persistent attempts to lose weight.

You'll read more about the study later in the book, but let me share with you one story that will show you how life-changing this book and its program can be.

Kelly was one of the quieter participants that first night. Although highly motivated to make changes in her life, she was also dubious about our approach. Like the other women, she very much wanted to lose weight and had a long and painful history of fruitless attempts. She'd often felt that initial hope and enthusiasm at trying something new, only to be disappointed in the end. She was pessimistic that we could provide anything significantly different than what she'd already tried (and failed at) countless times before.

It wasn't until the end of the session that Kelly finally spoke. Slowly at first, then with increasing intensity and emotion, she described the ways in which her inability to lose weight and the subsequent self-hatred controlled much of her life. Other group members nodded in recognition as Kelly admitted that she rarely ate at restaurants because she dreaded the looks of other diners as she ate, feeling their judgment and disapproving looks at her body and the food she chose.

She described how her self-hatred led to isolation, how she'd sometimes cancel plans with friends because she couldn't bear to be out in the world in such a fat body. She kept returning to the refrain that she had tried to lose weight, she had *really* tried, but she was just too weak to keep up the regimen of dieting or exercise.

I suggested to Kelly—to all of us—that perhaps we hadn't failed. Maybe, I said, we had successfully tested many weight-loss regimens and *they* had failed *us*. Had it ever occurred to them that maybe we did everything right, but the techniques we tried just weren't capable of delivering on their promise?

They all looked at me blankly. This possibility was clearly something they hadn't considered. They had spent years viewing their weight as evidence of their own personal failing.

The women were provided with a rough draft of this book and met weekly to discuss the personal meaning of its contents. As they learned more about the science behind weight loss, why some bodies naturally weigh more than others, why conventional recommendations to diet or exercise may not have much impact on weight in the long run, and that weight is not such an important factor in measuring one's health or worthiness anyway, an incredible transformation occurred.

In the end, the women participating in the Health at Every Size program emerged with better physical health, higher self-esteem, and a relationship with food that's as healthy as their cholesterol and blood pressure levels. The women participating in the diet program experienced none of these benefits and regained the weight they initially lost.

You'll read more about the Health at Every Size study later in the book. I bring it up now because I want you to know that even if you picked up this book looking for a weight-loss solution, you may want to stick with it, even though you know up front that you won't be getting the prescription you seek.

I want you to read what Kelly wrote in her journal shortly after that first meeting:

> It was powerful to realize how hard we had all tried to lose weight, how humiliating some of those attempts were, to feel one another's desperation. I so empathized with the other group members as we shared stories of our hopes getting dashed again and again.
>
> What motivates us to keep trying? I'm short and I don't like that, but I don't read growth books, attend heightening groups, or consider going to a salon to get stretched. That's because I just don't see my height as changeable. But weight is different: It seems like I *should* be able to change it.
>
> When I start a diet, I have a feeling of hope. I was on a real high on my way to that first meeting, I let the fantasies run wild. This is an actual government-sponsored university study, state-of-the-art. I'll finally lose weight: Guys will notice me as I walk

down the street, my mom will tell me how proud she is, I can have confidence when I apply for a job.

And then I heard Dr. Bacon say that weight loss may not be possible and would not be a goal. I felt like I had just been popped, like she inserted a needle into my big balloon, and my insides were leaking out. Life didn't seem worth living without the hope that I could be thin.

But as this thought crossed my mind, it helped me to see the extent of my magical thinking, how much I have riding on the fantasy, why I keep trying so desperately to lose weight. Inside, I believe that weight loss is the only thing standing between me and happiness. So *if I never get thin, I can never be happy*, I can never become the person I want to be.

In that moment, I understood: It was the dream of weight loss that clouded my ability to be happy with myself—not the weight itself. Perhaps Health at Every Size can finally help me feel better about my life and myself?

The Health at Every Size program won't ask you to give up on your dreams; it will help you to actually live them. It will give you the tools to realize those dreams, to live in a body you love, and to focus on things like feeling good and enjoying life—no matter what your weight.

Decades of research—and probably your own personal experience—show that the pursuit of weight loss rarely produces the thin, happy life you dream of. Dropping the pursuit of weight loss isn't about giving up, it's about moving on. When you make choices because they help you feel better, not because of their presumed effect on your weight, you maintain them over the long run. You do it because you *want* to, not because you believe you *should*.

When you stop trying to control your weight through willpower, your body starts doing the job for you—naturally, and much more effectively. If you stop fighting yourself, achieving and maintaining a healthy weight is effortless. Consider Kelly's experience:

Before participating in the Health at Every Size program, I never truly enjoyed food. Either I felt compelled to steer clear of my favorite foods, like potato chips and ice cream, or I ate them and felt guilty. And I felt like I could never get enough. But it's different for me now. As much as I love pizza, when my body's had enough I just lose interest. I don't have to fight my desire to eat because I just don't want to eat any more.

Before, I didn't know that I could trust myself. My fear was that if I let down my guard, I would eat out of control and just keep gaining weight. But that never happened. I don't count my calories or limit fat, I don't feel guilty when I eat—and everything is okay. I'm not scared of food anymore. My weight has stabilized and it seems like my body is doing a pretty good job of taking care of me! More importantly, I can now say that I absolutely love food. I never knew chocolate was so amazing!

The Health at Every Size program was truly transformative for Kelly and the rest of the women in our study, and it is my hope that this book will also be transformative for you.

The research participants had the advantage of coming together as a group and supporting one another in engaging with the ideas presented in this book—an advantage that you, as a reader, may not have. I am not confident that this book—or any book about weight for that matter—can stand alone. Cultural attitudes about weight are so strongly embedded in you that you are unlikely to be changed by mere exposure to ideas: It will take active personal engagement for these words to take root.

With that in mind, I encourage you to pay careful attention to the emotional and personal significance of the ideas presented here, to try to make sense of the ideas by relating them to your own life experiences.

You may feel resistance as you read. When this feeling occurs, consider what it may threaten in you before dismissing the idea. If you examine your fears, they hold less power in limiting you.

My hope is that this book can offer you a fresh, transformative view of yourself, your body, and your value as a unique individual. This was certainly true for Kelly and the other participants of the Health at Every Size research study:

> I came to the program looking to make less of myself (lose weight); I left proudly taking up *more* space, feeling lighter and less restricted in my body. I came to the program looking for rules about what to eat or avoid and how to control my urges; I left trusting myself, confident that I am more competent than any outside expert in knowing how best to feed myself. Food, previously a trigger for shame, guilt, and fear, is now a source of great pleasure. Most importantly, I know that everything I want in life is available to me now, not twenty pounds from now, which has given me a tremendous sense of freedom to explore what's really important to me.

Kelly learned a whole new way of understanding herself and her relationship with food. And so can you.

The first half of the book sets up the theory, explaining the biological and cultural underpinnings of weight and giving you self-assessment tools to identify the stumbling blocks to achieving the weight that is right for you and appreciating wherever that may be. Armed with the science and knowing where you currently are, you are ready for part two, which supports you in adopting Health at Every Size.

COMMUNITY ACKNOWLEDGMENT

The concept of Health at Every Size has a long history that predates me and includes many diverse viewpoints. I am grateful
to the pioneers who helped us envision the possibilities of a
paradigm shift and to the many other freedom fighters who continue
to conceptualize and grow the movement to this day.

Choosing a book title was a conflicted process. As I intended to
bring attention to the Health at Every Size movement and share my
perspective on it, the main title "Health at Every Size" was a natural
option. The first edition of the book has been out for a year now, and
I'm thrilled to feel successful in both aspects.

The downside to using the words in my title, however, is that it
may give off the impression that this is THE treatise on Health at
Every Size, and the only way to articulate the movement. It's not.
There are many divergent viewpoints within the Health at Every Size
movement and this book represents my perspective.

PART ONE
Deconstructing Weight

ONE

We're Wired to Maintain a Healthy Weight

Suppose you had a "fat meter" that would send a loud "STOP!" message to your brain once you'd accumulated enough fat. Suddenly, you'd have no desire for pizza, ice cream, or potato chips. You'd look at these favorite foods, even smell their enticing odors, and wouldn't even be tempted. Or maybe you would decide to eat anyway, and your metabolism would just rev up to burn off the extra calories.

Nice fantasy, huh? Well, it's not so far-fetched. Believe it or not, you do have that built-in mechanism. Why, then, you're asking, do you always feel driven to eat, even though you consider yourself overweight or struggle to maintain your weight? And why do you gain weight when you aren't restraining yourself?

Well, maybe your meter is broken. Or maybe its alarm isn't loud enough to trigger a reaction from your brain. And that's too bad. Because this mechanism is so powerful that people for whom it works never have to fight the temptation to eat when they're not hungry. Remaining at a healthy weight comes naturally to them; it's not something they have to work at through deprivation diets and long hours at the gym.

Unfortunately, for too many of us this potent weight regulation system has gone awry. Food still tempts us long after our caloric need is satisfied. And extra calories result in packing on extra pounds. Our bodies no longer know how to regulate its "setpoint," the level that is biologically ideal for us.

But don't worry. By the time you finish this book, you will have learned how to reset this powerful mechanism so that your body can naturally achieve its healthiest weight. You'll be able to eat normally without thinking about calories, allowing your hunger/fullness/appetite levels to regulate what and when you eat in a remarkably efficient mechanism. Eating will be simple and enjoyable.

Setpoint: Your Ideal Weight

When it's working right, this weight-regulation mechanism is as precise as the most sophisticated scientific instrument. Don't believe me? Just consider a fifty-year-old woman who weighs about five pounds more than she did when she was twenty. If she eats about 2,000 calories a day, over the course of thirty years she takes in about 22 million calories. Since five pounds of body fat stores about 17,500 calories, that means that her body was just .08 percent off in balancing energy in vs. energy out. This amounts to a difference of about 50 calories per month—less than the calories in one egg!

In other words, her energy balance was regulated with a precision greater than 99.9 percent![5] How many things in life can you say that about? Certainly there's no way you can be as precise by trying to exert your own willpower over what you eat and how much you exercise.

Until recent decades, adult weight stability over long periods of time was the norm and was an effortless process. One 1970s research study showed that the average weight of a sixty-year-old man was only four to five pounds more than the average thirty-year-old man.[6] That kind of weight maintenance is no accident.

So why fight? Give up counting calories and trying to control your eating through dieting. Instead, let your body do the regulating for you. I promise you'll have far better results.

The healthy weight that your body aims for is called your *set-point weight*. Think of it as the preferred temperature on a fat thermostat. Like any thermostat, this one can be set at whatever point is most comfortable. The system then works tirelessly to do anything it can to bring your body into alignment with that point. It acts like a biological force: The further you go from the center, the stronger the pull to get you back to the comfortable range.

This system only works if we let it, however. If you keep "jiggling" with the thermostat via diets, the mechanism breaks down. This jiggling is like a power struggle to wrest control away from your body's innate weight-regulation mechanism, and in the end, it only makes your body fight harder to retain control. The result: Your body forces you to not only regain any weight you've lost, but you may even pay a penalty with extra weight gain—and a setpoint now set higher to protect against future diets.

Rather than continuing to engage in this weighty battle with your body, you could declare a truce and join forces with it to help achieve a healthy, natural weight. You'll find that you will become less interested in eating when you are full. And your body itself will make up for those occasional party overindulgences without you having to deliberately deny yourself.

Your Body: A Weight Control Freak

Let's look more closely at just what a control freak your body is when it comes to maintaining the "right" level of body fat.

To better understand this concept, we need to take a closer look at your body's weight-regulating bag of tricks.

Picture this: You're out for an afternoon stroll, enjoying the warmth of the sun on your back. It's actually a bit too warm, so your body's automatic cooling system kicks in and you start to sweat, which reduces your core temperature and you feel cooler. Suddenly, dark clouds cover the sun and you feel *too* cool. Again, your body's automatic thermostat kicks in. The hairs rise on exposed body parts to trap air, goose pimples appear, and you begin shivering, all of which increases your temperature.

Do you control any of this? Of course not. Like breathing and digestion, these regulatory actions are governed by your autonomic nervous system, which works in the background without any conscious thought. All these systems are designed to maintain *homeostasis*, or balance, throughout your body.

Your body's attempt to maintain homeostasis is one of the most fundamental concepts in biology. Many physiological variables—such as oxygen levels, carbon dioxide levels, blood volume, and blood sugar—are tightly regulated under this system. For each, your body accepts a certain range with various physiological mechanisms preventing disastrous dips or curves.

The amount of body fat you have is similarly tightly regulated. More than fifty years of research proves that your body tries to maintain your fat at the level at which you are designed to function best (not necessarily a size 4 or even 24, however).[7] Your body is strongly invested in helping you maintain this healthy and relatively consistent weight, and it has amazingly efficient mechanisms in place to pull off this feat.

Unfortunately, recent lifestyle and environmental changes mess with this programming. We further throw the system off when we try to take control through dieting. The result: escalating weight.

Understanding Homeostasis

The chief ruler of your weight setpoint is your hypothalamus, a small region of the brain that acts as an intermediary between your brain and body.

The hypothalamus is a kind of all-knowing sensor. It picks up on sensations like the delicious smell from a just-baked cheese pizza, the burn you got on the roof of your mouth from biting into that pizza too quickly, and that overstuffed feeling from scarfing down too many pieces of said pizza. It's also tuned in to body states you're not aware of, like how much body fat you have at any given moment.

The hypothalamus reacts to the messages it receives by signaling other body tissues to release hormones, enzymes, and other chemicals to push you back into homeostasis.

For instance, if you're losing weight and you are below your setpoint, your hypothalamus might direct other body systems to regulate your eating and activity levels as well as your metabolic efficiency, the rate at which you burn calories, to get you to regain the weight.

At first the hypothalamus enlists your help. It can initiate the release of particular hormones that influence your appetite and mold your drive to eat, including changing how food tastes and how much it appeals to you. It can also lead you to actually crave higher-fat food if it wants you to get concentrated energy and gain weight. It can even decrease your drive to move, leading to serious couch potato behavior.

These actions are particularly strong if the hypothalamus senses that body fat levels are dropping too far below the setpoint. Undereating sets you up for brain activity that produces an urge to eat way beyond the ability of food to satisfy your hunger.

Of course, sometimes we're able to temporarily override the hypothalamus's efforts to restore homeostasis. For instance, if you're trying to lose weight, you may be able to consciously overcome feelings of hunger through your own willpower. People on diets manage this—albeit not for long. Or perhaps you don't want to cancel on your friend, so you make it to the gym despite your feeling of lethargy.

So then your hypothalamus gets more aggressive, affecting systems beyond your conscious control. You may feel cold, a sign your body is trying to conserve energy by sending less blood to the periphery, reducing your metabolic rate. Or you might feel sluggish, another sign that your metabolism has slowed. Conversely, you may feel hot after a big meal because your brain has boosted the metabolic effects of food to help your body burn off the extra calories.

Need some convincing that your body—not you—is really in control? Consider some of the following studies.

Of Rats and Setpoints

Some strains of rats have higher weights than others. Observing their growth, scientists determined that genetically heavier strains of rats ate more than thinner rats during adolescence and early adulthood, until they settled into a stable, setpoint weight. Once they reached their setpoint, they ate amounts similar to the thinner rats.

Ordinary adult rats, given unlimited access to food and opportunity for exercise, maintain stable setpoint weights. If food is restricted and then provided again, the rat knows just how much to eat to return to its setpoint weight. Fat, thin, or somewhere in between, it didn't matter: The rat returned to its setpoint weight once food was accessible again.

When a Rat Is Hungry

To examine the role of the hypothalamus in setpoint control, early researchers used two sources of evidence. Both involved placing an electrode directly into the brain of a laboratory rat. The electrode either damaged that section of the brain so it no longer functioned or stimulated that section of the brain to produce more neural activity.

The researchers focused on two sections of the hypothalamus they identified as playing a large role in eating behavior: the lateral hypothalamus (LH) and ventromedial hypothalamus (VMH).

When the LH was damaged and dysfunctional, the rats refused to eat and eventually died.[8] But when the LH was electrically stimulated and turned on, the rats ate, even if they were full, and got fat.[9] This behavior led scientists to conclude that the LH housed the "hunger center." Turn it on and we want to eat; turn it off and we're no longer hungry.

In another experiment, the scientists again created lesions in the LH, damaging the appetite center. Although the rats again stopped eating and lost weight, this time the scientists force-fed them to keep them alive.[10,11] Eventually, the rats started eating on their own. At some point their weight stabilized, although at a much lower level than before the lesion. In other words, they now had a lowered setpoint.

In other experiments, scientists examined how the rats expended energy after losing weight due to the destruction of the LH. They hypothesized that if a rat's setpoint was reduced, the rat's body would try to maintain the lowered setpoint and resist weight loss or gain.

In fact, that's just what happened. When the rats with the LH lesions were force-fed to gain weight to their previous levels, their metabolic rate increased substantially so they burned more calories.[12] In other words, restoring their old weight caused their body to use mechanisms to get them back to their new setpoint weight. Conversely, reducing their weight from the lower levels they were already maintaining caused a sharp decline in their metabolic rate so they could conserve calories and return to their setpoint. Fat or thin, it didn't matter: All rats returned to their setpoints.

The scientists concluded that the LH must not be the only hunger center, because if it were, the rats wouldn't have regained their drive to eat. Instead, they suggested, the LH must work in concert with other areas of the brain to regulate hunger and determine setpoint. Further research determined they were right.

When a Rat Is Full

If the LH is the hunger center, then the ventromedial hypothalamus (VMH) is the "fullness" center.

Again using rats and probes, scientists discovered that damaging or destroying the VMH caused the rats to eat more and gain weight.[13] Eventually, however, their eating habits and weight stabilized. In other words, they still maintained a setpoint; it had just risen higher. Kind of like what happens when we diet.

Alternatively, when the researchers stimulated the VMH, the rats stopped eating.[14] A hungry rat in the midst of a meal would drop the food pellet and ignore the food following a brief burst of stimulation. The researchers concluded that when the satiety center is activated, it produces a feeling of fullness, even overfullness. More than an absence of hunger, this stimulation drives the animal to avoid eating any more food, even if it tastes good.

These experiments suggested that while damaging the LH seems to lower the weight setpoint, damaging the VMH seems to "loosen" the setpoint, making it easier to reset.[15] It turns animals (including humans) into "finicky eaters," meaning they're more responsive to certain influences of food.[15] For example, if a rat with a damaged VMH is given food it likes, it eats more than a normal rat.

Sooner or later, however, it settles at a stable weight, and, as long as its diet doesn't change, it remains at that weight and responds to the usual tests of setpoint by doing what it can to remain at that level.

Likewise, if the VMH is damaged and the rat is given food it doesn't like, it loses weight until it stabilizes at the lower weight.[16] (By the way, normal rats that are force-fed until they become quite fat become just as finicky as those with damaged VMHs, suggesting that finicky eating is not a direct result of VMH lesions, but occurs when one is above his or her setpoint.)

From Rats to Humans

All this information simply underscores what scientists had already suspected: We have a setpoint and our setpoints can be manipulated.

Even as desperate as many people are to lose weight, sticking an electric probe in your brain and damaging parts of it is going a little too far. That's why scientists are now hard at work figuring out how to change the signals that go to and from your brain to turn *down* signals to the LH and turn *up* the signals to the VMH via drugs or lifestyle changes rather than surgery.

In fact, as you'll see in chapter 4, there are even specific compounds in foods that can alter these messages, partially accounting for raised or lowered setpoints.

Still skeptical? Well, consider this study in humans.

Researchers pulled together 100 volunteers who had effortlessly maintained a stable weight for six months, an indication they were within their setpoint range.[17] The volunteers agreed to live in a special hospital ward where their food intake and activity levels were carefully monitored and manipulated.

First they had to gain weight until they weighed 10 percent more than their original weight. Then they had to lose weight until they tipped the scales at 10 percent less than they originally weighed. Whether they started out fat, thin, or somewhere between, the results were consistent: When the volunteers ate so much that they gained an extra 10 percent of their body weight, their metabolism increased by 15 percent. Their bodies were clearly trying to drive their weight back down! And when they ate so little that their weight fell to 10 percent below their starting point, their metabolisms slowed by 15 percent.

Now, how can you possibly doubt the existence of your own setpoint?

Identifying Your Setpoint

Your setpoint is:

- The weight you maintain when you listen and respond to your body's signals of hunger and fullness.
- The weight you maintain when you don't fixate on your weight or food habits.
- The weight you keep returning to between diets.

Leptin . . . Your Fat Meter

Now you understand the role the hypothalamus plays in maintaining fat homeostasis, or your own setpoint. But just how does the hypothalamus learn what's going on in the weight department? After all, it's not like it forces you to weigh yourself every day.

To answer this question, scientists turned to a strain of mice, called ob/ob mice, with a genetic mutation that kept them fat, eating too much, exercising too little, and burning calories very slowly. If you put them in cages with other mice living under the same environmental conditions (all had the same opportunities for eating and exercise), the ob/ob mice stayed fat while the others stayed slender.

To find out why, a scientist sewed an ob/ob mouse to a "normal" mouse (an experiment called parabiosis), allowing the mice to share the same blood. The result was that the fat mouse returned to average weight, suggesting that something in the blood of the thinner mouse played a role in weight regulation.

Suspecting that few humans would want to be stitched to a thinner human to lose weight, scientists set their sights on isolating the gene that kept the thin mice thin. In 1995, Jeffrey Friedman and colleagues at Rockefeller University in New York located the gene. Turns out this gene was responsible for the production of a hormone called leptin.[18] Mice that lacked the gene—and didn't make leptin—were extremely fat.

Friedman hypothesized that the hypothalamus was sensitive to leptin and that when the mouse reached an appropriate weight, leptin traveled to the brain and either turned *on* the LH or turned *off* the VMH, causing a release of chemicals that helped maintain the setpoint.

The initial research was exhilarating. When the fat mice were injected with leptin, they lost 30 percent of their body weight in two weeks with no apparent side effects. Their metabolism sped up, they ate less, and they ran around more, suggesting that leptin affected many aspects of the energy balance equation simultaneously. When average-sized mice were given extra leptin, they also lost weight.

Since then, we've learned that when fat cells increase in size in a healthy person, they produce more leptin, signaling the hypothalamus to do what it needs to do to slow your eating, increase your activity level and metabolism, and return your fat cells to their previous size.

In other words, leptin acted as the "fat meter" fantasized about in the beginning of this chapter.

As you might imagine, the weight-loss industry went wild over the leptin research, certain that a weight-loss pill was finally within reach. Hello leptin, goodbye dieting.

After all, it made sense: If mice got fat because they didn't make enough leptin, and mice are genetically similar to humans, then wouldn't it stand to reason that fat humans also didn't make enough leptin? Inject them with leptin, the thought went, and the fat would melt away.

The biotech firm Amgen quickly bought the rights to Friedman's discovery for more than $20 million, with the promise of subsequent payments if leptin proved to be the magic bullet some anticipated. The day after announcing the acquisition, Amgen's stock sky-rocketed.

Scientists in the know were amazed at this reckless cash outlay as it hadn't been determined—and didn't seem likely—that many humans had a gene mutation similar to the ob/ob mice. As any scientist worth her rat pellets can tell you, what's true in mice isn't always true in humans.

The clinical trials on leptin were disappointing to say the least. In one, for example, seventy-three fat volunteers injected themselves with leptin or a placebo for twenty-four weeks.[19] Nearly everyone experienced skin irritation and swelling, and many withdrew from the study because of these problems, leaving just forty-seven to complete the study. Although there was an extreme amount of individual variability, of those who stayed in the study, the eight receiving the highest dose of leptin (which also caused the greatest irritation and swelling) lost an average of 16 pounds (though some individuals actually gained weight), while the twelve taking the placebo lost an average of 3 pounds. Low doses had virtually no effect.

Further studies in both rats and humans showed that weight returned to baseline levels after the leptin injections ended. The euphoria over leptin crashed like a lead balloon.

Yes, leptin is produced in humans, and yes, just as in the mice, leptin travels to the brain where it triggers the release of various chemicals to turn down your appetite, speed up your metabolism, and get you moving more. But, researchers learned, fat people were *already* producing plenty of leptin, even more than their thinner counterparts. The amazing results seen in the ob/ob mice only worked in the few humans with a similar genetic mutation.[20] Less than a dozen people have since been discovered to have this mutation.

The difficulty for many humans lies in the decreased sensitivity of the brain to leptin's effects. In other words, your fat meter is working fine: Your fat cells send leptin to the brain to initiate the steps to turn off your appetite and speed up your energy use, but it's as if the part of your brain that receives the message is swathed in cotton batting—it can't "hear" the message very well. Thus, your brain doesn't do its part by triggering the cascade of effects to reduce appetite, increase physical activity, and supercharge metabolism.

Leptin's main role appears to be protecting against weight loss in times of scarcity. When your fat stores shrink when you're dieting, so does leptin production. In response, your appetite increases and your metabolism decreases and you gain the weight back.

The opposite, however, is not as strong. Beyond a certain point, increased weight and the resulting increased leptin production do little to blunt appetite or increase metabolism because you hit a limit in your ability to sense the leptin. In other words, your brain is relatively less concerned with preventing weight gain in times of plenty.

This point is very important to understand, so let me explain it in others terms. Weight gain is relatively easy, but the human body is just not designed to support weight loss. This means that reversing weight gain habits will do a pretty good job of preventing weight gain, though they may not result in weight loss.

Another fact frustrating to many is that people with a history of repeat dieting send out less leptin than they would without that history.[21,22] This decrease is one of the mechanisms that explains why many chronic dieters tend to be heavier than those who haven't attempted weight loss. Your body has reset your setpoint to a higher level. Lucky you—you now have an extra layer of protection so you won't wither away next time you go on a diet (which the body perceives no differently than a famine). Very effective if you lived in another era, but perhaps not so appreciated amidst today's plenty.

Beyond Leptin

Though it isn't the magic weight-loss panacea it was initially envisioned to be, the discovery of leptin was a big advance in understanding weight regulation. We learned that it has an extremely powerful effect on our weight and is the cornerstone of our setpoint mechanism, even if we aren't sure how to harness this power.

The thousands of studies on leptin also spawned even greater research on the neurocircuitry underlying metabolism and on other hormones and neurotransmitters that support leptin. For example, we discovered that insulin, best known for its role in regulating your blood sugar (more on that in chapter 4), is an important ally, informing your hypothalamus about the amount of energy circulating in your bloodstream from your recent meals. Insulin's message gets amplified by several other gut hormones and nerves that respond to the volume and type of food you eat and other chemical messengers that are sensitive to sensations such as the stretch of your stomach or the texture or temperature of the food you eat.

In 1999, researchers discovered another particularly powerful hormone, ghrelin, that contributes to strong feelings of hunger. All day, ghrelin concentrations rise and fall in our bodies. Although we're not aware of these ups and downs, they help drive our behavior on a deeply subconscious level, either moving us toward the table or away from the plate. In recent years, research has also begun pointing to the various diet and lifestyle factors that modify the body's production of ghrelin and other eating-related signals.

Although many scientists glibly refer to ghrelin as the "hunger hormone," it's got plenty of partners when it comes to making people eat or stop eating. In fact, more than twenty chemical messengers have been found to stimulate eating, and a similar number suppress appetite.

While ghrelin plays the starring role as an appetite trigger, leptin, insulin, and another gut hormone, PYY, turn down the dial on ghrelin response. These hormones, and others, travel through the body carrying their indulge-or-don't messages. They also trigger nerve messages to the brain and are influenced, in turn, by messages returning from the brain.

To complicate the picture, other events occurring in your body mediate these messages. Your emotions, for example, generate chemicals that send potent messages to the same sites that respond to leptin and insulin. Your sleep patterns also influence this system.

With such a degree of complexity, it's no wonder that we're struggling with the question of how to influence our weight in a meaningful and lasting way!

Feast or Famine Genes

To understand just why our modern lifestyles throw our internal weight meters out of whack, you first have to understand this genetic compulsion we have to hang on to every calorie, and why that is so at odds with the world we live in today. For that, I'd like to introduce you to your great-great-great-great-great-great-grand-mother.

Her picture might not be hanging in your living room, but you—like every other human on this planet—descended from early humans to whom "dinner" might come just once every few days. Given the scarcity of food and the tremendous amount of calories expended catching it (think running after mammoths with spears), it's no surprise that our bodies evolved to be super-efficient at energy conservation, genetically wired to hang on to every calorie while they urge us to seek out the highest calorie food we can find. All long before the first food court, of course, where high calorie food is easily obtained.

Today, even though we can eat dinner all day long if we want and expend no more calories than it takes to breathe, digest, and click the remote control, this genetic propensity has remained largely unchanged.[23]

In fact, through evolution we've created a population more likely than not to have these "thrifty genes." That's because throughout human history, those at greatest risk of starving to death were those who burned energy quickly and could not store fat—like that size 4 woman you may know who never diets or exercises and eats what-ever she wants. Because women (and men) like her couldn't survive during lean times (no body fat to burn), their numbers dwindled in our gene pool. We just didn't need the skinny folks!

The rest of us, then, descended from the survivors, those with a very efficient system for storing fat whenever food was available. Given today's environment, you can see how our genes set us up to pack on some padding.

To put it in the proverbial nutshell: Our internal weight regula-tion system remains ideally crafted for the environmental condition of the past—food scarcity—helping us pack on pounds and thwart hunger and has yet to evolve for the environment of today, where food is everywhere and we're more likely to burn a CD than a calo-rie. The advent of cooking and the ability to strip certain nutrients (like sugar or fat) from other more nutritious and filling components (like fiber) also made it a lot easier to get calories into our bodies.

Add to this the increased dieting of today which, in our genetic memory, feels an awful lot like the famines of yore. Combine changes in the *types* of foods we're eating; and changes in *how* we're eating, and you have a recipe for, you guessed it, higher setpoints and creeping weight gain.

Type 2 Diabetes and Our Genetic Heritage

Throughout most of our evolutionary history, food shortages were common. When food was abundant, people who produced lots of insulin (a hormone that helps you get glucose—and fat—into your cells) could gorge since this insulin enabled them to store excess energy as body fat. This was an evolutionary advantage, since they could live off their fat during famines. Those who couldn't produce as much insulin starved.

Fast-forward to today and our typical American diet in which we're challenged to pour out insulin all the time (more on that soon). What happens? The abundance of insulin overwhelms our cells to the point that they react less to its message. What was once an evolutionary advantage given frequent famines and inconsistent meals now leads to insulin resistance, particularly in hardworking muscles that could potentially burn that extra energy. Our fat cells, on the other hand, don't develop this insulin resistance. Instead, they readily respond to insulin's storage message and extra glucose gets converted into fat and stored as fat. A fine evolutionary safeguard for the past when fat storage was valued, not so well appreciated today.

What Does It All Mean?

I know I've given you a lot of information in the preceding pages. If you need a little help assimilating it all, here's a cheat sheet:

- Your fat cells are not just dumb sacks of lard. They are active organs and send chemical messages that help to regulate many body functions.
- Your brain receives moment-to-moment messages from your fat cells so it is well informed about how much energy is in your fat stores.
- Your brain also receives moment-to-moment messages from your digestive tract, making it well-informed about your overall nutritional status.
- Your brain also receives signals stimulated by physical activity, emotion, sleep patterns, and other goings-on.
- Your brain assimilates this wealth of information and, in response, produces chemical messengers and nerve responses that regulate your appetite and metabolism, affecting not only when you experience hunger but also what foods appeal to you and how much food it takes to make you feel full. Although you're not aware of these chemical changes, they drive your behavior, moving you toward the table or instructing you to turn down seconds.
- Your body likes to maintain the status quo and keep your weight relatively stable; this range of stable weight is called your "setpoint."
- Your body strongly protects against dipping below your setpoint, though most people's bodies are relatively less aggressive at preventing them from rising above their setpoint. In

other words, weight gain is relatively easy at the same time that weight loss may not be possible.

■ When you lose weight and threaten this system, your body may react by raising your setpoint, protecting against future threat.

The Final Result?

Your body maintains whatever it perceives as an adequate amount of fat storage to protect itself. How much fat protection your body requires (your setpoint) is the result of a complex interplay of genetics and the lifestyle choices made today as well as in the past—and is intimately linked to your current weight.

This, in turn, leads to the catch-22: Your body wants to maintain the status quo and is stubbornly resistant to change. When you lose body fat, the very loss of fat triggers processes to reclaim it. So losing weight in and of itself is counterproductive to maintaining weight loss. We shouldn't be too surprised that weight loss is so rarely maintained.

What's My Setpoint?

Unfortunately, there's no magic formula or laboratory test to determine your setpoint. Nor is there any objective way to figure out how tightly yours is regulated. (Scientists estimate that the average person has a setpoint range of about ten to twenty pounds, meaning at any given time, there is a ten-to-twenty-pound range at which your body will be comfortable and not resist attempts to change. So losing/gaining small amounts of weight may not be difficult and won't be met by compensatory actions, if you are within your setpoint range.[5])

But you *can* find your own setpoint. How? By listening to your body and eating normally. You'll learn more about how to do that throughout this book.

Are You Above Your Setpoint?

Wondering if you're above your own setpoint? Then answer these questions:

■ Do you have difficulty recognizing when you're hungry and when you've had enough?

■ Do you routinely eat beyond a comfortable level of fullness and feel lethargic, stuffed, and uncomfortable after meals?

■ Do you go through periods where you eat out of control, anticipating that you will soon start to diet?

■ Do you skip meals in an effort to lose weight, then overeat because you are so hungry?

■ Do you skip meals to "save up" for a big feast?

■ Do you often eat as a coping mechanism? For example, when you're tired, angry, or nervous? How about killing time when you're bored?

■ Do you often feel guilty about some of the foods or the amount of food you eat?

■ If you overeat, do you figure you've blown your "diet" and end up eating even more?

■ Do you often eat quickly without taking the time to focus on the taste of your food or to savor and enjoy it?

■ Do you fluctuate between periods of sensible, nutritious eating and then eating out of control?

If you answered "yes" to any of these questions, you are likely above your setpoint. Don't feel bad! Most people aren't at their setpoint. This book will help you find it.

Warning: Many of these conditions may also be symptomatic of an eating disorder or other concerns. Be sure to discuss these symptoms with a trusted health professional.

Are You Below Your Setpoint?

Some people are chronically below their setpoint. You'll know this is you if:

■   You're often cold.
■   You feel like you're constantly preoccupied with food and often feel desperately hungry.
■   You wake up with an overwhelming urge to eat.
■   You have difficulty sleeping because of gnawing hunger.
■   You have a very low sex drive.
■   For females, you have infrequent periods or skip them entirely.
■   You suffer from any of the following: apathy, fatigue, irritability, and/or depression.

If you are below your setpoint, learning how to respond to your body's signals will help you to normalize your eating habits and feel better. It may result in a slight weight gain, but this is a good thing, I assure you!

Warning: Many of these conditions may also be symptomatic of an eating disorder, a thyroid dysfunction, or other concerns. Be sure to discuss these symptoms with a trusted health professional.

Achieve *Your* Setpoint!

This book is going to help you get to your natural setpoint, the weight that is healthiest for you. By the end of the book, you'll be answering "yes" to these questions:

■   Do you eat naturally in response to signals of hunger, fullness, and appetite without fixating on your weight or food habits?
■   Is eating effortless and enjoyable?

Soon, your body will be guiding you in making nutritious, pleasurable choices. No more counting calories, totaling fat grams, or weighing broiled skinless chicken breasts!

TWO

We're Emotionally Starved

Okay, so you know you have an internal weight regulation system that is predisposed to maintaining your individual body weight setpoint. If it's so powerful, you're wondering, how come our waistlines have been expanding over the last few decades?

Two reasons: First, we no longer allow the process to work. We don't trust our own judgment anymore. External rules, such as belief systems about good foods, bad foods, or appropriate amounts or times to eat, drown out our innate ability to respond to setpoint cues. We eat not because we're hungry, but because we're sad, guilty, bored, frustrated, lonely, or angry. And because food can't take care of our emotions, we eat and eat and never feel satisfied. We'll tackle these topics in this chapter.

Another part of the deal is that we're physically hungrier due to rising setpoints, the result of changing lifestyle choices. How we live our lives and what we eat *do* matter. Those are weighty topics that deserve their own chapters.

What Drives Your Hunger?

Have you ever thought about *why* you eat? Sure, sure, part of the reason is because your stomach is growling and that steaming bowl of pasta with marinara sauce is making your mouth water.

Imagine traveling back many millions of years to pose this question to Nate the Neanderthal.

"Why eat? I eat to survive, dummy. Now pass me that bison leg and quit bothering me with such silly questions."

Without the distractions of modern life, Nate is able to home in on the simple but profound answer to our question, an answer that often eludes us post-Neanderthals. The most basic reason we eat is to provide fuel for our bodies. Without food, obviously, we'd die.

In fact, hunger is at the foundation of our biological programming that ensures our survival as a species. Every cell in our bodies is so invested in making sure we eat and provide fuel, that not only are our bodies designed to make us feel miserable when we're hungry (lightheaded, irritable, headachy, weak, etc.), but they are also designed to reward us when we *do* eat, triggering pleasure centers in our brains that make the act of eating so much more appealing than simply stuffing our mouths. This pleasure is our reward for listening to our bodies' signals and it plays an important role in the setpoint mechanism.

If only hunger and eating remained that simple! Today, few of us view food as a means of fueling our bodies. Nor is it a source of true pleasure for many of us. In fact, the pleasure we get from eating is too often viewed as indulgent or sinful, rather than as valuable support for nourishing ourselves. We've learned to deny or control our hunger, rather than honor and celebrate it.

As you already know from the first chapter, denying your hunger doesn't lead to weight loss or better health. And eating when you're hungry won't make you fat. In fact, the opposite is true: eating when you're hungry helps maintain your setpoint and keep you at the weight that's right for you, and denying your hunger leads to compensatory mechanisms that trigger fat storage and weight gain.

Yet today there's simply too much noise around the issues of food, hunger, and eating for us to listen to our own bodies. We live

The Pleasure Principle

An interesting cross-cultural survey of food attitudes in the United States, France, Belgium, and Japan found that Americans associated food with pleasure the least and health the most.[24] When asked what came to mind upon hearing the words "chocolate cake," Americans were most likely to say "guilt" while the French connected it with "celebration." Overall, the researchers found, we derive less pleasure from eating than others.

What a shame. Even though we are biologically wired to find pleasure in food, we've become so obsessed with the hidden meanings of food in this country that we've forgotten what it is supposed to do. Nourish us. Provide pleasure. The French haven't; nor have the Italians, the founders of the so-called "Slow Food" movement. These cultures (and many others) honor food, savor it, spend hours preparing and enjoying a meal, rather than grabbing a burger at a drive-through and scarfing it down in the car as ketchup drips onto their laps.

Another study asked 282 people from France and the United States how they decided it was time to stop eating after a meal.[25] The French reported that they stopped when they were full. The Americans? They stopped when their plates were empty. Also interesting, the heavier the person was, regardless of whether they were French or American, the more likely they were to rely on external cues, like a clean plate, as opposed to how they felt.

For years we've automatically assumed that the reason the French weigh less and have a lower incidence of heart disease is because of the types of foods they eat and the red wine they drink. Maybe it's *how* they eat that really makes the difference.

in a world that's decided to define food as "good" or "bad," a world that encourages us to ignore our hunger and fullness signals in favor of continually seeking out that Holy Grail of thinness, or to use food to fill needs that have nothing to do with sustenance.

If you don't trust and respond to hunger, after a while the self-regulatory setpoint mechanism that controls your fat stores breaks down. You weaken your innate ability to hear your hunger and fullness signals. When this happens, you start to gain weight. No ideas you (or anyone else) may have about how to maintain a healthy and appropriate weight can be as effective as listening to your body. Losing weight is not about finding the perfect proportions of carbohydrates, protein, and fat or tricking yourself into feeling satisfied. Rather, maintaining the right weight for you is about respecting your hunger and trusting your body to guide you in doing what's best. And that's hard to do if you're *regularly* eating for reasons other than hunger and making choices that don't give you pleasure.

As you continue reading, you'll come to understand how we often try to nourish ourselves emotionally with food. See if you recognize yourself in these pages. Perhaps it can help you become more conscious about why you crave donuts.

I Hurt, Therefore I Eat: The Truth Behind Emotional Eating

We live in a culture in which food has become inextricably bound up with emotion and situation. We eat because we're bored, because we're sad, because we're happy. When we want to celebrate, we go out to eat. When we're grieving over a romantic breakup, we drown our feelings in ice cream. When someone is sick or someone dies, food becomes the way in which we show our sorrow and support—great amounts of casseroles and cakes and salads.

I'm not saying this is all bad. While food has inherent limitations in meeting our emotional needs, an emotional connection with food *is* part of a normal and healthy relationship with food. Food can and should bring us pleasure and comfort. Just think of the associations certain foods and aromas stir up for you: the sense of "home" you feel when you smell cinnamon and vanilla; the sense of safety a meatloaf and mashed potato dinner can provide; the sense of longing you get when your sister makes your grandmother's famous broccoli casserole at Thanksgiving. On rainy Sundays, a cup of hot cocoa is a wonderful accompaniment to reading the paper, while the ritual of a celebratory cake adds meaning to birthdays.

But too many of us have come to view food as a blanket for our emotions, numbing them as we turn to food to provide the love and comfort we crave. Food is reward, friend, love, and support. We eat not because we're hungry, but because we're sad, guilty, bored, frustrated, lonely, or angry. In doing so, we're ignoring those internal hard-wired hunger and fullness signals. And because there's no way that food can really address our emotions, we eat and eat and eat, but never feel satisfied.

Unfortunately, at this point most of us get stuck. We recognize the short-term comfort or pleasure we get from food, and without other skills to take care of ourselves, we come to depend on it for an instant feel-better fix. Then we get stuck in a downward spiral: Eating to feel better doesn't help us feel better in the long run; instead it adds guilt and anger about our eating habits and their ramifications on our weight. In fact, studies show that although you might receive immediate emotional comfort from eating, the associated guilt overpowers any emotional support you receive.[26, 27]

What too few of us understand is that food doesn't fix feelings. It may comfort us in the short term, or distract us from our pain, but in the long term it only makes our problems worse and keeps us from making substantive changes that could lead to greater fulfillment and a healthier life.

What this means is that if you feel driven to eat for emotional reasons, you don't have an eating problem. Nope. You have a *caretaking* problem. You're not taking proper care of yourself. I know this to be true because I was once an emotional eater. I ate because there was something I wanted, but that something wasn't food. Eating kept me from feeling lonely, got me through tough times, and, unlike people, was always there for me.

But then my obsession with weight surfaced. And suddenly food didn't do the trick anymore. Instead of long-term comfort, I would get a short-term fix followed by a more intense and longer lasting guilt. The more weight I gained, the more evidence I saw of my failings. The more I felt like a failure, the more I ate. And so on and so on.

Where did this thinking all come from? From the way we were raised.

I remember soon after my son was born. When he was hungry, he cried. He nursed until he was full, then dropped off to sleep, sated. Only when his stomach emptied again—typically in a couple of hours—did he cry again for food. He was in perfect touch with his hunger/satiety signals.

But as he got older and moved on to solid food, things changed. Not in how he approached food, but in how we (well, my mother, for one) taught him to view food. I remember one time when Isaac was a year old and my mother was feeding him strained carrots. He happily ate a few spoonfuls, then stopped opening his mouth. The message was clear: "No more!"

But my mom ignored the message. "Come on, Isaac," she crooned, "just a few more bites." She held the spoon temptingly in front of his mouth. When that didn't work, she pushed it against his lips. Still no luck. So she got more creative. "Here comes the airplane, into the hangar," she said, playfully waving the fork near his mouth, attempting to capitalize on his fascination with planes. "Open the hangar, Isaac."

He would have none of it. Isaac was full and no longer interested in food. He was a smart kid and knew what he needed. My mom was essentially telling him that he wasn't a trustworthy judge—that she, not he, knew how to manage his food intake. It was then that I understood where it all began for me!

But I don't blame my mom. My mother wasn't trying to do this on purpose; she was just unconsciously transmitting eating attitudes entrenched in our culture. If Isaac (and I) didn't get them from her, we'd certainly get them from somewhere else.

Our culture teaches us that there are appropriate times and places for food that, more often than not, have nothing to do with feelings of hunger and satiety within our bodies. Think of the messages we get: "I went to all that trouble to cook, and you're not even going to eat?" "You can't be hungry. You just ate dinner!" "It's not time to eat." "Clean your plate, children are starving in India." "You got an A? Let's bake some cookies to celebrate." "Poor thing, you fell off your bike? Will some ice cream help make it better?"

These external cues, then, dictate our eating for much of our lives. As a result, we stop listening to our internal cues about hunger and fullness. Instead, we eat because we think we should; to stuff feelings we don't want to have; to mark important moments in our lives; to fill a void we can't even clarify.

After years of turning to food for nonphysical reasons, our ability to perceive those internal signals has weakened, like the leg muscles in someone bedridden. Then, when we find we're gaining weight, we try to impose our own will to eat less over our appetite.

Scientists have a term for this. "Restrained eaters" are people who regulate their eating through external cues, often in an effort to manage their weight. Conversely, "unrestrained eaters" are those who still rely on internal body cues to determine when and how much to eat.

Extensive research suggests that restrained eaters are much less sensitive to hunger and satiety than unrestrained eaters.[28] In other words, it takes more food deprivation to get them to feel hungry and greater quantities of food to get them to feel full, compared to unrestrained eaters.

Are You a Restrained Eater?

So what kind of eater are you? Restrained or unrestrained? To find out, indicate how strongly you agree with each of the following statements by putting a number after each statement in the "Response" column. Leave the "Score" column blank for now.

1: Strongly disagree
2: Somewhat disagree
3: Neutral
4: Somewhat agree
5: Strongly agree

Intuitive Eating Scale	Response	Score
1. Without really trying, I naturally select the right types and amounts of food to be healthy.		
2. I generally count calories before deciding if something is OK to eat.		
3. One of my main reasons for exercising is to manage my weight.		
4. I seldom eat unless I notice that I am physically hungry.		
5. I am hopeful that I will someday find a new diet that will actually work for me.		
6. The health and strength of my body is more important to me than how much I weigh.		
7. I often turn to food when I feel sad, anxious, lonely, or stressed out.		
8. There are certain foods that I really like, but I try to avoid them so that I won't gain weight.		
9. I am often frustrated with my body size and wish that I could control it better.		
10. I consciously try to eat whatever kind of food I think will satisfy my hunger the best.		
11. I am afraid to be around some foods because I don't want to be tempted to indulge myself.		
12. I am happy with my body even if it isn't very good-looking.		
13. I normally eat slowly and pay attention to how physically satisfying my food is.		
14. I am often either on a diet or seriously considering going on a diet.		

Intuitive Eating Scale	Response	Score
15. I usually feel like a failure when I eat more than I should.		
16. After eating, I often realize that I am fuller than I would like to be.		
17. I often feel physically weak and hungry because I am dieting to control my weight.		
18. I often put off buying clothes, participating in fun activities, or going on vacations (hoping I can get thinner first).		
19. When I feel especially good or happy, I like to celebrate by eating.		
20. I often find myself looking for something to eat or making plans to eat—even when I'm not really hungry.		
21. I feel pressure from those around me to control my weight or to watch what I eat.		
22. I worry more about how fattening a food might be, rather than how nutritious it might be.		
23. It's hard to resist eating something good if it is around me, even if I'm not very hungry.		
24. On social occasions, I feel pressure to eat the way those around me are eating—even if I'm not hungry.		
25. I honestly don't care how much I weigh as long as I'm physically fit, healthy, and can do the things I want.		
26. I feel safest if I have a diet plan, or diet menu, to guide my eating.		
27. I mostly exercise because of how good it makes me feel physically.		

Scoring

This scale was developed by researchers[29] and has been used in many studies that examine people's eating habits. To help make sure you didn't bias your results based on what you thought you *should* respond, the questions were set up so that agreeing with some indicated that you were a restrained eater and agreeing with others indicated the opposite.

For the following questions, copy your response into the scoring column: 1, 4, 6, 10, 12, 13, 25, 27. (In other words, if you chose "1" [strongly disagree], copy the "1" into the scoring column; if you chose "2," copy the "2"; etc.) Now, go back and reverse score the following questions: 2, 3, 5, 7, 8, 9, 11, 14, 15, 16, 17, 18, 19, 20, 21, 22, 23, 24, 26. Here's what I mean by reverse score: If you chose "1," give yourself a "5," etc. (1=5, 2=4, 3=3, 4=2, 5=1).

Low scores in the score column (1 or 2) indicate attitudes of a restrained eater, and help you to identify areas for potential growth. This book is going to help you become an unrestrained eater, moving more toward higher scores of 4 or 5.

Restrained Eating: Danger, Danger!

What's the danger in restrained eating habits? If you are a restrained eater, you try to control your body weight and don't trust your body to do it for you. You're likely to be gaining weight or—at the very least—frustrated in your efforts to lose.

Why? Because attempts to control your food intake through willpower and control require that you drown out the internal signals, leaving you much more vulnerable to external signals. This approach is a problem because unless you lock yourself in a closet, there's no way to control the constant exposure to food we face in our world. Food or food images are *everywhere*. Food companies are the second largest advertisers in the U.S. economy (trailing only automobile manufacturers).[30] Drive by a fast-food restaurant and the smell of frying meat and potatoes suddenly makes you ravenous; see a commercial for pizza and before you know it your fingers are speed-dialing Pizza Hut; whether you're hungry or not, dieting or not, you suddenly have to eat.

But if you're an unrestrained eater, those cues don't faze you. Sure the pizza smells good, but one piece may be enough; if your needs are met, you lose your desire for more. Meanwhile, the restrained eater is already on her fourth piece.

Check out the research to see how this plays out. Say you've just had a fabulous dinner at one of the top restaurants in town. It's dessert time, but you're really full. Nonetheless, the waitress insists on handing you a dessert menu, or describes in glowing terms the apple tart she's sure you'll love, or brings the dessert tray around to *show* you the tempting pastries. When researchers tested these scenarios with real people,[31] they found that unrestrained eaters were much less likely to order dessert regardless of what type of persuasion the waitress tried, while restrained eaters were much more likely to order dessert if they heard about it or saw it.

This research plays into the issue of dieting, too. In one study, women were told they were going to rate the quality of certain foods.[32] Some women got a milkshake followed by three bowls of ice cream; some just got the ice cream. The restrained eaters who *didn't* get the milkshake ate very little of the ice cream (trying to be "good"), but those who drank the milkshake also ate most of the ice cream. (The "what the hell" effect[33]. . . i.e., "I drank the milkshake, I ruined my diet, what the hell, I'll eat the ice cream, too.") The idea that there will be a restriction in the future paradoxically motivated these women to act counter to their internal restriction, "to get it while I can."

Overall, more than seventy-five studies have been conducted to examine the effects of various situations that disturb the restrained eater's self-control. The results are consistent: Restrained eaters react to emotions and external cues in a nearly totally opposite manner of unrestrained eaters.

Emotions such as depression, anxiety, anger, fear, and excitement or disinhibitors, such as alcohol, cause a restrained eater to overeat. Conversely, they turn off the appetite of an unrestrained eater. As long as things go well, the restrained eater can maintain control. But if anything gets in the way or changes, she can't maintain that control. The reason is clear: Restrained eaters don't rely on the normal signals of fullness to regulate their eating, so there are no brakes in place.

Also disturbing: Restrained eaters burn fewer calories after a meal than unrestrained eaters, and more of the calories they burn come from carbohydrates as opposed to fat.[34, 35, 36, 37, 38, 39]

Becoming an Unrestrained Eater

I hear you, I hear you. You want to know how you can become an unrestrained eater. Be patient: Chapter 9 will guide you in learning how to "hear" your body's signals of hunger and fullness and finding new ways to address those emotional issues that once drove you to the refrigerator. The next few chapters help you understand the stumbling blocks, how you got here, and why your setpoint dial is set where it is.

THREE

We Resist
Weight Loss

Are you still looking for the right diet or exercise plan to help you permanently lose weight? It may be hard to believe that there just isn't scientific evidence to support *any* theory of how to lose weight and keep it off. No matter how many times or how authoritatively the message is repeated that diet, exercise, and discipline can get you what you want, it doesn't change the fact that it has not proven true for any but a tiny minority of people.

This chapter examines why dieting backfires, why exercise fails to deliver on its weight-loss promises, and how sleep habits and how you manage stress complicate weight regulation. It also details a few other surprising environmental factors that contribute to your weight. And before you go looking for a shortcut to weight loss, be sure to read the discussion on pills and bariatric (weight-loss) surgery.

If you are focused on weight loss, you may be hesitant to read this chapter. After all, believing in these techniques provides the conviction to suffer through that diet or exercise plan. You may be concerned that losing faith in weight loss is tantamount to giving up, condemning you to being forever disappointed, stuck in a body you don't want. Why read this chapter?

Because first you need to understand that failed weight-loss attempts aren't your fault. Lightening up on the self-blame will make you more effective at achieving what is possible.

In Greek legend, the gods condemned Sisyphus to ceaselessly roll a rock to the top of a mountain, where it would tumble to the bottom, forcing him to start uphill again. Sisyphus's efforts are not unlike the weight-loss cycle of dieting, regaining, and dieting again that many of us have experienced firsthand. Or the New Year's resolutions to exercise regularly, which are quickly abandoned when weight-loss goals are not accomplished, only to be tried again the following year.

Why subject yourself to such a tragic fate? Who wants to be stuck interminably repeating the same painful task if it doesn't accomplish what you want and serves no useful purpose?

My wish is that this chapter will provide you with a sense of relief and renewed hope. The fact that your body can so powerfully resist weight loss is a sign that it *can* control your weight, much better than you can—meaning you don't have to fight your desires through conscious control. There is no need to watch your food intake or force yourself to "work out."

Imagine that. You can enjoy eating and moving your body. No more rice cakes when you really want that buttery biscuit, no more bicycling to nowhere as punishment when you do indulge. Future chapters support you in learning just how to trust and honor the weight-regulation system that is packaged inside you.

Putting Calories into Perspective

You may already know this plain fact: Weight loss is simply a matter of taking in fewer calories* than you spend. Conventional weight-

---

*For all the attention that's been paid to the calorie over the years, we never got it right. A calorie is actually a very small measure of energy, and its generic use is technically incorrect. The correct term is "kilocalorie," which refers to 1,000 calories. For the purposes of this book, though, I will continue to use the word "calories" because that's the term people understand best.

loss ideology exploits this fact, prompting you to diet (reduce calorie intake) or exercise (increase calories spent). On the surface, this seems logical.

The problem is it doesn't work—at least not in a lasting way. All you folks who have dieted or exercised with gusto, only to regain the weight, listen up! You did not fail to keep the weight off because you are lazy, weak, or undisciplined. It's not because you didn't want it badly enough. You regained that weight *because the contributors to your body weight, such as what, when, and how much you eat, as well as how you expend energy (including your inclination to move), are not completely under conscious control.*

Sure, on a short-term basis you can do a pretty good job of manipulating your food or exercise habits—and that's why short-term weight loss is relatively easy. On a long-term basis, however, your body can undermine your best efforts to control your weight.

What Are Calories Really

Calories are a measure of energy. Energy is a difficult term to understand as it takes on such different forms. To put energy in perspective, if you could harness food energy and put it to work, there is sufficient energy in five pounds of spaghetti to brew a pot of coffee. Or you could light a 60-watt bulb for ninety minutes with a piece of pie.

The energy contained in 2,000 calories is just about enough to fuel everything I like to accomplish in a day, but it might exceed someone else's ability to make use of it. The unused energy gets stored on his or her body and shows up as weight gain on the scale. For another person, those same 2,000 calories may not be enough to fuel his or her activities, and his or her body has to take some energy out of storage. His or her scale registers weight loss.

My Hypothalamus Made Me Do It

Do you think you can choose to eat or not, or skip dessert? The extent to which we have free will when it comes to eating—and even moving—is a lot more complicated than commonly believed. Sure, you can make choices at an individual meal. Likewise, the motivation to show up for your running buddy may override your temptation to hit the snooze button and go back to sleep.

But here's what's confusing. Weight-regulation mechanisms act over the course of weeks, months, or years, not meal to meal, nor do they dictate daily decisions to exercise. Over the long run, you just don't have that kind of control. Biology lurks behind the urge to eventually cheat on your diet or to go back to sleep.

This is how it works. As discussed in chapter one, a section of your brain, most notably your hypothalamus, helps regulate your weight. It accomplishes this regulation through many different mechanisms, such as sending out chemical messengers that control the rate at which you burn energy. Conceptually, it probably makes sense to most people that the body controls unconscious processes like this.

What's harder to understand is that signals from the hypothalamus also regulate conscious behaviors, such as eating, by increasing or decreasing the appetite. Those unconscious signals influence how appealing food is to you, contributing to actions such as ordering a pizza or having a second piece of pie. Just because an action is conscious and requires your complicity doesn't mean that all aspects of it are voluntary.

Sometimes your hypothalamus might just be giving you a little nudge, saying I'm hungry, feed me, and boy those corn chips look tempting. But you can resist with a strong will to lose weight. Yes, you are in control. You can conquer hunger. Willpower works— short term.

But other times the deck is stacked against you so strongly that it's way too hard to "just say no." Those chips are so compelling that you can't resist.

Always remember this. *It's not your fault!* Biology is so powerful it can "make" you break that diet.

A rare few individuals can muster up an extraordinary amount of willpower to conquer even the most intense hunger drive. Think of the political conviction of someone on an extended hunger strike. Careers in the public eye, like modeling or acting, which require individuals to maintain a certain body type, can also sometimes provide enough incentive for people to "just say no." But I don't recommend you try, as your body doesn't give up without a good fight.

When your body can't get you to comply with its demand to break your diet, it asserts even more control by toning down certain metabolic processes. As a result, people who do succeed at conquering the drive to eat are miserable. Experimentally underfed people experience lower energy levels, apathy, dizziness, intolerance to cold, slower metabolism, preoccupation with food, intense hunger and cravings, decreased sex drive, general irritability, and depression, among other characteristics.[40] Not a pretty picture—though incredibly effective at helping you conserve body energy. In today's context, it may not be so reassuring to know that you're well equipped to survive food shortages. But this survival instinct sure was a valuable trait in the past!

Eat Less, Weigh More

If you sometimes feel that dieting has surpassed baseball as the national pastime, you're not alone. So many of us are dieting, coming off a diet, or feeling guilty that we're *not* dieting, that the word "diet" has morphed from a noun to a verb.

Yet here's the thing: Not one study has ever shown that diets produce long-term weight loss for any but a tiny number of dieters. Not one.

Consider the Women's Health Initiative, the largest, longest, and most expensive randomized, controlled dietary intervention clinical trial, designed to test whether the prevailing wisdom actually works. More than 20,000 women tried out a low-fat diet, reportedly reducing their calorie intake by an average of 360 calories per day. After almost eight years on this diet, there was no change in weight from starting point, and their average waist circumference, which is a measure of abdominal fat, had *increased*![41]

Consistent with the research conducted on thousands of other diets, including my own study, the dieters lost weight at the beginning, but gained it back.

Commentators often attribute weight regain to people's inability to maintain their diets over the long run: the old "no willpower" problem. Yet this study was well controlled to support the women in maintaining their diets. *Weight regain occurred despite maintaining their reduced-calorie diet!*

And lest you think these results are particular to low-fat dieting, check out the data from this study of other popular diets.[42] After twelve months, Atkins dieters were eating 289 fewer calories compared to when they started the diet, Zone dieters were eating 381 fewer calories, LEARN dieters were eating 271 fewer calories, and Ornish dieters were eating 345 fewer calories. Yet all were steadily regaining weight over the last six months of the first year. And this despite an accompanying increase in exercise!

Imagine this: You spend eight years denying yourself foods, feeling virtuous as you successfully restrict yourself—all that pain and discomfort—and, at least from the perspective of weight, nothing to show! Wouldn't you rather have been among the 29,000 women in the control group of the Women's Health Initiative who were encouraged to continue their usual eating habits? They didn't lose weight either, but at least they didn't endure the misery of dieting!

It's not just that dieting doesn't work. Diet enough and it may actually push your setpoint up, so you wind up weighing more after the diet than if you'd never started the darn thing to begin with![43, 44, 45, 46, 47, 48, 49]

Dieting interferes with your weight regulation system in several ways.

Recall our discussion of the hormone leptin from chapter 1. When you diet, your body produces less of this appetite-suppressing hormone.[21, 50, 51] This, in turn, jump-starts your appetite, making that chocolate cake look as tempting as a stack of unattended $100 bills. No wonder you want to break your diet! Leptin also slows your metabolism. Combine the two and you find yourself on the Weight Gain Express.

But that's not all. Over time, as you diet, stop dieting, diet, stop dieting, your body gets sick of it all and simply sets the leptin-meter to permanent low, producing less of the hormone regardless of which part of the diet cycle you're in.[21, 22] Less leptin means your body isn't working as effectively as it should to tame your appetite and stoke your metabolic machinery. Your setpoint has now been pumped up a notch.

In addition to the reduced leptin during diets, your body pumps out *higher* levels of lipoprotein lipase, an enzyme that increases fat storage.[52] And, if the studies in rats translate to humans (and there is strong evidence they do), yo-yo dieters are compelled to choose foods higher in fat.[53, 54] Some reward for trying to be "good," huh?

So here's a review of the above, with a few other choice tidbits added in. Dieting:

- Slows the rate at which your body burns calories.
- Increases your body's efficiency at wringing every possible calorie out of the food you do eat so you digest food faster and get hungrier quicker.
- Causes you to crave high-fat foods.
- Increases your appetite.
- Reduces your energy levels (so even if you could burn more calories through physical activity you don't want to).
- Lowers your body temperature so you're using less energy (and are always cold).
- Reduces your ability to feel "hungry" and "full," making it easier to confuse hunger with emotional needs.
- Reduces your total amount of muscle tissue (and you may know that a pound of muscle burns more calories than a pound of fat).
- Increases fat-storage enzymes and decreases fat-release enzymes.

The message here? Don't blame yourself when you "break" your diet. It's not about gluttony or a failure of willpower. In fact, most dieters show extraordinary self-restraint, persistence, determination, and willpower. You didn't fail; the diet did.

Numerous animal studies verify this simple fact: After a diet, an animal will regain the weight *without overeating*. Reflect on your own history: how much were you really eating when you regained the weight?

The first step toward recovery: Do no more damage. In other words, quit the diet habit cold turkey. Since most dieters are likely to be above their setpoints, simply kicking the diet habit and restoring control to your body may result in a bit of weight loss. But regardless of whether your weight changes, I do promise that there's even better stuff in store for you.

Sounds too good to be true, doesn't it? No more cutting calories and going hungry. No more guilt about what you eat. All you need to do is lighten up and put your body in charge. Well, perhaps there's a little more to it than that. After all, it's been a long time since you trusted your body, and, like any damaged relationship, it will take a while to begin communicating clearly again. Chapter 9 guides you in becoming attuned.

Of course, diet attempts are not the only contributor to your weight. Plenty of other lifestyle behaviors and environmental exposures affect that number on the scale: activity habits, stress, even the toxins we're exposed to. Let's tackle the "activity makes you skinny" assumption next.

The Couch Potato Syndrome

Though more people are acknowledging that diets don't work, there is rarely any challenge to the concept that exercise can produce weight loss. We hold very tenaciously to our beliefs that "fat = lazy" and "if people would just get off their butts and get moving, they'd be much thinner." The problem with these ideas? There's no evidence to support them!

In theory, exercise should help moderate your setpoint. Physical activity (whether in the gym or in the garden) increases your sensitivity to signals of hunger and fullness[55, 56] by increasing leptin sensitivity[57] and production, increasing insulin sensitivity, and affecting numerous other hormones, neurotransmitters, and cellular receptors involved in weight regulation.[58]

In fact, burning calories is just a tiny part of the many ways physical activity affects your weight. Check out the different ways physical activity can rev up your metabolism and affect your weight. It:

- Speeds up your metabolic rate, not just while moving/exercising, but for many hours afterward.
- Reduces your hunger drive.
- Increases your body temperature so you burn more energy.
- Increases your energy levels so you burn more energy.
- Improves your sensitivity to hunger and fullness.
- Increases your amount of muscle tissue so you burn more energy.
- Increases fat-burning enzymes and decreases fat-storing enzymes.
- Improves cell sensitivity to insulin (you need less to do the same job), allowing you to burn more energy.
- Uses more fat and less carbohydrates for energy (which helps stabilize blood glucose levels).

Last—and maybe least important—is that while doing many of these, it burns calories.

Given all these dramatic effects, will a dedicated exercise routine help you to lose weight, or more precisely, body fat? The answer may surprise you.

Exercise Is Not the Ultimate Weight-Loss Panacea!

Contrary to popular belief and despite the exercise effects listed above, long-term studies do *not* show that people lose significant weight on exercise programs.

Before we examine this, first note that weight differences between those who exercise regularly and those who don't aren't very dramatic. Most studies find that people who regularly exercise are only about five to ten pounds lighter than those who are sedentary. The Women's Health Study, for example, evaluated almost 40,000 women and determined that the difference in body mass index between those at the highest level of exercise and the lowest was only about 0.4. For a 5'4" woman, that amounts to about three pounds![59] The Harvard Alumni Study compared more than 12,000 men who regularly participated in various intensities of exercise and, similarly, found a difference of less than five pounds.[60] These results are consistent with many other studies.

Since good health habits tend to travel in packs, it's difficult to definitively attribute even these slightly lower weights to exercise. The same people who exercise may also eat their leafy green vegetables, have better stress management techniques, or maintain other habits that may explain some or all of the weight difference. Also, perhaps the causality operates in the other direction; after all, heavier people may be less inclined to exercise given the lack of social support. Gyms, for example, are rarely friendly to those in larger bodies. And comfortable exercise clothing is harder to come by if you've got a larger body.

But what happens when people try to lose weight through exercise? When formerly sedentary people regularly participate in exercise programs, the research is not showing dramatic weight loss. In fact, a meta-analysis of twenty-five years of exercise programs indicated that training programs only result in loss of 0.2 pounds per week.[61] Consider the Heritage Family Study as an example, in which 500 men and women participated in a twenty-week endurance training program.[62] On average, the men lost less than a pound, and the women lost nearly nothing! In another study, the large women participating in an intense six-month resistance training program also did not exhibit any body fat loss or change in body composition.[63] The Midwest Exercise Trial put men and women on a sixteen-month intensive endurance exercise program.[64] The men were quite successful, losing, on average, about 11 pounds; the women, on the other hand, *gained* a little over a pound, while losing less than a half pound of body fat!

Surprisingly, many studies have found women actually *gain* weight and body fat with exercise. One study that monitored large women who did six months of aerobic exercise four to five times a week found that a third of them gained 15 pounds of body fat, and that the gainers averaged an 8-pound weight gain.[65]

If exercise affects so many aspects of your setpoint mechanism, you may be wondering, why hasn't it proven to support weight loss?

No one has the answer to this question, but I suspect there are two explanations. The first relates to the point raised earlier that your body is very protective at making sure you don't lose too much weight, but is relatively lax about supporting weight loss. Consider our discussion of leptin. Remember that you reach a saturation point where more leptin doesn't have a correspondingly stronger effect? This fact suggests that exercise (which helps you produce more leptin and improves leptin sensitivity) is very effective at preventing weight gain, even if it is less effective at promoting weight loss, and could explain why people who exercise regularly are just a little lighter than those who don't.

Here's another theory that may simultaneously be true. Many people believe that exercising gives them permission to eat more than they are actually hungry for. They never allow themselves to experience the more important weight-lowering benefits, such as reduced appetite (relative to the increased energy spent) and increased sensitivity to hunger/fullness signals. Because they do not respond to their body signals, the improvements stimulated by exercise do not have a noticeable effect on eating habits, and they may even eat more to compensate.[66]

In support of these theories, one research study monitored large women on an exercise program.[56] They noticed that as the women participated in the exercise program, their leptin output increased and their appetites correspondingly decreased. Despite this decrease in appetite, however, their food intake didn't change. In other words, appetite was reduced—evidence that their bodies were trying to support them in weight loss—but they weren't paying attention to it, with the result that their increased exercise habits never showed on the scale.

Perhaps individuals who exercise regularly while simultaneously taking advantage of their heightened sensitivity to hunger and fullness signals will have better success lowering their weight through exercise, if that is what their bodies are meant to do. In other words, exercise may only be a weight-lowering technique when coupled with dumping the diet mentality and replacing it with internally regulated eating habits.

While it is unclear whether being regularly active reduces one's setpoint, there is no doubt that increased activity, in addition to being fun, is the single most important thing you can do to improve your health and well-being. Active people are much healthier than sedentary ones, *regardless of weight*.[67] Exercise can cure, prevent, or minimize most of the major chronic diseases and disturbances, including diabetes, insulin resistance, hypertension, high cholesterol levels, cancer, digestive disorders, circulatory disorders, etc.

Also important, being active can help you feel better about yourself. Several studies have shown that when people increase their activity they also increase their self-confidence, self-acceptance, and sense of personal worth and feel more comfortable in their bodies. As chapter 8 will make clear, these are exactly the tools you need to be successful at implementing all the other health-promoting strategies detailed in this book. Chapter 10 gives you a game plan to get you up and moving.

Beyond Food and Activity

So I've shot down dieting and exercise as sure-fire weight-loss techniques. Few people think beyond these two pieces of the puzzle, but there's a much bigger picture that's less self-evident, much of which is poorly understood. For example, a pregnant mom's nutrition and other habits affect the offspring's body weight later in life. It's also well established that stress, sleep deprivation, even viral infections, microbes in your gut, and environmental toxins also play a role. Let's take a look at some of these additional contributors to weight. We'll keep our focus on lifestyle and environmental factors, rather than pre-birth or genetic factors.

Stress

Uh-oh. Job interview coming up. The mere thought of it stimulates your nervous system to get charged. When the body is challenged by almost anything, from getting out of bed in the morning to running up a flight of stairs or having to stand up and give a talk, the brain activates the sympathetic nervous system, the so-called "flight or fight" response, which causes the release of the stress hormones, among them cortisol and epinephrine. Their net effect is to make a lot of stored energy (glucose and fat) available to cells. Cells are then primed to help the body get away from danger.

If you were a caveperson innocently picking berries when suddenly you come nose to nose with a saber-toothed tiger, you'd appreciate this. The flood of energy might help you scamper up that tree.

Couch Potatoes Created in the Womb?

You are not only what you eat, you may also be what your mother ate. Several studies find that if your mother dieted during her pregnancy, you're more likely to be heavier as an adult. One study found that the adult children of dieting pregnant women were less likely to be physically active than the adult children of women who didn't diet. This suggests that conserving energy to protect against the food insecurity you experienced in utero may now be "hardwired" into your genetic memory.[68]

However, with mental stress, the body pumps out these hormones to no avail. Fighting or fleeing won't help when the "enemy" is your own mind. Nonetheless, your bloodstream is flooded with nutrients, and sugar storage mechanisms are suppressed. With nowhere to go, the unused sugar in your bloodstream gets converted to fat.

Cortisol acts both to pack the fat away into storage and as a powerful appetite stimulant, prompting you to eat more and get even more nutrients into your bloodstream. Stress also results in suppression of the release of growth hormone, which would have reduced fat storage and sped up your metabolism. It's not surprising that we see links between chronic stress and higher weight.[69, 70] Also, more stress results in less nutritious eating, which contributes to the higher weight.[69]

It may be that stress doesn't act alone. In one very interesting experiment, scientists subjected mice to stress by locking them in a cage with a more aggressive mouse. Some of the mice were given standard feed, and the others were fed the mouse equivalent of a processed food diet. The stressed mice eating the processed foods gained a significant amount of weight, much more than the stressed mice fed the standard feed. They also gained significantly more weight than mice consuming the same processed food diet that were not subject to stress. If this translates to humans, it suggests that it's not just the stress, but the combination of stress and a nutrient-poor diet, that does you in.[71]

In another interesting experiment, researchers injected a virus that replicates in neurons with receptors for leptin. The virus was engineered to carry a gene for a green fluorescent protein. The presence of the protein enabled researchers to trace the path of the virus as it moved through the brain. It turns out that in addition to sensing leptin levels, the neurons with leptin receptors also received input from a region of the brain that plays a role in emotion.[72] In other words, the brain section that modulates emotion was, just like leptin, influencing appetite and energy expenditure.

Sleep

Can you dream your way to maintaining a lighter weight? As wild as the idea sounds, the relationship between sleep deprivation and weight gain is actually well established.[73,74,75,76,77] Several studies also detail the link between sleep loss and the metabolic hormones.[78,79]

Have you ever had a restless night followed by a day when no matter what you ate you never felt full or satisfied? If so, you probably experienced the workings of leptin and ghrelin. Insufficient sleep drives leptin levels down, which means you don't feel as satisfied after you eat. Lack of sleep also causes ghrelin levels to rise, stimulating your appetite so you want more food.

That's what happened to the twelve men in this research study.[79] When sleep was restricted, leptin levels went down and ghrelin levels went up. The men's appetites also increased proportionally, as would be expected. Also interesting was that their desire for high-carbohydrate, calorie-dense foods increased by a whopping 45 percent!

Strange but True: Viruses, Bugs, and Toxins

Is weight gain contagious? Can you blame it on the bugs in your gut? How about the pesticides in your food? Turns out there's scientific evidence supporting all these factors playing a role in some people's weight gain. There are many different—and surprising—factors that influence our eating habits and fat deposition. Here's the scoop.

A Weight-Gain Virus

Scientists were surprised to find that heavier people were four to six times more likely to have a cold-like virus, called adenovirus-36, than leaner people. Inoculating mice, rats, chickens, and monkeys with the virus results in the animals gaining weight and body fat—without eating more.[80, 81]

Researchers didn't try to infect humans, but they did expose human stem cells—the blank slate of the cell world—to the virus and found that they turned into fat cells.[82] They didn't just change, they stored fat, too.

Certainly we have a history of blaming several diseases and conditions on diet, only to find out later that a microbe was to blame. Consider ulcers. Long thought to be a product of high stress and a poor diet, most ulcers are now known to be caused by the bacterium H. pylori. Or consider heart disease: To date, three different microbes have been discovered that are thought to contribute to clogged arteries. There is also a well-established association between periodontal disease and heart disease that is attributed to certain bacteria.[83] Strong evidence associates several viruses with weight gain.[84]

Bugs Making Us Fat

You might not be out of line to link a burgeoning belly to the bugs in your tummy. The three to four pounds of bacteria swilling around in our bellies not only play a central role in our digestion, but are also important energy regulators.[85] And it turns out that some microbes are better at wringing calories out of your meals than others. Transferring these high-octane bugs from fat mice into lean mice causes the lean mice to plump up.[86]

Fatter people tend to have a significantly greater proportion of one of the two main types of bacteria found in the gut, known as Firmicutes, than the other, known as Bacteroidetes. Detailed molecular analyses show that the Firmicutes are much better at extracting calories from food.[87]

When researchers spent a year meticulously measuring the gut flora of the heavier volunteers as they tried to lose weight by eating low-calorie diets, they actually discovered that the proportion of Firmicutes in their digestive tracts rose and the proportion of Bacteroidetes fell.[87] This discovery could easily explain why it becomes harder and harder to lose weight through dieting.

Think about this. The same bowl of pasta yields a different number of calories for each eater. Rodents raised in a sterile environment and lacking in gut flora need to eat 30 percent more calories just to remain the same weight as their normal counterparts.[88]

What causes an individual to have their particular mix of gut flora isn't clear. But perhaps some change, such as a food additive or antibiotic use, has caused a fundamental shift in these bugs, making it easier for many people to gain weight.

The Fattening Effect of Pollution

The jury is out on the relationship between pollution and weight, but the connection is certainly plausible, and it's a hot topic in research.[89] It is well established that dioxins, pesticides, and other compounds disrupt hormonal function. Since your hormones play a large role in weight regulation, it's not a big leap to assume that toxins also disrupt your ability to effectively regulate your weight.

Compounds that change hormonal function are called "endocrine disrupters," and those that are known to increase fat production are more specifically labeled "obesogens."[90,91,92] Tributyltin chloride, or TBT, is an example of an obesogen that has been well studied in animals.[91,93] Frogs and mice injected with miniscule doses of TBT got very fat. And prenatally exposed mice are 10–15 percent heavier than control mice.

TBT is ubiquitous in our environment. Originally part of marine paints, it is now used in fungicides, wood preservatives, and in the manufacture of PVC plastics (used in water pipes and food packaging). A limited study pegs the average human TBT blood concentration at 27nM, or just slightly higher than what has shown to affect laboratory animals.[94]

Although a causative effect has yet to be established, production of industrial chemicals in the United States, including TBT, closely parallels the weight increase observed in the United States.

Most environmental toxins are fat-soluble compounds that resist breakdown. Once they're absorbed into your body, they get stored in fat tissue, and fatter people have been observed to have higher concentrations than leaner people.[89] That may not be a problem when the toxins are locked into fat tissue, which is relatively inert. However, think about what happens during repeated cycles of weight loss: Those toxins get released into the bloodstream where they have another opportunity to do damage.[95] Makes you question whether weight loss is a positive goal, doesn't it? No doubt part of the reason why studies show higher incidence of certain diseases in larger people can be explained by the damage caused by repeated dieting.

Looking For a Shortcut?

Perhaps by now you got the message that dieting and exercise haven't been proven to support sustained weight loss and that many factors beyond your control contribute to your weight. Maybe you're considering outside help?

Weight-Loss Drugs, Supplements, Surgery, or Other "Aids"

It's easy to get caught up in the fantasy that a pill or a scalpel can give you what you want. Advertising for weight-loss "aids," whether supplements, drugs, surgery, acupuncture, or metals that change your body's polarity, manipulates your emotions and reinforces and exploits your insecurities. Fearmongering about the dangers posed by "excess" weight and false promises of benefits allow you to rationalize these weight-loss aids as promoting good health and increased longevity. Inspirational success stories and celebrity testimonials lead you on. That physicians, dieticans, and other "experts" back the aid provides added permission to buy in to the fantasy.

But do weight-loss dreams really come true? Has anyone figured out how to effectively short-circuit setpoint mechanisms? Of course not. If something seems too good to be true, it is. While numerous "aids" may support short-term weight loss, there is no convincing evidence that anything can help you maintain weight loss over the long run without the risk of seriously compromising your health. Here's a quick look.

Selling Hope in a Pill Bottle

That there are pharmaceutical weight-loss treatments on the market is more about the pharmaceutical industry's power to persuade regulators to obliterate barriers intended to keep consumers safe, than about their success in generating maintained weight loss.

Yes, you can temporarily curb your appetite or boost your metabolism with an amphetamine or similar supplements, but you may also be nervous, jumpy, and subject to insomnia and addiction and a host of other problems. Plus, once you stop taking the supplement, your lost weight comes right back, if not more.

Then there's Alli, the FDA-approved, over-the-counter weight-loss drug, designed to keep your body from absorbing fat. The problem is you also miss out on absorbing many fat-soluble nutrients essential for good health.[96, 97] You are also unlikely to lose much weight.[98] Plus, soon after taking Alli, your weight may ratchet back to where it started, if not higher.*

And let's get graphic about what blocking fat absorption means: Instead of entering your body where it might actually be useful, that

---

*No long-term studies have been conducted, but this is a reasonable assumption given that prolonged use is contraindicated and it stops working after use.

fat dribbles out the end of your digestive tract. Alli-oops, as some people say. "Anal leakage" and "dumping syndrome" are the official medical terms. The drug company that makes Alli even issued an advisory: "You may feel an urgent need to go to the bathroom. . . . It's probably a smart idea to wear dark pants, and bring a change of clothes with you to work."[99]

The two Food and Drug Administration–approved prescription drugs, orlistat (which is prescription-strength Alli) and sibutramine, are not showing exciting results,[98] even though almost all the testing has been industry-funded. First, 30 to 40 percent of the research participants drop out of the studies (presumably because they are not successful?) and are not included in the final analysis. Of the remaining subjects who do complete the trials, weight loss is small: on average between 6 and 10 pounds. And each drug carries adverse cardiovascular effects.

The fact that such supplements are useless over the long run makes sense. First, your body systems are intricately entwined. Upset one and it has multiple reverberating effects on others. We may call the unwanted effects "side effects" but they are no less a part of the mechanisms of action than the effect we are looking for.

But more importantly, all supplements work on changing one aspect of your weight-regulatory system. If the principal effect of a drug is to suppress your appetite and reduce the amount you eat, then your body will perceive the caloric deprivation and compensate accordingly. For instance, it will slow your metabolism so you expend less energy, and any weight loss will be temporary at best.

A supplement that works in the brain to increase metabolism will be similarly ineffective, since your body will eventually turn up your hunger signals to compensate. Just as we see long-term weight regain result from diet and exercise, expect the same from supplements. You can't trick your body for too long.

So don't fall for the hype. There is no "magic pill" that will melt the pounds away. No doubt by the time this is published there will be new drugs and supplements on the market. But I'm not optimistic that we can expect anything different in the near future. It is unlikely that thin bodies will ever come from a bottle.

Dreams on the Operating Room Table (Bariatric Surgery)

Bariatric surgery refers to operations that help promote weight loss. It's among the highest-paying surgical specialties, which perhaps partially explains why accuracy and integrity in research and reporting go by the wayside. Combine that with our vulnerability—desperation to lose weight is not conducive to good judgment—and it's a setup for disaster.

People are misled about the extent and severity of the health risks associated with being fat and told that bariatric surgery is a solution. It's not. It would be more appropriately labeled high-risk disease-inducing cosmetic surgery than a health-enhancing procedure. And unlike a diet, you usually can't abandon it when you realize you made a mistake.

The ads for bariatric surgery make it sound so easy. Go to the hospital, gently breathe into a mask until you are lulled into unconsciousness, wake up thinner, and watch the pounds continue to drop off over time.

What's the other side to the story?

Bariatric surgery is nothing more than a forced diet: The various techniques reduce your stomach's capacity to hold food and/or damage your organs so that they can't absorb as many nutrients. The goal is to intentionally induce malnutrition, and post-surgical nutrition deficiencies are the norm.[100,101,102,103,104,105]

Dying is a distinct possibility. One study published in the *Journal of the American Medical Association* followed more than 16,000 people who underwent bariatric surgery and found that 4.6 percent died within a year.[106] (Men had higher death rates than women: 7.5 percent versus 3.7 percent.)

Other sources indicate lower mortality rates, but even the American Society for Metabolic and Bariatric Surgery, which presents the most optimistic picture, indicates that two to five out of every thousand individuals die within a month of gastric bypass, the most commonly conducted surgery.[107] Reported results are likely to be deceptively low: One investigative report found that deaths directly attributable to gastric bypass surgery were recorded as deaths from other causes, resulting in many never being accounted for.[108]

The largest examination of mortality rates[109] following bariatric surgery found chilling results: nearly 3% of the patients died after the first year and 6.4% at the end of the fourth year. Of those who had surgery in 1995 and had at least 9 years of follow-up, 13.0% had died. Of those who had the surgery in 1996 and 8 years of follow-up, 15.8% had died, and of those who had surgery in 1997 with 7 years of follow-up, 10.5% had died. Sandy Swarzc, on the Junkfood Science blog, compared these rates to the U.S. National Center for Health Statistics of the Centers for Disease Control and Prevention data, matching Americans of the same age and BMI and concludes: "By best estimates, bariatric surgeries likely increase the actual mortality risks for these patients by 7-fold in the first year and by 363% to 250% the first four years."[110]

"Complications" are likely. A few other possible complications that the ads usually forget to mention, as compiled by Dr. Paul Ernsberger and Sandy Swarzc: adhesions and polyps, massive scar tissue, advanced aging, anemia, arthritis, blackouts/fainting, bloating, body secretions (odor like rotten meat), bowel/fecal impaction, cancer (of the stomach, esophagus, pancreas, and bowel), chest pain from vomiting, circulation impairment, cold intolerance, constipation, depression, diarrhea, digestive impairment due to heavy mucus, digestive irregularities, diverticulitis, drainage problems at incision, early onset of diabetes, early onset of hypertension, electrolyte imbalance, erosion of tooth enamel, excessive dry skin, excessive stomach acid, esophageal contractions, esophageal erosion and scarring, feeling ill, gallbladder distress, gynecological complications, hair loss, hemorrhoids, hernia, hormone imbalances, impaired mobility, infection from leakage into body cavities (peritonitis), infertility, intestinal atrophy, intestinal gas, involuntary anorexia, irregular body fat distribution (lumpy body), iron deficiency, kidney impairment and failure, liver impairment and failure, loss of energy, loss of muscle control, loss of skin integrity, low hemoglobin, lowered immunity and increased susceptibility to illnesses, malfunction of the pituitary gland, muscle cramps, nausea, neural tube defects in your children, neurological impairment (nerve and brain damage), osteoporosis, pancreas impairment, pain along the left side, pain on digestion, pain on evacuation, peeling of fingernails, potassium loss, pulmonary embolus, putrid breath and stomach odor, rectal bleeding, shrinking of intestines, stomach pain, sleep irregularities, suicidal thoughts, thyroid malfunction, urinary tract infection, vitamin and mineral deficiency, vitamin and mineral malabsorption, violent hiccups that persist daily, vomiting from blockage, vomiting from drinking too fast, vomiting from eating too fast, vomiting from eating too much (more than 2 ounces) . . . and best of all—weight regain.[111]

It's hard to understand the justification for intentionally damaging healthy, functioning organs and voluntarily assuming the risk of death and "complications." Apparently, the rationalization is that the dangers of carrying "excess" weight are much worse than the dangers posed by the treatment. Yet the evidence just isn't convincing. Even the American Medical Association has raised serious doubts about bariatric surgery's effectiveness and safety, noting that ethical and scientific questions abound and that the long-term consequences of these surgeries remain uncertain, both in terms of health outcomes and whether significant weight loss is maintained.[112] The developer of gastric bypass, Dr. Edward Mason, also voices concern: "For the vast majority of patients today, there is no operation that will control weight to a 'normal' level without introducing risks and side effects that over a lifetime may raise questions about its use for surgical treatment of obesity."[113]

The most comprehensive independent review of bariatric surgery, conducted by the Emergency Care Research Institute, a nonprofit health services research agency, examined evidence from seventy studies.[114] The investigators reported that while significant weight loss occurred, patients still remain obese. However, they noted that the evidence demonstrating that associated diseases improved was weak, and it was not evident that surgery resolved heart disease or extended life span. They report that claims of improved "quality of life and long-term health impacts are less conclusive."

There is a remarkable paucity of long-term data, but emerging data suggests gradual weight regain and return of co-morbidities during the long term.[115, 116, 117]

It is also logical to expect that because the post-surgery weight loss occurs quickly, most of the weight loss is valuable muscle tissue, not fat, which typically occurs in other weight-loss studies in which the type of weight lost is monitored.

Following surgery, patients are still fat, though less so, and may not have improved prospects for health or longevity. Some may never be able to eat normally again, and may be limited to eating small amounts (about 1,300 calories per day) and forever avoiding certain foods, like milk and sweets. Even if they follow their post-surgery diet, they are still likely to experience pain, vomiting, and an inability to control stool ("dumping"). The American Society for Metabolic and Bariatric Surgery reports that 85 percent of patients experience dumping[118] while a study conducted by Brazilian surgeons found 64 percent experience vomiting five to nine years after their surgery.[119] Research also shows a high rate of depression and suicides among those who have undergone the surgery.[109, 120]

Patients are complimented on their weight loss after surgery. The increased social approval makes them unlikely to admit the painful side effects publicly or acknowledge that the quality of their lives is far worse. Even patients who experience complications often report improved quality of life post surgery.[121] As one post-surgery client explained to me: "We're ashamed to talk about the negatives. After all, we've failed all our lives and now we've failed again. So we pretend that it's all rosy. We accept the compliments and quietly soil our pants, quietly tolerate the hours of excruciating pain that results from one poorly chewed piece of food, the ongoing hospital visits to treat our nutritional deficiencies. But what scares me most is the denial. Scratch a 'success story' and you find someone having numerous complications, but they are so brainwashed to believe they were going to die from fat, and so desperate for social approval, that they actually believe they are healthier and better off for having the surgery. Of course, their doctors support them in that view. And they're the ones raving about the results and recommending surgery to others!"

We don't get the full story. And you can't predict *your* outcome when you're considering the surgery.

Wouldn't it be amazing if bariatric medicine shifted its focus to helping fat people get or stay healthy rather than thin?

Bringing It Home

As this chapter illustrates in exhaustive detail, there is no magic solution to losing weight and keeping it off in a healthy manner. If you continue to seek the Holy Grail of weight loss, you may be feeling depressed right now. There are no guaranteed solutions—and the commonly recommended methods just aren't showing results.

But fantastic news lurks beneath: *You don't have to worry about your weight!* Just trust yourself and everything's going to be okay. Your body can take good care of you. It did this instinctively from day one, and with a little effort, you can re-engage with these powerful mechanisms so they take good care of you once again.

So be patient. A little more background will be helpful, and then part 2 will give you strategies to put your body back in the driver's seat.

Of course, we can't leave food out of a discussion about weight. Not surprisingly, the highly processed, calorie-dense, nutritionally bereft foods that make up the modern diet also play a role in our difficulty maintaining a healthy weight. Let's talk about nutrients next.

FOUR
We're Eternally Hungry

Now you understand that dieting is more likely to encourage weight gain than sustained weight loss. You aren't falling for the common perception that exercise is the magic weight loss panacea either. Maybe you're wondering whether you can lose weight if you just change *what* you eat.

Let's cut to the chase. *What you eat—at least from the perspective of weight loss—probably just doesn't matter a whole lot.* Nobody has yet proven that any particular dietary habit results in sustained weight loss. This statement makes sense: Our weight regulation system was designed to encourage weight gain rather than support weight loss. In other words, while it may be true that what we eat has contributed to a small degree to the raised setpoints we see today compared to the past, changing your diet won't necessarily result in lowering your setpoint and weight loss. This observation may seem downright unfair in our current cultural milieu, but it is where evolution has taken us.

Of course, what you eat does matter for good health.

Let's look more closely at how certain dietary styles may contribute to ratcheting our weight up.

It's the Food!?!

Clearly what we eat today—and many other details of our lives—differs significantly from foods commonly consumed in the past. Many foods common on today's menu don't activate our weight control system as readily as the foods we used to eat, leaving us hungry despite getting sufficient—or more than sufficient—calories.

We first started seeing Americans gaining weight in the late 1970s. That's also when our food supply underwent a significant shift and we started eating more. Not just a little more: Between 1970 and 2000, according to the USDA's Economic Research Service, our daily calorie intake jumped over 500 calories per person, a 25 percent increase*.[122]

But don't make the assumption that heavier people are responsible for this caloric leap. Interestingly, studies show that large people eat no more than lean people, despite a popular misconception that large people consistently overeat.[123, 124, 125] In the words of the National Academy of Sciences from their report on Diet and Health: "Most studies comparing normal and overweight people suggest that those that are overweight eat fewer calories than those of normal weight."[126]

One review examined thirteen studies and found the intake of heavier people to be less than or equal to thin people in twelve of those studies.[124] In one interesting study, investigators unobtrusively observed customers at fast-food restaurants, snack bars, and ice-cream parlors and found that the fatter customers ate no more than the thin ones. These are only casual observations, of course, and this particular study may be obscured by differences in what people eat in public versus what they eat in private, but many studies support these results, and few show otherwise.[127] What's likely is we're all eating more on average—and some are more genetically predisposed to hang on to it.

You also don't want to make the assumption that our dietary habits play a large role in weight gain. As we'll see in chapter 6, the weight gain we've experienced over the past few decades is not as

---

*While there are many compelling arguments that challenge these actual numbers and the degree of the increase, it does seem evident that we're eating more.

dramatic as we've been led to believe. All told, our current lifestyle probably only accounts for an increase in weight of less than 10 pounds or so for the average person (but significantly more for a small subset of the population that is particularly genetically vulnerable). That weights appear to have leveled off now may mean that our regulatory system has recalibrated to adjust to this dietary change.

Also, there are many other contributors to our collective weight gain. Ironically, the 1970s also marks a time period when more people turned to dieting.[2] As discussed previously, dieting is another likely contributing factor to our collective increase in calories, as restrictive behavior frequently triggers overeating in the short term and may cause the body to preferentially store more body fat in the long term.

Along with the increase in calories has come a shift in the type of food we're eating. If foods could be scientifically engineered to encourage weight gain, our modern food processing industry has done it. It does not surprise me that the introduction of high-fructose corn syrup, trans fats, fiber-free carbohydrates, and super-sized menus directly mirrors increases in weight.[128]

The Changing Tide of Nutrition

It used to be that the only foods available to us were generally nutritious. Their nutrients registered on our weight control monitors, turning off our appetites after we received sufficient calories.

Modern food processing has changed that. It's easy now to get concentrated calories that bypass our weight regulation system, adding calories without necessarily sending comparable signals that trigger feelings of fullness or satiety and otherwise register on our weight control meters. And many of us consume fewer foods that do register in that weight regulation system and turn off our hunger drive.

The problem? Our high-fat/high-sugar diet, rich in processed foods and animal foods.

For, it turns out, *what* we eat seems to be more important when it comes to keeping our weight regulation system functioning optimally than *how much* we eat. For instance, several studies find that vegetarians get the same amount of or significantly more calories than their meat-eating counterparts, yet remain slightly slimmer.[129, 130, 131] In part, this observation is because what we eat influences our metabolic efficiency and how much energy our bodies expend. What we eat also drives hunger and satiety signals, thus influencing how much we put in our mouths.

Myth Buster

Eating less will not help you to live longer. In fact, the 17-year NHANES I study found that exercise and eating *more* were better defenses against heart disease deaths than exercise and restricting calories.[132]

This fact became clear when researchers studied data from almost 10,000 participants in the first National Health and Nutrition Examination Survey (NHANES I).[132] They concluded that eating less did not necessarily make people thinner, and eating more did not necessarily translate into heavier weights.

Then there are the Chinese. Studies find that people in China take in about 20 percent more calories per person than Americans (about 270 additional calories a day) but are much slimmer than Americans.

While the sedentary American lifestyle may account for some of this difference, there is more to it than exercise alone. For instance, one study compared American and Chinese office workers—both with similar couch potato tendencies—and found pretty much the same results.[131]

There's no doubt about it: Continually eating certain foods increases the drive to eat and reduces the energy spent, while eating other foods has the entirely opposite effect.

Precisely controlled animal research demonstrates this point well. You may think it's just common sense that rich or good-tasting food would result in overeating, leading to becoming fatter than would occur on blander food. Research does support this theory. For example, human research shows that with more variety, people eat more.[133, 134] But how this happens defies common sense.

One experiment divided ordinary rats into three groups.[135] One group was fed rat chow mixed with vegetable shortening (kind of like a rat's version of cheesecake); these rats grew fatter than normal rats do. The second group received rat pellets that look and smell a little like condensed straw; these rats maintained a typical weight. The third group received rat chow that was made to taste bitter; these rats lost weight. After a brief period on these diets, the rats all stabilized at their new weights.

Next, the researchers tried to force the rats to change their weight, to see if this would be met with resistance. Rats were kept in refrigerated cages, and they had to eat more to compensate for all the heat they were losing; all three groups increased what they ate by the same amount, to avoid losing weight. In another trial, they had a chance to eat less: They were given a rich food solution through a stomach tube. (The food wasn't given through the mouth to ensure that the sensory input didn't alter results. This is obviously not an experiment many humans would volunteer for!) All of the rats ate less on this regimen; again, they ate precisely enough to maintain a constant weight. Essentially the researcher was asking, "Do you care more about how fat you are, or how much you eat?" The rats' response was clear: how fat we are.

The chain of causation is not what we accept as common sense: tasty food stimulating appetite, and overeating leading to weight gain. Instead, it works like this: Tasty food raises the setpoint, and the rats eat enough to maintain the new setpoint; unappetizing food lowers the setpoint, and these rats also eat the precise amount to maintain their new setpoint. (Be sure to read on—I wouldn't want you to jump to the conclusion that eating delicious food makes us fat; it's a lot more complicated than that!)

More precise research identifies the specific nutrients in foods that ramp up the setpoint. In the rest of this chapter, I'll show you how your food choices may affect your setpoint. As you consider these ideas, be sure to keep them in the context of what you have already learned: Your body has a competent internal system that can guide you in choosing the types and quantities of food that will best nourish you. I want you to have the information from the field of food science that enables you to work with this internal knowing all the more easily.

Respect, Not Rules

Many people are already afraid of eating certain kinds or amounts of food. They often restrict their eating or feel guilty when they're not following a detailed food plan. If this is true for you, the information in this chapter may fuel your fears, tempting you to create a new set of rules about what and what not to eat. Be careful. If you do, you'll only be sabotaging yourself and your ability to learn how to truly satisfy your physical hunger.

For example, you will learn that high-fructose corn syrup doesn't activate your weight regulation sensors to the degree that some other foods do. How are you going to apply that information? Will you use it to label soda and cookies as "bad," to be avoided in your quest to lose weight? Or, can you use it to become more aware of how you feel as you consume them, noticing whether it takes more soda or sweets than you would expect to feel satiated?

I'll say it now and I'll be saying it again: Please do not use this information to create or justify self-punishing rules for demonizing food or restricting your intake. If you find yourself doing that, stop reading this chapter and skip ahead to the next one. You can come back to this chapter at a later time, if and when it's appropriate. If a Health at Every Size professional suggests that you bypass this chapter and go on to the next, trust his or her advice.

Given the potential for misuse, why do I include nutritional information in this book? I do so because I believe that you have the right to accurate information as you make your food choices. Information—like food—is not dangerous in itself. The question is: How do you choose to use it? You can grab a knife to chop your garlic or to slit someone's throat; it is *you* who gives the knife its character. If we wish to create a happy relationship with food and enjoy a well-nourished body, then clarifying the intention that informs your food choices is of the utmost importance. Let me provide an example that will make this more evident.

Later in this chapter you'll learn about some benefits to a high-fiber diet. If a dieting mindset kicks in, eating high-fiber foods becomes one more "should." And if your preferences run more to hot dogs and potato chips, that new rule will probably make you feel guilty. Feeling guilty won't allow you to sustain good health habits.

What's the alternative? Suppose your intention is to develop your ability to eat intuitively, a practice that I'll encourage and describe in detail in later chapters. Instead of viewing food choices in terms of their potential effect on your weight, you'll be tuning in to how various foods make you feel. With that purpose in mind, you can use the information in this chapter to help you connect what you eat with how you feel.

If your diet is low in fiber, for example, you're probably all too accustomed to the discomforts of constipation. As you read this chapter, you may begin to suspect that your discomfort relates to getting insufficient fiber. With this new awareness, you begin to experiment with including more high-fiber foods in your meals and snacks. You notice that your stack of bathroom reading is gathering dust as you're spending significantly less time in the bathroom. You continue to choose high-fiber foods, not because some diet plan is calling the shots, but because doing so results in feeling better. You're learning through experimentation that your own body can guide you toward food choices that truly feel nourishing.

As you tune into your body's wisdom, you may end up eating some of the same foods that one diet plan or another prescribes. But it's coming from a different place. You're no longer ignoring what you want and need in favor of some external authority's dictates. Instead, you're acting on your own desire to nurture yourself. You're making your choices from the inside out, following the guidelines of your internal nutritionist. Because it helps you to feel good, it's easy to sustain. Over time you'll find that it becomes natural and effortless to make choices that leave you feeling good.

Bottom line? You don't need food rules to guide your choices. You don't need to fight your desires. All you need is to respect your body, by listening and responding to its signals. Information about how foods affect you can support your process of tuning in to your body and feeling ever more at home.

Embrace the Ambiguity

Before we jump into our discussion of specific nutrients, though, here's another cautionary note to consider. People often have strong defense mechanisms that keep them rooted in their old habits. Defense mechanisms can operate below the level of conscious thought, allowing you to dismiss information before it threatens your world view.

Having taught nutrition for years, I've observed a very powerful defense mechanism that often gets in the way of positive change: black and white thinking, in particular, difficulty in tolerating and embracing ambiguity and contradiction.

Here's an example of how it gets played out. Research suggests that substantial health benefits come from reducing consumption of conventional animal foods from the typically high consumption seen in industrialized countries. This proposition is not particularly radical. In fact, most nutritionists today accept this idea; Even following the USDA's "food pyramid" recommendations will naturally lead to decreased consumption of animal foods. Still, a call for reducing consumption of conventional animal foods may seem threatening to many people. It frequently gets lost in translation, resurfacing as the assertion that "animal foods are bad" and that you need to be a vegan to be healthy (or thin), which in turn provokes resistance from many individuals.

But such a statement simply isn't true! Many animal foods are loaded with beneficial nutrients. Many fish, for example, are rich in beneficial omega-3 fatty acids, a nutrient that is otherwise difficult to find in modern diets. Or consider hamburgers. The iron packed into that patty is particularly easy for your body to absorb, a boon to the many individuals who would otherwise suffer from iron deficiency.

Consuming moderate amounts of animal foods provide you with valuable nutrients that may otherwise be difficult to obtain. Yet the same fish that is rich in omega-3s often contains mercury, a toxin that poses a serious health risk when it accumulates in your tissues.

And a diet primarily based on hamburgers and similar foods—and lacking variety—puts you at risk for a long list of health complications. Nonetheless, these foods might be just the ones that titillate your taste buds and give you some of the nutrients you need. I say, go for it!

We need to acknowledge and accept the contradictions and ambiguities that accompany our concerns for good nutrition these days. No particular food is out-of-bounds in the context of generally sound nutrition. Know that your body's innate intelligence can help you make choices that support your well-being—and can help you appropriately moderate them. It's also helpful to remember that many of the deleterious effects of certain compounds result from their accumulation, not from occasional or moderate consumption. That risk is minimized when you use your body's signals to guide consumption.

Vegetarianism and veganism can be wholesome and admirable dietary styles when approached with the right intentions, but they can also be troubling restrictive behaviors, or markers for eating disorders. *What* you eat is less important than why you eat it.

Besides, we need and want food for many reasons. On the most basic level, food supplies us with energy. That means that even soft drinks provide nourishment. Of course, we need more than just energy from foods, and living on Cokes alone won't fully nourish you. But you can't subsist on a diet of only carrots and broccoli either: Variety is essential to ensure that you get the full range of nutrients your body needs.

As you learn about how foods affect you, always remember: As valuable as academic research may be, your intuition is much more effective in guiding you to feed yourself well. What's "true" in the field of nutrition changes as research continues and our culture changes. Nutrition research is also severely hampered by scientific reductionism, as nutrients act very differently depending on the context in which they are consumed. A dictum we learn from one particular study may not hold true if you alter other aspects of your diet not considered in that study. And lastly, we can't ignore individual differences: Your particular genetic make-up may result in certain nutrients affecting you differently than that "average person" that the research describes. I encourage you to take the advice of the external authorities with a grain of salt. Use it to help you experiment with different foods, and then reap the benefits of trusting your body's wisdom.

With these cautions in mind, take a moment to reflect on what's best for you. What's your intent in learning about nutrition? Can you use your knowledge to help you tune in to your body, rather than creating food rules? Can you challenge yourself to be open-minded and accept the ambiguities? If you have any concerns about how you're going to use the information that follows, again, I advise you to jump to the next chapter. You can always come back to this chapter another time.

Now, let's begin our journey into understanding the possible impact of nutrients on your setpoint.

Carbohydrates

Some carbohydrates are more quickly digested and absorbed, contributing to a quick increase in blood sugar. Most of the increase in our calories over the past twenty years has come from those types of carbohydrates, called "high-glycemic carbohydrates."[136] Simply put: We're gobbling huge amounts of sugar and heaping plates of white rice, and we just can't leave that bread plate alone.

When consumed in excess, these foods cause a large spike in insulin production—the hormone that allows cells to use glucose for energy. Repeated large spikes can eventually overwhelm your cells, making them less sensitive to insulin. In scientific terms, this decreased sensitivity is called insulin resistance. (Genetic susceptibility also plays a large determining role.) Many scientists suspect that insulin resistance is the most important factor in determining susceptibility to weight gain.[137]

Insulin also helps other energy nutrients—like fat—get into cells. But unfortunately, the muscle cells get insulin resistant, not the fat cells, making fat storage easy at the same time that your hungry muscles are crying out for energy.

Insulin resistance leads to weight gain as the glucose we can't use gets converted into fat and stored. This extra fat tends to settle in the abdomen, where it is more volatile and more likely to contribute to diabetes, heart disease, and other illnesses.[138] Type 2 diabetes, the name given to the severe form of insulin resistance, is more common among heavier people, in part because of this process: Insulin resistance drives weight gain. Many large people have at least a moderate degree of insulin resistance, even if it's not severe enough to be labeled diabetes.

But insulin does much more than enable your cells to use glucose for energy or to store fat. It also signals your hypothalamus to send out less neuropeptide Y. Reducing the supply of this neurotransmitter turns *down* your appetite switch while *increasing* your metabolism. Insulin also stimulates the release of leptin, which amplifies this effect. That's why normal insulin production and use is so important for weight regulation.

Avoiding insulin production isn't helpful; it's the insulin spikes that are disconcerting. While most people put the blame for insulin spikes on excess consumption of sugar, it turns out that refined grains, like those found in many breads, cereals, and rices, are equally at fault. Ironically, the U.S. government's attempt to deal with obesity by encouraging people to build their diets on the old Food Guide Pyramid's base of "bread, cereal, rice, and pasta," seems to have backfired. (Note that the pyramid comes from the U.S. Department of *Agriculture*. A primary purpose of this agency is to promote agriculture—and its recommendations are designed, in part, to support agribusiness. More on the politics of food and weight in chapter 5.)

These refined products spill into your blood quickly: From your body's perspective, there's not much difference between a slice of refined bread (even if they call it "wheat bread") and a tablespoon of white sugar. While the government insists that manufacturers "enrich" refined breads, grains, and pastas by adding back certain vitamins and minerals, this does nothing to slow the rate of glucose entering your bloodstream, nor does it completely restore valuable nutrients.

Will eating high-glycemic foods cause you to gain weight or develop health problems? Despite the concerns evoked when one considers their actions in the body—and the media hype—there is very little consistency in the epidemiologic research that examines the association between high-glycemic eating habits and increased risk for diabetes, cardiovascular disease, or weight gain.[139] The ambiguity in the research probably reflects the limits of scientific reductionism: that overall dietary patterns play a much larger role in weight and health and the impact of individual nutrients is only apparent when part of a larger trend. In other words, you may be able to get away with a high-glycemic eating style if your other dietary choices support good health.

The difficulty with a high-glycemic eating habit may have more to do with what it's missing than what it contains: fiber. Fiber plays a large role in how your body handles other carbohydrates. It acts as a dense filter, slowing the rate at which other carbohydrates are digested in much the same way a sand bag slows the rate at which rainwater enters the ground. This filtering, in turn, results in a slow, steady release of insulin, instead of that abrupt spike. Fiber also provides a sustained feeling of fullness, magnified by the water it absorbs. In fact, foods high in fiber will make you feel fuller than the same amount (or more) of any other kind of food.[140]

Yet less than one of the 10.6 servings of grain products we eat in an average day is made up of fiber-rich whole grains.[136] And the typical American diet contains *two to three times* less fiber than that of our (thin) Paleolithic ancestors.[141]

In the studies that suggest high-glycemic foods increase diabetes risk, that risk disappears when the diet is otherwise rich in fiber.[142, 143, 144, 145, 146]

Fiber-rich foods include whole, unprocessed vegetables, grains, beans, fruits, nuts, and seeds. One study found eating just three extra apples or pears a day led to significant weight loss in "overweight" people.[147] (The study just measured short-term weight loss, so don't take it seriously as a weight loss technique. My point in mentioning it here is that higher fiber eating appears to reduce calorie intake in the short run. This makes sense, given its effect on satiety. And rest assured, increasing fiber is great advice for general health improvement, regardless of its impact on weight.)

Instead of regularly drinking apple juice, perhaps you can occasionally enjoy a juicy apple? Unlike fruit, fruit juice is stripped of the fiber—and is lower in other beneficial nutrients as well.

Choosing Whole Grains

Whole grain products can typically be identified on a food label. Look for the word "whole" in the ingredients list. If you see the word "enriched," it's a sure sign it's not whole grain.

Food companies can sometimes make it difficult to determine which foods are whole grains. Many breads are colored brown and made to look like whole grain, but are not. Also, some food manufacturers make foods with whole-grain ingredients, but, because whole-grain ingredients are not the dominant ingredient, they don't give you the benefits of a whole-grain product. (Don't get tricked by small quantities of a whole grain—ingredients are listed in order of weight, so make sure the whole grain appears first.) Another way to identify whole grains is to look in the nutritional facts information and check whether it contains fiber. A significant amount indicates that it most likely contains a good amount of whole grain.

Some grains may not use the word "whole." Brown rice, for example, is the whole form of white rice, its refined and less nutritious counterpart. "Old-fashioned oats" are the whole form, while "quick" oats are the refined form. Popcorn is another example of a popular whole grain that doesn't use the word "whole." Some less common whole grains that may not use the word "whole" include amaranth, buckwheat, millet, quinoa, spelt, sorghum, and triticale.

Bulgur, barley, and couscous are grains that come in both forms, although whether or not they are whole is not always indicated. Pearled barley is refined (not a whole grain).

Another study, this one from Harvard that followed 75,000 women for ten years, found the more fruits and vegetables the women ate, the less likely they were to gain weight over time.[148] And researchers at the National Cancer Institute who followed nearly 80,000 people for ten years found those who ate the most vegetables had the lowest amount of abdominal fat (the type of fat that is more readily implicated in causing harm[149]).

The same thing shows up in research on whole grains: Ten of the eleven studies on this topic reported that the more whole grains an individual consumed, the lower his or her weight.[139] Let me repeat a point made earlier: I am not reporting this research to suggest that a high-fiber diet will result in weight loss—that has not been proven. What I am suggesting is that a high-fiber diet helps you feel satiated on fewer calories. When a food is stripped of fiber, it loses some of its ability to say "enough." Without this brake in place, you may feel driven to eat more calories than your body needs.

Whole grains haven't had their bran and germ removed through processing, making them better sources of fiber and other nutrients. Refined grains, on the other hand, such as white rice or white flour, have both the bran and germ removed from the grain. Although vitamins and minerals are added back into refined grains after the milling process, they still don't have as many nutrients as whole grains do, they don't provide as much fiber, and they speed through your digestive tract, raising your blood sugar quickly.

Rice, bread, tortillas, cereal, flour, and pasta are all grains or grain products. It's to your advantage to switch to whole-grain versions, rather than consuming the more accessible refined grains.

Don't like the taste of whole grains? Future chapters will help you change your tastes. I want you to eat that apple because it's what you're craving—not because you think you *should*.

Understanding the different effects refined carbohydrates and whole grains have on your body gives you valuable information to use as you move toward becoming an intuitive eater. Remember that no one food will make or break anything, and the goal is not to deprive yourself of foods you love. If you only like white rice with Chinese meals, enjoy it! Look for other places to include fiber-rich foods. And while it might sound like an oxymoron, the moral is that by *adding* foods to your diet—fruits, vegetables, whole grains, beans, and other fiber-rich foods—you are more likely to keep your weight regulation system functioning at its optimal level.[150]

How do you know if you are getting sufficient fiber? There are two easy body clues to be attentive to. The first is having comfortable bowel movements; fiber has the amazing ability to make your stool the right consistency and can help prevent diarrhea as well as constipation. The second clue is having consistent energy and moods throughout the day, as a result of fiber's role in stabilizing your blood sugar. If you often find yourself on edge and moody, it may just be the result of too little fiber!

High-Fructose Corn Syrup: How Sweet It Isn't

Now consider the super-sized Cokes that some of us are drinking. Twenty years ago, those Cokes might have been sweetened with a 50-50 mix of sugars made from sugar beets or sugar cane and those made from corn syrup. Today, however, 100 percent of its sweetening comes from high-fructose corn syrup (HFCS). In 1966, we had never heard of the stuff; by 2001, we were annually consuming an average of 62.6 pounds a person.[151]

Why? Because it's plentiful, cheap, and shelf-stable. Not to mention heavily subsidized by the U.S. government and supported by trade restrictions.

High-fructose corn syrup is what helps breads brown and stay soft on the shelf. That's why you'll even find it in hot dog buns. It lurks in condiments like ketchup and mayonnaise, in most crackers, even in cough syrup. Since it helps prevent freezer burn, it can be found in most frozen foods—even non-sweet foods like TV dinners. Check your pantry and refrigerator shelves: Chances are HFCS is on the label of every processed food in there, from pasta sauces to bacon, from beer to protein bars and so-called "natural" sodas.

This tremendous jump in high-fructose corn syrup consumption also mirrors the increase in weight, and some scientists put much of the blame for our expanding waistlines on HFCS.[151] That it plays a large role is doubtful, but it does seem likely to be one of the many contributing factors. Three short-term studies found that the more

HFCS in the diet, the more people weighed. One possible reason: They didn't compensate for the extra fructose calories by reducing calories from other sources. Instead, they just kept eating.[152, 153, 154]

Fructose vs. Glucose

How can two sugars act so differently in your body? Though similar, each has a different chemical makeup.

Drink a soda sweetened with glucose—as most are in Europe and other countries—and insulin production increases, allowing the glucose in your blood to be transported into cells and used for energy. The increased insulin production increases production of leptin, which helps regulate appetite and fat storage, and suppresses production of ghrelin, a hormone that increases feelings of hunger. The insulin also travels to receptors on the brain, where it helps regulate appetite and fat storage.

Drink a soda sweetened with fructose—as most are in the United States—and it acts in a totally opposite manner. Because it doesn't stimulate as much insulin secretion, it doesn't increase leptin production much. Thus it doesn't suppress production of ghrelin or activate brain cells to regulate appetite and fat storage.

It seems that while glucose and other sweeteners trigger a "stop-eating message," fructose doesn't have the same effect on our hunger/satiety signals. So we may add a few hundred fructose calories a day on top of our regular calorie intake without feeling overly full. As you learn to tune into your own signals for hunger and fullness, pay attention to whether this is true for you. Notice if you need more than you would expect when eating large quantities of foods containing HFCS. (This isn't a foolproof system for knowing what's going on in your body as the weight regulation mechanisms that HFCS bypasses also play a role in long-term weight regulation, not just meal-to-meal satiety.)

Researchers are not unified in implicating high-fructose corn syrup, noting that old-fashioned sugar is already half fructose, and even high-fructose corn syrup is generally no more than 55 percent fructose. The issue may be related to quantity. Today, about one-sixth of all our calories and 13 percent of all carbohydrates come from HFCS.[155]

Wondering how plentiful high-fructose corn syrup is in your diet? Just check the ingredients list on food labels: It should be clearly specified.

Fat = Fat?

Another nutrient that affects your weight regulation system is fat. Fat consumption has clearly increased over the years: Americans ate an average of 523 more calories in 2003 than in 1970.[157, 158] Interestingly, while the *percentage* of fat in our diet has dropped (given our overall increase in calories)[159] much of the fat we're eating today is *added* fat, as opposed to naturally occurring fat in foods. Average consumption of added fat jumped from 53 pounds per person in the 1970s to over 74 pounds in the year 2000, a 40 percent surge.[157]

Why does this matter? Well, consider that most dietary fat—especially the stuff that gets added—has even less of an impact on leptin secretion than fructose. Ergo, it doesn't trigger those sensors that tell us it's time to stop eating, so it may contribute to that higher setpoint.

Need proof? Consider a study from my colleagues at the University of California, Davis. They found that women consuming a high-carbohydrate, low-fat diet released 40 percent more leptin than those consuming a high-fat, low-carbohydrate diet.[160]

Other research finds that, ironically, consuming a high-fat diet can increase your desire for more food![161] Why? Well, if high-fat diets don't stimulate leptin release, you're not getting the appetite-suppressing effects of leptin. Fat is also less effective than protein or carbohydrates at suppressing ghrelin's hunger call.[162] So it may take more fat calories to satisfy you. Numerous other studies suggest this decreased leptin production from high-fat diets leads to increased eating and weight gain.[163, 164, 165, 166, 167]

Artificial Sweetners: No Panacea

Okay, you're thinking. I'll just make sure I minimize my consumption of high-fructose corn syrup by focusing on foods with artificial sweeteners. Not so fast. There's some evidence that artificial sweeteners like aspartame (Equal), saccharin (Sweet 'n' Low), and sucralose (Splenda) may also increase setpoints in non-diabetics.

In one study, researchers fed two groups of rats sweet-flavored liquids for ten days.[156] One got sugar-sweetened liquids while the other got liquids sweetened with sugar and saccharin. After ten days, both groups received a sugary, chocolate-flavored snack and regular rat chow. While both groups of rats ate about the same amount of the chocolate snack, those previously fed sugar and saccharin ate three times the amount of rat chow than those rats fed only the sugar-sweetened drink.

Scientists think that artificial sweeteners could interfere with our natural ability to regulate how much we eat*. It doesn't change our drive for sugar (that's always appealing), but it does increase the drive for calories.

---

*Artificial sweeteners trigger the cephalic phase of insulin secretion, which could actually be good for diabetics, helping their bodies to better prepare for absorbing nutrients, but for others could trigger hunger and favor weight gain.

As you learn how to become attentive to your body's signals for hunger and fullness, stay aware of whether higher fat foods satisfy your appetite. Do you seem to need more than you would expect to feel full? (The previously mentioned caveat is true here too: Since leptin plays a role in long-term weight regulation, not just meal-to-meal satiety, your satiety level may not give you the full picture, though it's a pretty good indicator.)

It's quite complicated to figure out what really drives your eating behavior, however. High-fat foods are typically "forbidden" foods for dieters. If you hold onto the idea that "high-fat is bad" and deprive yourself, you make yourself vulnerable to what scientists call "deprivation-driven eating" and the usual brakes that stop eating stop working effectively. In other words, dietary rules—like the low-fat admonishment—may contribute to the over-eating that some people experience. Giving yourself permission to enjoy high-fat foods may just be the secret that supports you in enjoying them in a moderate and healthy manner.

High-fat diets may also lead to insulin resistance,[168] which increases the potential for weight gain. Reduce the dietary fat, and insulin resistance reverses.[169]

Additionally, the body converts food fat into body fat quickly and easily, which also may contribute to higher weight in people who overeat: One hundred excess calories of ingested fat can be converted to 97 calories of body fat. One hundred excess calories of protein or carbohydrate, however, are converted to only 77 calories of body fat because more calories are burned in the conversion process.[170] (If you don't overeat, this imbalance may not exist since you probably won't convert as many calories into body fat.)

Here's another surprising fact: Some animal studies suggest that repeated and frequent exposure to fatty foods reconfigures the brain to crave still more fat![171] One study even found that fatty food can override whatever leptin signals do manage to get out. In this study, researchers force fed rats until they had gained a significant amount of weight, then injected leptin directly into their nervous system. The result? The rats continued to eat less of a standard rodent diet and more of the high-fat diet.[172]

There Is No "Free" in Fat-Free

In the past ten years, grocery store shelves have seen an explosion of fat-free and low-fat foods, all designed to play into our fears of fat. There's only one problem: Reduce the fat and you reduce the flavor. To compensate, manufacturers dumped in plenty of flavor enhancers. Thus, most processed fat-free foods are filled with sweeteners (usually high-fructose corn syrup). That may boost your setpoint, leading to weight gain.

And how about this finding: One eight-month study found slashing the amount of fat from the typical 30 percent most Americans get to 15 percent enabled participants to eat an average of 120 *more* calories and still maintain their body weight.[173]

While the evidence supporting the effect of dietary fat on weight is compelling, most of this research doesn't distinguish between types of fat—which is really important and may explain some of the ambiguity in the research. For example, unsaturated fats (the kind primarily found in plant foods) trigger more leptin production than saturated fats (found mainly in modern animal foods) or trans fats (found in processed foods), which trigger barely any. High-fat diets are typically high in saturated and trans fats, which may explain why they do a poor job in activating your weight regulation system.

Within unsaturated fats are the monounsaturated fats, found in high amounts in olive oil and oils made from some seeds and nuts, polyunsaturated fats, like those found in vegetable oils, and a specific type of polyunsaturated fat called omega-3 fat, also found in high amounts in some nuts, seeds, and fatty fish. Monounsaturated fats and omega 3 fats stimulate the most leptin release (thus stemming hunger), followed by the other polyunsaturated fats, with saturated and trans fats trailing far behind.[174, 175, 176, 177, 178]

Given all this evidence about fats, here's another interesting observation—the major source of saturated fat in our diet is meat. And meat consumption reached record highs in the 1990s. That includes red meat and poultry, both of which are high in saturated fat compared to other protein sources.[136, 159] Between 1909 and 2000, consumption of chicken quintupled from 10 pounds per year per person to 54 pounds; beef jumped 24 percent and pork jumped 15 percent.

Unmasking the Fat Myth: Doesn't Fat Fill Us Up?

Most people believe that fat is the most filling form of food because it's denser in calories (one gram of fat contains 9 calories vs. the 4 calories in a gram of carbohydrates or protein) and it keeps your stomach from emptying too fast. Yet research shows just the opposite when compared calorie for calorie to protein or to fiber-rich carbohydrates.[140] Why? We can't store carbohydrates or protein calories as well as fat calories, so they get used immediately or turned into body fat. However, we can store endless fat, and since it doesn't need to be metabolized immediately, it provides a weaker satiety signal. Fat is also so calorically dense it's easier to eat too much before your "I'm full" signal kicks in.

No one—especially me—is suggesting you eliminate fat from your diet. Not only are some types of fat necessary for survival and healthy functioning, but it's clear that monounsaturated and omega-3 fatty acids have a weight-taming effect through their effect on long-term weight regulation. Not surprisingly, these were the types of fats in greatest availability during the time of our Paleolithic ancestors—and those we get the least of in our modern diets.[179] This fact may also partially explain the well-documented benefits of the Mediterranean diet: People in Greece get a higher percentage of fat in their diet than we do, but maintain lower weights and have less heart disease. Their diets are rich in the beneficial fats.

Fat is also important as the vehicle that delivers flavorful compounds in food to our taste buds, making foods much more pleasurable. And pleasure, as you'll see in future chapters, plays an important role in making us feel content because it actually activates satiety sensors in our brain.

So instead of eliminating fat from your diet, consider becoming mindful of the types of fat you're getting in your diet. You may want to experiment with increasing unsaturated fats and noticing the impact this has on your feelings of satiety and contentment. It may just be that this change leads to a greater sense of satiation and well-being—and is something you come to prefer. Remember, we're all a bit different: Check it out for yourself!

Protein . . . and the Meat Controversy

For all the hoopla around the high-protein diet craze, the gurus of this movement had one thing right: Protein is much more effective at filling you up than either carbohydrate or fat.[180, 181] If you were to go on a high-protein diet, you'd probably eat less at individual meals, and see a quick weight loss *in the short-term.*

However, this form of eating has minimal impact on longer term signals. Eventually—over the course of weeks or months—you may be driven to take in more calories—or spend fewer calories—than if your diet were composed of nutrients like low-glycemic starches and mono-unsaturated fats that activate satiety signals. For this reason, high-protein diets are unsustainable—and the real problem comes when you stop the diet.

In fact, the link between protein and weight goes in the opposite direction than is trumpeted—larger people tend to eat more protein than those that are slimmer.[182] Makes sense when you consider that high-protein diets are also high in saturated fat and low in fiber. Another problem is that even diets just a little high in protein (more than 10 percent of calories) can make you crave carbohydrates because of their impact on certain hormones.[183] Yet the average

American woman gets about 23 percent of her calories from protein; the average American man, about 18 percent.[157]

But wait, you say, sure that this time you've got me . . . didn't our thin Paleolithic ancestors subsist on a high meat diet? Yes, you may be right (this is controversial). *But* . . . and it's a big "but" . . . the meat they ate was very different from what's available today. They subsisted on wild game, not corn- and soy-fed domesticated cattle. Meat from wild game contains about 2 to 4 percent fat and relatively high levels of monounsaturated and omega-3 fats compared with today's grain-fed domestic meats, which can contain 20 to 30 percent fat, much of it saturated.[184]

Thus, in evolutionary terms the meat we eat today is a new food for us. To mimic the kind of (meat-based) diet our ancestors followed, we'd be better off concentrating our diet around unprocessed plant foods, using meat, if desired, as an accompaniment rather than the main attraction.

The research also shows that choosing plant foods over animal foods affects us in many ways other than weight, increasing longevity and reducing risk of heart disease,[185] metabolic syndrome,[186] and many other diseases. Despite the fantasy promoted by the Atkins camp and other supporters of meat-based diets, there is no evidence that it will get you thinner or healthier.[187]

Want to get the short-term, appetite-reducing benefits of protein without the negative long-term effects that may result from overconsumption? By having a little bit of protein with every meal, you are likely to notice that you will feel full longer. It will also temper the rise in blood sugar that results from the carbohydrates you eat with it, which is especially helpful if you feel a drop in energy after eating foods high in carbs. Plant proteins, like those found in vegetables and beans, serve this purpose well and come bundled with plenty of fiber and other great nutrients.

Drinks

Whether or not sweetened drinks affect weight gain is a matter of great controversy. A well-funded industry clouds the scientific analysis. When researchers analyzed 111 studies of beverages published over a four-year period, they found that studies entirely sponsored with beverage industry money were up to eight times more likely to result in industry-favorable conclusions than studies not funded by the industry.[188] Take the industry-funded studies out of consideration and there is a strong correlation between soft drink consumption and heavier weight.

Makes sense that drinks play a role in our weight. For most of our evolutionary history, the only beverages we drank were breast milk and water. Because water has no calories, our bodies didn't evolve to reduce food consumption to compensate for the drinks we were consuming. Though humans have been drinking wine, beer, fruit juice, and milk for thousands of years, the proportion of calories coming from beverages was relatively minor until about fifty years ago when soft drinks started to proliferate.

Thirst is an important drive that needs to be satisfied, and sometimes water just doesn't satisfy. The trick is to make sure you're not going extreme in calorie-laden drinks, as they can crowd other nutrients out of your diet. They also may not give you the satiety signals you need to help you stop. (The temporary feeling of fullness from the volume of liquid in your digestive tract doesn't last long.) But remember, dietary variety is good. You don't want to cheat yourself out of some of the nutrients that can come from drinks, like the anti-oxidants found in grape juice and wine, especially if these drinks are more appealing to you at times than the real deal grape. Most important is to learn to pay attention to what you are consuming and how it truly feels in your body. Doesn't matter if it's juice, a soft drink, or a "sports energy drink," if you overindulge, chances are it will show up unfavorably in your energy level and mood. Is this true for you? Remember the good old days when drinks were served in 8 ounce portions—not the gallon containers we now find in movie theaters?

Processed and Fast Foods

When is the last time you ate a meal made without opening a can, bag, or jar or handing over money at a drive-through window?

Just consider: In the last 30 years, our annual spending on fast food jumped eighteen-fold—from $6 billion to $110 billion a year.[189] Potatoes used for processed foods like frozen French fries (eaten mostly in fast-food eateries), potato chips, and shoestrings jumped from 8 percent of total U.S. per capita fruit and vegetable supplies in 1970 to 11 percent in 1996. Is it any surprise to find that this jump coincides with the same timeframe in which Americans have gained weight?

Also not surprising: Research from twenty-one developed countries found that girls who ate fast food at least twice a week were more likely to be heavier than those who ate fast food less frequently.[190]

Our fast-food culture represents the worst combination of factors I've described in this chapter. For those that are genetically vulnerable, consuming it as the major source of your food intake could raise your setpoint. Fast foods—burgers and fried chicken topped off with the high-fructose corn syrup found in everything from buns to special sauce to the coating on those chicken nuggets—lack fiber and many other beneficial nutrients but contain plenty of high-glycemic carbohydrates and saturated and trans fats.

You'll read more about this culture in chapter 5. For now, a message I want you to take away from this chapter is that the type of food we eat has an effect on the signals that increase or decrease appetite and fat accumulation. The food climate in which we live today clearly plays a role in our collective weight gain.

This fact is not to discount the role of genetics and other factors. To repeat an earlier point, fat people and thin people probably don't eat much differently from one another. It's just that some people are more genetically predisposed towards fat storage as a result of particular eating conditions while others burn those calories more efficiently.

Another important message to remember is that just because certain habits may raise one's setpoint doesn't mean that reversing those habits will result in weight loss. Differences in the regulatory pathways make weight gain relatively easy though weight loss is resisted. Improved health habits are more likely to result in preventing weight gain than in promoting weight loss.

How Do You Eat?

Now that you know how *what* you eat affects your hunger/fullness/
satiety signals, it's time to spend a bit of time looking at the effects of
how you eat on these important signals.

Ask yourself these questions:

- ■ Do I typically wake up in the morning and rush to work, not
  stopping to eat regardless of how hungry I am?
- ■ Do I nosh lightly during the day and then have a huge dinner because I am so ravenous?
- ■ Do I super-size whenever I go out, disregarding signals of
  fullness?
- ■ Do I love the overflowing plates I get in restaurants and eat
  until I've cleaned my plate, regardless of how full I feel?

None are helpful habits to follow if you're trying to maintain a
healthy body. Not surprisingly, the huge portion sizes we get today,
and our chaotic eating habits, contribute to difficulty regulating
blood sugar and weight.

For instance, several studies find that people who skip breakfast
are more likely to be heavy than those who eat first thing in the
morning[144, 191] and that people who eat four or more meals per day
are less likely to be heavier than people who eat three or fewer meals
per day.[191]

This finding is likely related to the "thrifty" gene concept discussed earlier. Missing meals and chaotic eating habits trigger your
"starvation defenses," in which your body does whatever it can to
hang onto whatever calorie it can, leading to poor insulin sensitivity
and increasing your setpoint. Researchers have also found higher
levels of stress hormone levels when people skip breakfast, compared to when they have it.[192]

Putting It Together: The Scoop on Food

We've evolved to eat the sorts of foods available to our ancestors, whose genes we've inherited and whose bodies we still (more or less) inhabit. Humans have not had much time (at least from an evolutionary perspective) to accustom our bodies to processed foods or the foods from animals raised as they are today. A diet built on a base of whole foods, rich in plants, will better mimic the ancestral diets we were designed for and best support us in maintaining good health—and a healthy weight regulation system.

This is not to suggest that you need to eat whole plant foods *exclusively*! Before you weep over having to abandon your mom's fried chicken and gravy, remember that there's no benefit to being extreme. Your body (and your weight regulation system) can effectively be fueled by hamburgers and donuts when they're consumed in moderation and in the context of an overall nutritious diet. Once you know how to listen to your body's signals, you'll get comfortable eating amounts that satisfy you without overdoing it. It's only in excess that they crowd out more nutritious options, and your body nudges you to get more calories in order to get its varied nutrient needs met. So instead of focusing on taking food away, think about what you want to add for an overall nutritious diet.

Here are a few exercises to help you recognize if *what* you're eating and *how* you're eating may be compromising your health and triggering your body's reaction to hold on to excess weight. Identify your challenges here, and future chapters will help you put wholesome habits into practice.

Is It a Good Food? A Bad Food?

There's one nutritional concept that seems to make a healthy relationship with food particularly difficult, and that's the idea that some foods are good while others are bad. Labeling a food good or bad stops you from questioning and discovery. If you label a Twinkie as bad, you are not able to observe its effects on you, and you lose the opportunity to learn from it. On the other hand, if you maintain a neutral attitude, you can watch your response to that Twinkie.

You can be more perceptive to its flavor, noticing whether it really tastes good to you or if it was just the idea that tasted good. Perhaps you learn that it doesn't satisfy your craving—that there was something else you really wanted that the Twinkie can't provide. Perhaps you become more sensitive to your taste buds toning down after the first few bites, making the next bites less pleasurable. Or perhaps you notice that half an hour after indulging in that Twinkie, your energy crashes and you start craving sugar again. This information will ultimately affect your taste for Twinkies in the future.

Is eating that Twinkie good or bad? It all depends on how frequently you eat it, how much you eat, what else you eat it with, whether you were attentive to it. . . . Rather than eliminating these variables, we need to listen to them. By staying connected to your body, some foods may lose their appeal or you may no longer feel driven to over-indulge.

So, in answer to the question, "Is [fill in the blank] bad?," the response is, "Of course not." We simply need to respect it. Let it teach us whether or not we want to indulge or when enough is enough.

How Do Your Eating Habits Drive Your Setpoint?

Complete the following charts to learn about your habits.

The Glycemic Rush . . .

How often do you . . .	Seldom or never	1 or 2 times per week	3 to 5 times per week	Almost daily	Several times a day
Drink soft drinks, fruit juices, or sweetened drinks?					
Eat sweet snacks, such as cakes, pies, cookies, and ice cream?					
Use canned or frozen fruits packed in heavy syrup or add sugar to cereal or other foods?					
Add sugar to coffee or tea?					
Eat candy?					
Use jam, jelly, or honey on bread or rolls?					
Eat refined breads, tortillas, or white rice?					
Eat low-fiber or sweetened cereals?					
Overeat? (Hint: felt uncomfortably full.)					

If you frequently choose the items listed above, your diet is high in foods that stimulate that quick increase in blood sugar, which may be followed by an over-release of insulin and resultant low blood sugar. While all of these foods can have a place in your diet, a *pattern* of eating these processed, sugary foods—or overeating—may result in increased risk for insulin resistance. You'll probably notice that it also results in moodiness and energy lows.

I'm not suggesting you cut out these foods. Just pay more attention to how your food choices make you feel. If you notice that making different types of choices stabilizes your energy and mood, it provides great incentive to make changes. You make these changes because you want to, not because you think you should.

Simple changes—like reducing the amount of these foods you eat, substituting whole grains for refined grains, sweetening cereals with sliced fruit rather than sugar, as opposed to giving up the foods you love—will support your journey. Always keep in mind that foods are not inherently bad: Moderation—which you'll find happens naturally once you learn to tune into you internal hunger cues—not avoidance, is all you need. Extremism won't be more effective—and is likely to even work against you.

Check Your Diet for Fiber . . .

To figure out how much fiber you consume in a day, write down the number of servings you eat in a typical day for each of the food categories below. Next, multiply by the factor shown—this number represents the average amount of fiber from a serving in that food group. Then add the total amount of fiber consumed.

Food Group	Number of Servings	Amount (g)
Vegetables (½ c cooked; 1 c raw)	_____ x 2 g =	_____
Fruits (1 medium; ½ c cut; ¼ c dried)	_____ x 2 g =	_____
Dried beans, lentils, split peas (½ c cooked)	_____ x 6 g =	_____
Nuts, seeds (¼ c; 2 tbsp		

peanut butter) _____ x 2 g = _____

Whole grains (1 slice bread; ½ c rice,
pasta; ½ bun, bagel, muffin) _____ x 2 g = _____

Refined grains (1 slice bread; ½ c rice,
pasta; ½ bun, bagel, muffin) _____ x 0.5 g = _____

Fiber in your breakfast cereal (check label) _____ x ___ g = _____

Total _____

What Does the Number Mean?

39+: According to U.S. government standards, this amount of fiber should keep anyone healthy. If you get more, that's great too. Some cultures show people routinely getting 75+ grams of daily fiber and enjoying excellent health.

38: If you are male, your fiber meets the U.S.-recommended goal. If you are female, this is great and in excess of what is recommended. But again, getting significantly more than the government recommendations is likely to be even better.

25-37: You consume more fiber than the average American. If you are female, this is good news since your fiber meets the recommended amount (25). However, if you are male, these numbers are below the recommended amount.

15-25: You consume more fiber than the average American (but not enough for optimal health).

10-15: Your intake is similar to the average American intake (but not enough for optimal health).

0-10: Uh oh!

If there is one simple rule of thumb for nutritious eating (supportive of a healthy weight regulation system), it is to follow the fiber. Fiber tends to associate with many other beneficial nutrients—

and steers clear of those that are less health-promoting. Fruits, veggies, nuts, beans, and whole grains are always a great idea. High-fiber eating is a great boon for energy and mood stability—and for keeping you satisfied between meals. You'll also find that it does a great job of supporting comfortable bowel movements. Do you keep magazines in your bathroom? That's a sure indication that you can benefit from more fiber!

Think about it: No more straining on the toilet! Incentive enough to make a change, isn't it?

Fat Consumption

How often do you . . .	Seldom or never	1 or 2 times per week	3 to 5 times per week	Almost daily	Several times a day
Eat trans fats (processed fats)?					
Eat saturated fats (animal fats)?					
Substitute mono-unsaturated fat like olive oil for saturated fat like butter?					

Best to get those trans fats down to minimal, which is getting easier to do these days with increased government regulation. You don't need them, and even in small amounts they increase your health risk. They're a marker for low-nutrient foods anyway.

Saturated fats? No need to avoid, just enjoy in moderation. (Saturated fats predominate in animal foods. The easy rule of thumb if your consumption is high is to reduce portion sizes when consuming animal foods, and consider using them as an accompaniment, rather than the centerpiece of your meals.) Also, look for opportunities to substitute monounsaturated fats for saturated fats. Perhaps you can use olive oil rather than butter when sautéing or try "butter-ing" your (whole grain) bread with ripe avocado.

Switch to a diet lower in saturated and trans fats, and you may also notice more comfort with bowel movements. Check it out!

Eating/Activity Habits

How often do you . . .	Seldom or never	1 or 2 times per week	3 to 5 times per week	Almost daily
Diet or watch your calories?				
Skip breakfast?				
Accumulate aerobic exercise that totals more than 30 minutes a day? (This could include short bouts of lifestyle activity, such as stair walking.)				

Remember that idea introduced earlier: dieting bad, movement good? Chapter 9 will support you in dumping the diet habit, and chapter 10 will give you some practical (and fun) tips to help you uncover your drive to shake it up.

Taking It Home

Take a few moments now to reflect on your reaction to this chapter. Did you find yourself feeling "bad" about your love for soda? Or self-righteous because you only drink water? Did you feel uncomfortable with the message that eating less meat is beneficial? Did you resolve to read food labels and limit your consumption of certain foods in the future?

I want you to consider this information in context. Don't latch onto anything you've learned as new commandments in the what-to-eat/what-not-to-eat game. That simply sabotages your ability to trust your body's innate system for taking care of you. Future chapters will help you read your body's messages, supporting you in making shifts because you feel better rather than because you think you should. Your understanding of the science can support you in tuning in.

Don't jump to the conventional conclusion that you need to carefully watch what you eat—or make dramatic or uncomfortable changes. Sound science supports that when we enjoy a variety of foods and trust our bodies, we naturally get the nutrients we need to keep us healthy. For now, put the focus on getting to know yourself better—and recognizing that there is a very complicated picture behind your drive to eat—or to push yourself away from the table.

And I also don't want you to give this information more power than it deserves. Truth is, that while environment and how you live your life play a role in directing the action, your genes are in the driver's seat. Chapter 6 helps you sort this out.

And hang tight, help is on the way. Part 2 helps you establish your game plan for what to do.

FIVE

We're Victims
of Food Politics

Previous chapters explained that our bodies drive us to eat and to store protective calories to keep us alive and kicking. This chapter shifts focus from our internal mechanisms that keep us eating to the external influences that may determine *what* we eat.

The purpose of this chapter is to increase your awareness of how outside influences can affect your current decisions about food. In the second part of the book, you'll learn how to use your internal cues to guide you in choosing when, what, and how much to eat. Knowledge of what happens behind the scenes can help you figure out what your body truly wants, as opposed to what big companies would have you believe. Use this information to think about what makes sense for *your* body and *your* lifestyle. My intent in drawing attention to these issues is not to scare you away from the foods you love, but to ultimately give you the power to reclaim your tastes and better enjoy your food.

Why is it that the mere aroma of frying food wafting from a McDonald's can start you salivating, making you crave French fries as if they were gold nuggets? Because the fast-food chain has spent millions in research, marketing, and public relations to ensure this

Pavlovian response. Because your choice may be a result of what the companies want you to want—as opposed to what's right for you. The fast food companies are not the only culprits. Today nearly every processed food manufacturer engages in activities designed to reshape your taste buds, cravings, eating habits, and attitudes toward food, and to co-opt others, like dietitians, researchers, journalists, physicians, and government officials, to deliver their message.

Their tactics have been remarkably successful. Ninety percent of the money Americans now spend on food is spent on processed food.[189] And most Americans prefer the taste of processed foods to whole foods from nature. Cook's Magazine, for example, found in a blind taste test that even chefs preferred vanilla flavoring to actual vanilla.[193]

Even more disturbing, this corporate manipulation of our palates and food attitudes is being conducted with active government support. In fact, the government, while giving lip service to health promotion, paradoxically encourages the consumption of processed foods (which are of lower nutritional value than whole foods) through farm subsidies and other economic policies.

To understand what's going on and how our culture—and you— has been manipulated, just follow the money.

Show Me the Money

Whether they're developing foods, promoting their products, or projecting an image, food companies are doing it for just one reason: the money. They're not in it to take care of our health, so don't trust them when they claim they are. We can hardly blame them; in fact, they're just obeying the law.

Economic laws dictate that for-profit corporations are obligated to maximize shareholder profits. They are not social service agencies, and they have no responsibility to foster public health or well-being. In fact, a corporate leader who willfully makes a decision to prioritize public health over profit can be sued by shareholders for breach of legal obligation.

This rule of business means that unlike people, corporations usually don't have a conscience. They're only obligated to do the right thing if they can justify it as a means towards increased profits.

Here's how it plays out when it comes to health: If a corporation believes that selling more nutritious food increases profits, they do it. That's why most food companies reformulated their products to remove trans fats when the federal government required that they list the amount of trans fats on their labels. Not because they wanted to improve their customers' health—if that were the reason they would have ditched the trans fats years ago—but because now that they had to show how much of this very-bad-for-you fat was in their foods, they faced reduced sales. Plus, by touting that their products were "trans-fat free," they could provide the perception that the products were healthier, possibly increasing sales to a more health-conscious public.

Call it "nutri-washing," a handy term coined by public health attorney Michele Simon.[194] It's what happens when General Mills boasts that its cereals are made with whole grains but doesn't bother to tell you they're still full of sugar with an often inconsequential amount of fiber. Or when Skippy touts its low-fat peanut butter but neglects to mention it still has as many calories (and substantially more sugar) than the full-fat version. Or when Slimfast adds some vitamin powder to its products and claims its shakes are a nutritious alternative to real food.

Simon alerts us to a particularly insidious form of nutri-washing: the food companies have even made their own nutrition seal programs to help you choose nutritious foods. You may be comforted to know that Diet Pepsi has been awarded the Smart Spot nutritional seal by PepsiCo. And for that extra turbo-charged nutrient-packed meal, be sure to enjoy it with Pepperoni Flavored Sausage Pizza Lunchables, which was awarded Kraft Foods' Sensible Solutions seal.

Where's the Money?

Food companies face unique challenges in their quest to increase profits. Competition is tough and they've got to work aggressively to make sure we consume their products—and that we choose their products over those of their competitors'. That justifies the $36 *billion* a year they spend trying to convince us to buy their products, making them the second largest advertisers in the United States.[30]

Of course, they don't promote all products equally. For example, you don't regularly see advertising, promotion—or even brand names—on foods like potatoes or apples. That's because there's little profit to be made from selling potatoes (as any farmer will tell you). But put a little (cheap) labor into transforming those potatoes into potato chips, and voilà! Mega profits. Just look at the math: Potatoes in their raw form sell for about 50 cents a pound. Once transformed into potato chips, they sell for about $4 a pound.

The industry calls its work of transforming potatoes into potato chips "added value." I call it profit, built at the expense of our health. There are lots of great nutrients in that original potato, but few remain in the processed potato chip. Just empty calories (that empty your wallet).

"But I prefer potato chips to baked potatoes," you protest. "It is added value for me, which is why I lay out the money." Yes, yes, I know. We'll talk about your taste preferences later in the chapter. It's none too surprising if your taste preferences have developed so that you prefer the stuff that generates higher industry profits. Industry has most of us right where it wants us. But for now, let's keep following the money.

Processed food provides such large profit opportunities because the raw materials they require are almost incomprehensibly cheap. A bushel of corn has more than 130,000 food calories. Enough, in theory, to sustain a person for over two months. A bushel of corn costs only about $4. That means that a full year's worth of corn calories costs less than $25.

Why so cheap? To put it simply, the government pays to keep it that way.

Unlike most industries, agriculture does not run on the free market basis of demand/supply = price. In the rest of the economic world, the higher the demand and the lower the supply, the higher the price. So if supply is high and demand is low, meaning prices are low, suppliers cut their production to increase price.

In agriculture, however, the opposite occurs because the government pays farmers for certain crops if they can't sell them at a fair price. This subsidy provides an incentive to farmers to grow more of that crop even if it's not selling and even if prices are low; they're still going to get paid for it.

The best example of this policy is what happened to corn production in the early 1970s, when a major agriculture bill provided subsidies to farmers to make up the difference between the cost of producing a product and the market price. For example, if it cost $1 to produce a bushel of corn and the market price is only 75 cents, the government pays the farmer the missing 25 cents, plus a little extra for profit. In 2005, the government distributed more than $22.7 billion in farm subsidies. Subsidy programs are projected to cost more than $190 billion over the next decade.[195] No wonder an estimated 50 percent of grain farmers' net incomes come from government subsidies.[196]

Yet barely any subsidies are earmarked for fruits, vegetables, beans, and nuts, making them relatively expensive in comparison. To make matters worse, the federal government purchases surplus foods that result from these subsidies (like cheese, milk, pork, and beef) for distribution to food assistance programs, including the National School Lunch Program, while veggies and fruits are much more expensive for the schools to acquire. The end result is that low-nutrition surpluses end up on the plates of kids and low income people (who are often feeding families).

The meat and dairy industries, conspicuously absent from overt subsidies, are probably the biggest winners in this economic landscape. Much of that extra corn gets fed to cows, chickens, and pigs (despite the fact that it sickens the animals to digest corn). This cheap feed grain helps keep animal-based foods relatively cheap, which means you can buy a $1 hamburger at McDonald's.

Given this economic incentive, farmers produce huge amounts of subsidized corn, way more corn than either we or livestock animals can eat. Well, in the 1970s we found a new use for it: High-fructose corn syrup, found in nearly every processed food on the market. Add tariffs plus quota restrictions on imports of foreign sugar, and you can see why high-fructose corn syrup is a much better buy than alternatives. The bottom line? Every $1 in profit on high-fructose corn syrup that manufacturers earn costs taxpayers $10.[197]

Plus, as you learned in chapter 4, high-fructose corn syrup doesn't activate sensors that regulate our setpoint to the degree that other sweeteners do, possibly contributing to our collective weight gain.

Cheap corn also provides the raw material for corn oil—another constituent of many processed foods.

In fact, nearly every menu item on a fast-food menu is derived in some form from cheap corn, from the chicken nuggets (corn-fed poultry and corn-derived binding agents) to the French fries (fried in corn-derived oils) to the sodas (high-fructose corn syrup).

The second most highly subsidized farm product is soybeans. Like corn, soybeans sound wholesome, at least on the face of it. But most soybeans are transformed into soybean oil, which is then hydrogenated, resulting in a surfeit of trans fatty acids in processed foods.

Industry has discovered a way to profit from every part of this (cheap) bean. Most vegetable oils are made from soy; soy lecithin is a common emulsifier; soy flour forms the base of many baked products; and various forms of soy protein (soy protein isolate, texturized vegetable protein, hydrolyzed soy protein) are added to everything from fast-food burgers to protein powders to animal feed and even cardboard.

Many of these same foods bypass your internal weight regulation system (and provide little nutritional benefit), as discussed in the previous chapter.

Bottom line: *By creating a system that maintains a cheap and plentiful supply of corn and soybeans, among other products, government policy has inadvertently favored the production of foods that promote weight gain (and damage health).* Does it make sense that a bag of orange-colored, laboratory-flavored puff balls—lacking in any nutritive value other than energy—is cheaper to produce than a peach? Does it make sense that between 1985 and 2000, there was a 40 percent increase in the price of fruits and vegetables and a 25 percent decrease in the price of soft drinks (adjusted for inflation)?[198]

This change in prices is part of the reason why the poor are more likely to be heavier than wealthier people: Processed food is cheaper and more accessible than food that comes more directly from nature, thanks to government subsidies. And an entirely new industry has sprung up to take advantage of these cheap natural resources to create those processed foods and, by the way, make an enormous profit in the process.

How Industry Gets Us to Eat More

Food companies have a vested interest in getting us to ignore our body signals. The more we eat, the more product they sell, and the more money they can make. If we stopped when we were full, it would be bad for business!

One way they do this is by marketing to our desire for value, super sizing everything for pennies a product. They can do this because the cost of the raw materials is so cheap compared to the labor and marketing required to get us to buy it. In other words, giving us more food for nearly the same money doesn't cost the industry proportionately more money. So they make larger portions "better buys," enticing us to buy more food and spend more money. A large portion of McDonald's French fries, for example, costs 40 percent *less* per ounce than a small serving. So even though a small order is probably enough to satisfy our appetite, why order it when we can get the large for just 10 cents more?

This super-sizing wouldn't be such a problem if we simply ordered the large and only ate half, or bagged half for lunch tomorrow. But studies find that if we get large servings, we eat more. For many of us, if you're given a medium serving of popcorn, you'll eat it and declare yourself full; but given a large serving, you'll also eat all of it, and declare yourself just as full. A study at Pennsylvania State University, for instance, found that diners given 50 percent more of a pasta dish ate 43 percent more than those with a smaller portion.[199] Similar results occurred with bigger portions of potato chips, deli sandwiches, popcorn, and soup.

Many of us eat what's in front of us because we've been taught to take our hunger cues from external cues (what's on the plate) rather than internal cues like hunger. That's why it becomes so important to use your internal signals to guide you, rather than relying on the amount served to you. (Remember, restrained eaters are much more vulnerable to external cues. Strengthen your "intuitive eating" skills [chapter 9] and you're less likely to be duped.) The food industry has done a great job of manipulating this reality to the point that many of us consistently exceed our body's need for calories. Great for profits, not so good for our health.

Of course, the calorie-conscious among us balk at the high-calorie super-sized meals and may not fall for the super-sizing. So industry instead exploits their fear of calories, getting them to pay a lot more for, you guessed it, a lot less. Take the 100-calorie snack packs, which are often more than twice as expensive per ounce than the products they imitate. Or the Lean Cuisine entrees, which sell for quite a bit more than the Hungry Man dinners, yet may contain half as much food. Yet there's no research to support that these products actually result in our eating less over the long run, nor in sustained weight loss.

Interesting how industry has found a way to profit, whether they sell us more or less! Don't be fooled by their claims. Instead, when you stay attentive to what truly satisfies your hunger, you will know what foods best meet your nutritional needs and satisfy your appetite.

How Industry Gets Us to Eat Processed Foods

We have evolved biologically to crave and love the very ingredients that make up the bulk of processed foods: sugar, fat, and salt. When food was more difficult to come by, foods high in fat and sugar (with its associated fiber) kept us full longer and provided more valuable calories; foods high in salt helped us maintain our body's water balance. A sweet succulent strawberry at the height of ripeness provided great fiber, vitamins, minerals, and phytochemicals, much more than in its less sweet, less ripe, or its processed form.

Industry has manipulated this biologic imperative, stripping the tastes that trigger our pleasure response from other valuable nutrients. When we eat processed foods, we get the joy without all the associated nutrients intended for us. Our taste buds have adapted to these new foods so that wholesome foods don't stimulate our appetites to the same degree they used to. Today, foods that aren't loaded with added fat, sugar, salt, or manufactured flavors taste bland and boring to us.

To understand this, it's helpful to understand how you perceive flavor. Consider what happens when you eat a piece of chocolate. Your saliva breaks it down so the individual molecules that compose that candy come in contact with your taste buds. This process activates nerves that send a message to your brain, leading to the release of certain chemicals, including opioids (pleasure-stimulating chemicals), into the bloodstream.

The more sugar and fat you consume, the more opioids released. Because the reaction is so pleasurable, you consume more of these foods to continue to receive the pleasurable reaction, creating a powerful, neurochemical drive to overeat those foods.

Meanwhile, these opioids and other pleasure chemicals enter the bloodstream and carry their messages to the hypothalamus, which sends out another set of chemicals to regulate appetite. One of these chemicals is called neuropeptide Y, which promotes feelings of hunger. Essentially neuropeptide Y and the opioids are telling you, "Yeah! Chocolate! Sweet, creamy, yummy. Eat more!"

That chocolate also releases volatile gases, some of which you can smell. As the chocolate melts in your mouth, more of those volatile molecules are released, flowing through your nose or mouth to nerve cells that transmit more messages to your brain. Surprisingly, the aroma of food plays a much larger role in your perception of flavor than the taste receptors in your mouth: perhaps as much as 90 percent! That's why when you have a cold, food doesn't taste very good. Your mucus-plugged nose prevents the volatile molecules from reaching nerves in the nose and sending the scent message to your brain.

Like most cells in your body, those involved in taste and odor perception aren't static. They only live about three weeks, so they're in a constant state of death and renewal. Similarly, the nervous system is continuously making new connections with these new cells and losing its connections with dying cells, even as the sites in your brain that receive messages from these cells are constantly dying and being regenerated.

While we all have genes that code for receptors specific to certain tastes, such as sweet, those genes work differently in each of us.

In some people, for instance, the gene is more active, creating more receptors for sweet tastes than others and thus lending credence to the phrase "sweet tooth." In others, the gene that codes for "salty" receptors is more active, explaining why some people will choose potato chips over pie any day.

Like all genes, the activity of your taste/odor genes is determined, in part, by the environment. And what is the environment? Why, it is what you eat! The more salty foods you eat, the more active the gene that codes for "salty" receptors; the more sweet foods you eat, the more active the gene that codes for "sweet" receptors.

Not only that, but studies find that diets high in sugar and fat also induce neurochemical changes in areas of the brain involved in appetite and reward.[200, 201, 202] Thus, you essentially re-wire your brain so it rewards you every time you eat these foods, inducing cravings in much the same way someone hooked on cocaine gets a "reward" every time they use the drug. Before you know it, you're hooked on high-fat, high-sugar tastes—exactly what the food industry was hoping for.

But change what you eat and you also change the activity of taste/odor genes, the types of receptors on cells, and the signals going to your brain.

This whole process works great when you're dealing with a strong flavor like chocolate, or coffee, or a fresh strawberry. Remember the last time you ate a just-picked strawberry? Its flavor molecules were at their peak, sending hundreds of powerful messages to your brain about the taste of the berry. In much the same way the flavor of a good wine changes over time in both the bottle and the glass, the messages change in depth and power as you eat, particularly if you eat slowly and mindfully.

The molecules that make up flavors are fragile, however. So the quicker a ripe strawberry gets from the plant to your mouth, the more flavorful it is. That's one reason why freshly picked produce from your garden or the farmers' market often tastes so much better than produce from the supermarket, which may be days or even weeks or months old.

When you process food, many flavor compounds are destroyed. As a result, unless processed foods are altered to improve their flavor, they just aren't going to taste as good as the real thing foods.

Take cherry juice, for instance. Once the cherries are shipped from the orchards to the processing plant, they've already lost some of their flavors. Put them through the crusher, bottle the juice, ship it to the stores, and you'd get a pale cousin of the real thing.

To make the juice more appealing, the manufacturer begins manipulating those flavor molecules. Good flavor chemists can work wonders with taste. A little chemical manipulation and they could even make this book taste like a sweet, just-picked cherry.

One problem, however, is that nature doesn't provide us with perfect consistency, which means that the food processors would have to treat each batch differently to make sure the final product was flavored appropriately. Way too much work. If, on the other hand, they have a blank palette to work with, they can just add the same flavoring each time without having to adjust the recipe. So they use masking agents to minimize the original flavor of the food.

Then they add flavor chemicals to create the flavor they want. They usually do this by identifying the dominant compounds that give the cherry its flavor, then reproducing those, rather than the hundreds or thousands of individual molecules involved.

That's why processed foods rarely taste quite like the original: the resulting flavor is much more one-dimensional. While "cherry flavoring" may be more intense than the flavoring in the actual cherry, it doesn't contain the original cherry's subtlety and complexity. It's like the difference between a jug of cheap Gallo wine and a fine Bordeaux.

As you learn to become attentive to your hunger, you'll want to pay more attention to the flavors that satisfy you. Do you notice the difference between a juicy orange and orange juice from concentrate? How about a chunk of real cheddar cheese versus a slice of processed American cheese? What's *your* preference? Chapter 7 will help you refine your attentive eating skills, so you can better appreciate the wider range of taste sensation found in "real" (unprocessed) food.

Given that 90 percent of our food budget in this country goes to buy processed foods, few of us even know what "real" food tastes like anymore. Instead, we—and our taste and odor receptors—have become accustomed to the lab cocktails produced by chemists. We've come to expect the one-dimensional flavor intensity in food and even require it if we're to perceive enjoyable flavor.

Watch Out for That "Natural Flavor"

Don't fall for the deception entailed in the words "natural flavor." The legal definition of "natural flavor" means the flavor is derived from plant or animal sources, not that the flavor came from the original food itself. Generally, the "natural flavor" is created by culturing bacteria, yeast, and molds and capturing the flavor compounds they generate when they ferment. "Natural apple flavor" was probably derived from compounds never seen on an orchard! Is this natural? Not to me! But the word "natural" apparently sells well.

So when we do eat a real apple, our senses are no longer attuned to detect the delicious subtlety and complexity found in the apple's hundreds of flavor compounds. And since we can't detect the intensity our tastes are looking for in that apple, it tastes bland and unappealing.

In other words, food manufacturers have gotten us hooked: We need the intensity they bring to processed food in order for food to taste "good" to us. Meanwhile, we've turned away from unprofitable "real" (unprocessed) foods.

No wonder so many of us prefer fast food to whole fruits and vegetables!

The Insidious Food Industry

Food manufacturers go to great lengths to promote positive images of their foods to influence us to buy them. One way they do this is by claiming nutritional benefits to their foods—or, at least, claiming that they're not bad for us. Some have been remarkably successful at manipulating public belief.

It starts with advertising. Advertising costs for any single, nationally distributed food product often exceed government spending on *overall* nutritional education by ten to fifty times.[203] For example, the average advertising budget for a nationally advertised candy bar is $50 million and for a nationally advertised soft drink is $100 million. Compare that to the $2 million a year the government spends promoting fruits and vegetables.

Of all the money spent on advertising, only 2.2 percent goes to promote fruits, vegetables, grains, or beans. Contrast that fact with the 70 percent spent to sell convenience foods, candy and snacks, alcohol, soft drinks, and desserts.[30]

But advertising is just a small part of the way the food industry influences our tastes and ideas about nutrition. They also act behind the scenes to get health organizations and professionals to deliver their message.

Industry Manipulation of Health-Related Organizations and Professionals

The food industry is also a strong contributor to nonprofit health organizations, like the American Diabetes Association and the American Heart Association. Awareness of these financial ties help you become more savvy when considering nutritional claims. For instance, Nestle contributed more than $100,000 to the American Diabetes Association in 2003.[204] Not surprisingly, the American Diabetes Association sends out information about Nestle products to its members and others seeking advice. And when the American Heart Association launched its FRESH Steps Initiative, the chief executive officer of Subway was there for the announcement. And why shouldn't he have been? Subway has donated $4 million to the American Heart Association since 2002 and committed to an additional $7 million through 2007. In exchange, Subway can use the American Heart Association "fighting heart disease and stroke" logo on its materials.

Do you really think Kellogg's Cocoa Frosted Flakes is "heart-healthy" while the Post equivalent is not? No, but Kellogg's "paid" for the American Heart Association heart-healthy label, while Post didn't. The Center for Science in the Public Interest estimates that the American Heart Association received more than $2 million for use of the "heart-healthy" label in 2002.[204]

In 2003, the American Academy of Pediatric Dentistry (AAPD) accepted $1 million from Coca-Cola.[204] AAPD President David Curtis defended accepting this money by saying, "Scientific evidence is certainly not clear on the exact role that soft drinks play in terms of children's oral disease." Huh? Sounds pretty different from the group's previous statement that ". . . frequent consumption of sugars in any beverage can be a significant factor in the child and adolescent diet that contributes to the initiation and progression of dental caries [cavities]."

Apparently Coca Cola also finds these partnerships good for business. The American Academy of Family Physicians (AAFP) proudly announced on their website formation of "a corporate partnership with The Coca-Cola Co., in which the beverage giant will provide a grant for the Academy to develop consumer education content related to beverages and sweeteners for the AAFP's award-winning consumer health and wellness Web site."[205] Is comment even necessary here? (Kudos to those individual physicians who ripped up in their membership cards in protest!)

Even nutritional experts have been co-opted by industry. Go to an American Dietetic Association (ADA) conference, as most nutritionists do, and the funding is obvious. Any major corporation that manufactures food is likely to be found here. They apparently find attendees useful conduits to market their products.

Check out the ADA's nutrition fact sheet on chocolate, which says, "Chocolate is no longer a concern for those wary of saturated fat, and . . . in fact, chocolate can be part of a heart-healthy eating plan." Sponsor? Mars, manufacturer of M&Ms and numerous other chocolate candies.

The ADA's fact sheet on beverages notes, "Regular carbonated soft drinks contain calories; milk and juice contain calories, vitamins and minerals—all beverages can have a place in a well-balanced eating pattern."[206] Sponsor? The National Soft Drink Association.

Check out this statement from the ADA fact sheet on canned foods: "Recipes using canned ingredients are as nutritious as recipes prepared with fresh or frozen ingredients." Sponsor? The Steel Packaging Council.

McDonald's sponsors a fact sheet called "Nutrition on the Go," while Ajinomoto, which makes the flavoring MSG, sponsors a fact sheet on "Food Allergies and Intolerances." In reality, the fact sheets typically are written by corporate public relations departments or firms and are intended to improve the image of certain products or practices.[204]

While I'm not disputing that chocolate and soft drinks can have a place in an otherwise nutrient-dense diet, do we really want Mars and the National Soft Drink Association educating us on nutrition, hiding under the auspices of the world's foremost nutrition education organization?

Co-opting professionals is an important corporate strategy. Corporations routinely provide money and information to academic and research institutions and professional organizations and support meetings, conferences, and journals. In fact, it is hard to "excel" and get recognized as an expert in most fields without corporate ties.

Profits are a logical expectation of industry funding, and it is well-established that this investment pays off. For example, industry-sponsored research is much more likely to show positive results than independent research. Take drinks, for example. One review showed that scientific articles about drink consumption were four to eight times more likely to be favorable to the financial interests of the sponsors than those that didn't receive industry funding.[207] And none of the intervention studies with industry funding had an unfavorable result!

Another example of industry's influence on research came out of Harvard, where researchers surveyed all U.S.-accredited medical schools to evaluate relationships between researchers and sponsors.[208] Half the schools said they would allow pharmaceutical companies and makers of medical devices to draft articles about their products to appear in medical journals, and a quarter would allow them to supply the actual results reported in those articles.

Which professionals do most Americans look to for nutrition advice? Physicians. This trust is often a dangerous mistake. Doctors get very little training in nutrition. A report by the National Research Council found that physicians received an average of twenty-one classroom hours of nutrition education throughout their entire training, with most schools providing less.[209]

Take a look at where some of this education comes from. Many medical schools use the curriculum provided by Nutrition in Medicine and the Medical Nutrition Curriculum Initiative.[210] These organizations are supported by the Egg Nutrition Board, The Dannon Institute, National Cattleman's Beef Institute, National Dairy Council, Nestle Clinical Nutrition, Wyeth-Ayers Laboratories, Bristol-Meyers Squibb Company, and Baxter Healthcare Corporation. Do you think a coalition of people who sell animal foods or pharmaceuticals will present an unbiased approach to nutrition? No wonder little emphasis is given to encouraging plant foods in our diets, and pharmaceuticals are so frequently prescribed in situations in which lifestyle changes have proven effective.

Now that I've taken on the non-profit organizations, professional organizations, academia, and physicians, who is left to challenge? How about the federal government?

Suppose there were a food that:

■ Contained as much saturated fat and cholesterol as red meat
■ Was highly associated with increased risk of ovarian cancer[211, 212, 213, 214]
■ Contained a protein that *may* (research is inconclusive) trigger type 1 diabetes in genetically susceptible children[214, 215, 216, 217]

■ Contained a hormone (IGF-1) that is strongly linked to increased risk of breast[218] and prostate cancer[219, 220, 221]*

■ Promoted gas, stomach cramps, bloating and/or diarrhea in most people, particularly in African Americans, Native Americans, and Asian Americans[222]

■ Was contaminated with ammonium perchlorate,[223] a component of rocket fuel, at a level five times higher that the Environmental Protection Agency's standard for safety[234]

Would you make it a required product for all children in the federal lunch programs? Would you recommend that every child drink three glasses of it daily? Would you allow Donna Shalala, at that time the Secretary of Health and Human Services, to appear in advertisements for it?[225]

Well, that describes milk—and it's precisely what our government does! Makes the slogan, "Milk—it does the body good," sound a little hollow, doesn't it?

Surprisingly, there is no evidence to support the commonly held belief that milk builds stronger bones.[226] When scientists reviewed all the studies that examined the relationship between dairy consumption and bone health published between 1985 and 2000 and narrowed them down to those that were well-controlled and provided strong data, they found that 57 *percent showed no significant relationship between the two*, while 29 percent showed a favorable relationship and 14 percent showed that dairy consumption was actually detrimental to bone health.[227]

One large study followed 78,000 women and found no evidence that higher intakes of milk reduced bone fracture incidence or osteoporosis.[228] In fact, researchers found a higher risk of hip fracture in women drinking two or more glasses per week compared to women who drank one or less per week.

It is true that milk contains calcium, an important component of bone strength, but it also contains acidic amino acids that cause your

---

*Note that IGF-1 is a protein hormone and many suggest that it should be broken down during normal digestion. However, there have been several studies documenting that IGF-1 levels are boosted in people who drink milk.

body to excrete calcium, which may partially explain why people who consume large quantities of dairy products don't show lower rates of osteoporosis. Reducing calcium loss may play a larger role in promoting strong bones than increasing calcium consumption. Milk is also low in some nutrients that promote calcium absorption.

I grew up believing that consuming dairy products is essential for a strong and healthy body and that every child should drink milk daily. I now know these to be myths; they are promoted by health officials primarily because the National Dairy Council is extremely powerful at lobbying. They are also smart marketers. The Dairy Council is one of the leading suppliers of materials used to teach nutrition education in the schools. In this way, the Dairy Council shapes our beliefs under the guise of public service.

My point here is not that milk is poison and to be avoided—just that it doesn't do the job it is promoted for. If our government wants to promote a certain food, there are other foods that would do a better job of supporting the health of a broader spectrum of our population. Politics, not scientific data, dictate dairy promotion and our staunch, almost religious, belief in its health-promoting qualities.

Currently, most child nutrition programs (such as the National School Breakfast Program and the National School Lunch Program) require that milk be offered. Not only does the government mandate its inclusion in programs and promote milk, but it subsidizes the industry, essentially guaranteeing profits for dairy owners.[229] These subsidies are in large part due to the strong lobbying efforts by the dairy industry, which is one of the most influential industries in Congress.[229]

One reason the government is so vulnerable to industry influence is the conflict of interests that exist within the primary governmental body responsible for public nutrition education, the United States Department of Agriculture (USDA). Note the *Agriculture* in their name. Another purpose of this agency is to promote agriculture, and its recommendations are designed, in part, to support agribusiness. These dual roles sometimes conflict with each other, which is why public nutrition education is often a compromise between what is best for industry and what is best for the consumer.

For example, the USDA halted publication of the 1991 Eating Right Pyramid after meat and dairy trade groups objected to placement of their products in the pyramid. They then issued a watered-down version, the Food Guide Pyramid, revised to take into consideration industry's objections.[203]

It would be pretty difficult for the government to give a recommendation like "eat less meat," which is advice well accepted by those who study nutrition, without offending a powerful industry. The word choice in the Food Guide Pyramid is more palatable to the meat industry—"choose lean meats"—though less scientifically meaningful.

The USDA runs the National School Lunch Program and the School Breakfast Program. These programs allow millions of low-income students to receive a free or reduced-price lunch or breakfast every day. The bad news? The nutritional quality of those meals.

As discussed earlier, the USDA buys millions of pounds of surplus beef, pork, and other meat products to distribute to schools, but it does not subsidize more nutritious alternatives. That poses a tough dilemma for schools on a tight budget. It can cost a school district more than twice as much to provide a veggie burger instead of a hamburger. As a result, the government's own School Nutrition Dietary Assessment Study has found that an astonishing 80 percent of schools serve too much artery-clogging food in the lunch line to comply with federal guidelines. This situation is quite profitable for the meat industry, especially when you consider that taste preferences are strongly established in childhood. Hook 'em while they're young and get repeat customers for life.

The revolving door between the USDA and private industry has done much to inhibit sound nutrition policy. President George W. Bush, for example, appointed more than 100 top officials who were once lobbyists, attorneys, or spokespeople for the industries they oversee.[230] In many cases, former industry advocates have helped their agencies write, shape, or push for policy shifts that benefit the industries they used to work for.[230]

Even if not officially in public office, members of the agricultural industry serve on government committees that help draft nutrition policy. Suppose you need accurate information about the health impact of cigarette smoking. Would you call a tobacco company? Not a chance, right? Should the committee that helps the government draft nutrition recommendations be dominated by people who work within or have financial ties to the food industry? Of course not.

But that's what happens. The USDA and Department of Health and Human Services (HHS) formulate the Dietary Guidelines for Americans, including the Food Pyramid and other guidelines that make up the basis for all federal food programs, such as the National School Lunch Program. More than half the committee's members have extensive ties to the meat, dairy, sugar, processed food, egg, and supplement industries.

The Nutrition Transition

Calorie consumption has increased dramatically in the last few decades[159] and much of the increase is attributed to processed and animal foods.[136] It is not a coincidence that these foods are most profitable to the food industry.

Years ago, before the advent of modern food manufacturing, most available foods were nutritious, farm-grown or farm-raised foods that sent messages to our weight regulation system. Our body read those signals, driving us to get calories in proportion to our needs.

However, modern food processing has changed that. Today, the cheap calories found in the saturated fats, trans fats, and high-glycemic carbohydrates common in today's "industrial diet" don't register as strongly in our weight regulation system and don't turn off our hunger drive, thus pushing many of us to eat more despite getting sufficient calories. It is not surprising that much epidemiologic research shows a strong relationship between consumption of low-cost, processed foods and weight.[231]

The impact of industrial foods extends, of course, well beyond our weight. Indeed, many of the chronic diseases common today can be traced directly to the industrialization of our food. Data shows that simply by moving to America and adopting the industrial diet, people from nations with low rates of the "diseases of affluence" such as diabetes, cancer, and cardiovascular disease quickly acquire them.

Of course, the United States is not alone in this trend. Indeed, most modern societies seem to be converging on the same dietary pattern. Most countries in Asia, Latin America, Northern Africa, the Middle East, and the urban areas of sub-Saharan Africa have all experienced a similar dietary shift—with related increases in these diseases (and weight)—over the last few decades.[232]

The more commonly recommended solutions merely reinforce industry's interests. "Health foods" are typically even more processed versions of the same old industrial foods: they just reduce the fat, substitute artificial sweeteners for the sugar, bump up the fiber or soy protein, or fortify foods with added nutrients.

Shifting Blame

Industry defends itself by laying blame on the individual. Indeed, the key tactic for the Center for Consumer Freedom, the food industry's front group and spin-maker, is "to promote personal responsibility and protect consumer choices."[194] The general idea is that "No one forces the consumer to buy cheese puffs." Government supports this strategy with a focused campaign on encouraging individuals to make better, more informed choices.

I care deeply about individuals' freedom of choice and informed consent. I expect government agencies to serve the public good rather than corporate profit. I hold business and industry to a standard of social responsibility.

If you think I'm angry that corporations and government agencies have co-opted the production and distribution of food at the expense of our health and well-being, you're right. I value the sensation of hunger as a sign of the body's wisdom, not as a commercial asset to be manipulated for market share. I value food as nourishment, not as a unit of sales. I value our bodies as gifts of life, not as product-consumption devices.

While it is clear that our food choices are a matter of personal responsibility, it is important to recognize that we do not make our choices in a vacuum. We select our foods in an environment toxic with government policies that encourage cheap prices for foods with low nutrient value, and in which billions of dollars have been spent to convince us to distrust ourselves, to overeat, and to eat foods laced with ingredients that raise our setpoints and damage our health.

Taking It Home

Don't let industry and government distract you from their responsibility in providing good food and accurate information and promoting a healthy attitude towards eating. We have been deceived by faulty ideas, policies, and greed. Clearly, our current food environment needs a major overhaul. While we can't fully legislate the problem away, we can certainly get muckraking and insist that industry and government do much, much better.

And the good news is that you can also make change on a personal level. You can relax. You don't have to leap from your seat every time a new carcinogen or miracle food is hyped. Be cynical about the fads, headlines—and even the latest research findings. Develop your "media literacy" skills so that you are less likely to be suckered in. Become a more educated consumer so that you are less vulnerable to the myths and disinformation. When in doubt, a back to basics approach—getting your foods from nature, with less human interference—will serve you well. Most importantly, you can reclaim enjoyment of nutritious foods and reengage with your body's ability to maintain a healthy weight. Future chapters show you how.

SIX

We're Victims of Fat Politics

ichard Carmona, formerly the surgeon general, the highest government health official, described obesity as "the terror within, a threat that is every bit as real to America as the weapons of mass destruction."[233] Six months before he made that grave pronouncement, terrorists had destroyed the World Trade Center. The country was on high alert and the fear of continued terrorist action was at the forefront of our minds.

At your next family get-together, when your mom ladles that glop of gravy on your mashed potatoes, when she urges, "Eat, eat! It's good for you!" and especially when she puts that second helping of apple crumb pie with whipped cream on your plate, call 911. Get that woman detained.

Then reflect on the craziness that underlies this "obesity epidemic": Terrorists not only in our airports and cities, but in our kitchens. Cheeseburgers and French fries as weapons of mass destruction. Fat people as the living repository for American shame.

Manufacturing the Obesity Epidemic

More than 400,000 Americans die of overweight and obesity* every year, so many that it may soon surpass smoking as the leading cause of preventable death.[234] At least that's what the Centers for Disease Control and Prevention (CDC) told us in the prestigious *Journal of the American Medical Association* (*JAMA*). Their report grabbed headlines, helped along by dramatic, well-distributed press releases from the CDC and *JAMA*, and resulted in tens of thousands of citations in the popular press and thousands more in scientific journals.

But an updated federal report acknowledged that the analysis suffered from computational errors.[235] Using better methodology and newer data, CDC epidemiologists *reduced the estimate fifteen-fold*, determining that obesity and overweight were only associated with an excess of 26,000 annual deaths, far fewer than guns, alcohol, or car crashes.[235] (Later in this chapter, we'll discuss the behind-the-scenes politics that led to these reports.)

Separating overweight from obesity reveals further interesting information. First, *"overweight" people live longer than "normal" weight people.* (In the year 2000, there were 86,000 fewer deaths in the overweight category relative to what was expected if people were in the normal range.) Next, the excess deaths in the obesity category were clustered in the more extreme range (body mass index [BMI] greater than 35), which is not where the majority of obese Americans fall (BMI 30 to 35).

Most striking is that the CDC did not publicize the new results, nor change their public health message. After all, they used the original study to justify their war on obesity. Why not stop the war now that the evidence has disappeared? And if they are so concerned about the health of "overweight" people, why isn't this news cause for celebration? Interestingly, the study found slightly more total annual U.S. deaths in the "Underweight" category than in the two

---

*Body mass index (BMI) is defined as weight (in kilograms) divided by height (in meters) squared. A BMI between 19 and 25 is considered "normal," between 25 and 30 is considered "overweight," and 30 and above is classified as "obese."

heaviest categories ("Overweight" and "Obese"), suggesting a stronger case for shifting public health attention to the dangers of thinner weights.

The CDC didn't just overhype a crisis, they helped invent it. With only 26,000 victims, we don't have an obesity/overweight epidemic; our epidemic is one of fearmongering and ignorance. Consider the following statements:

1. Overweight and obesity lead to early death.
2. Overweight and obesity lead to disease.
3. We are gaining weight at epidemic rates.
4. Weight loss improves health and longevity.
5. You control what you weigh.
6. Anyone can keep lost weight off if she or he tries hard enough.
7. Thinner is more attractive.
8. We can trust the experts to provide accurate information.

For most of us, these statements seem like basic truisms. However, much of what we believe to be true about weight—*including all of the statements above*—is in fact myth, fueled by the power of money and cultural bias. Public health officials, health advocates, and scientists are complicit (often unintentionally) in supporting and encouraging the lies. The campaign against obesity is not about science or health; its misconceptions about the most basic research are astounding. If you suspend your preconceptions and open yourself to the scientific evidence, a very different picture emerges.

1. The "Death by Fat" Myth

No obesity myth is more potent than the one that says obesity kills. It gives us permission to call our fear of fat a health concern, rather than naming it as the cultural oppression it is.

That "obesity kills" has been the backbone of the federal public health campaign. Yet that is not supported by evidence examined by federal employees. Their research found that "even severe obesity failed to show up as a statistically significant mortality risk"[236] and suggested that overweight may actually be protective.[235]

About Terminology

Nowadays, you don't have love handles, puppy fat, curves, or a spare tire—you're overweight or obese. Throughout this chapter, I use the terms "overweight" and "obese" because they are commonly understood medical terms, and I am describing research and attitudes that rely on these terms. However, these categories are meaningless in determining someone's health status, and the terms "overweight" and "obese" miss the mark. Over what weight? There is no precise weight beyond which you will definitely be unhealthy! And the etymology of the word "obesity" mistakenly implies that a large appetite is the cause.

Using these terms medicalizes and pathologizes having a certain body, which is why these words are rarely found elsewhere in this book. Instead, I use a more appropriate term: fat. There is a growing movement that seeks to reclaim the term "fat" as a descriptive term, stripped of its pejorative implications. This change is supported by many fat-acceptance activists and the National Association to Advance Fat Acceptance (NAAFA), a "human rights organization dedicated to improving the quality of life for fat people." NAAFA argues, rightfully so, that fatness is a form of body diversity that should be respected, much like diversity based on skin color or sexual preference.

This finding is not new news, but entirely consistent with the bulk of the literature.[237] All of these well-respected studies cited below, for instance, determined that overweight people were living at least as long as, and frequently longer than, normal weight people:

- The Established Populations for the Epidemiological Studies of the Elderly investigation (included more than 8,000 senior citizens)[238]
- The Study of Osteoporotic Fractures investigation (included more than 8,000 women)[239]
- The Cardiovascular Health Study (included almost 5,000 individuals)[240]
- Women's Health Initiative Observational Study (included 90,000 women)[241]
- An investigation of almost 170,000 adults in China[242]
- An investigation of 20,000 German construction workers[243]
- An investigation of 12,000 Finnish women[244]
- An investigation of 1.7 million Norwegians[245] (Yes, you read that right: 1.7 million people! In this, the largest epidemiological study ever conducted, the highest life expectancy is among individuals who are overweight by our current standards and the lowest life expectancy is among those defined as underweight. What's more, individuals who fit into what is deemed the ideal weight range had a lower life expectancy than some of those who were obese.)

These are not a few errant investigations, but representative of conclusions that dominate the research. The most comprehensive review, for instance, pooled data from 26 studies and concluded that overweight individuals were living slightly longer than those of normal weight.[246]

Even the definitive National Institute of Health Clinical Guidelines on Identification, Evaluation and Treatment of Overweight and Obesity in Adults concludes that the weight associated with the *lowest* death rate is considerably *above* a BMI of 25.[247] (Yet that doesn't stop them from recommending weight loss for overweight individuals—nor from defining their mandate as "evidence-based.")

The scientific evidence is clear: *Body fat is not the killer it's portrayed as.*

2. The "Disease-Promoting Fat" Myth

The idea that weight plays a large causal role in disease is also unproven. Little evidence supports that weight is the primary cause of many diseases for which it is routinely blamed, except osteoarthritis, sleep apnea, and possibly a few cancers. In contrast, there are several diseases for which high levels of body fat provide a distinct, though rarely acknowledged, advantage.

"The current generation of children is the first generation in modern American history projected to have a shorter life span than their parents."

This proclamation was drawn from an opinion piece[248] published in the prestigious *New England Journal of Medicine* and offered *no* statistical evidence to support its claim, though you would never know it from the authority it has been granted in the media. Consider this before you buy into the hype: Life expectancy has increased dramatically during the same time period in which our weight rose (from 70.8 years in 1970 to 77.8 years in 2005) and continues to hit record highs.[249] That's right, government statistics predict that the average kid can now expect to live seven years longer than his or her parents! Not only are we living longer than ever before, but we're healthier than ever and chronic disease is appearing much later in life.[249] Death rates attributed to heart disease have steadily declined throughout the entire spike in obesity.[250] Both the World Health Organization[251] and the Social Security Administration[252] project life expectancy to continue to rise in coming decades.

Many "obese" people are healthy and don't suffer from the diseases that we tend to blame on weight, and a considerable proportion of "normal weight" people are prone to the cardiac and metabolic abnormalities that we blame on obesity.[253, 254]

Epidemiologic Studies Cause Statistical Deaths

The majority of knowledge regarding the relationship between health and weight is drawn from epidemiological research. Epidemiological obesity research compares groups of overweight and obese individuals with a control group of normal weight individuals. It is intended to uncover associations which then need further examination. It cannot tell us whether a variable causes or even influences another.

Consider this: It is well established through epidemiological research that bald men have a higher incidence of heart disease than men with a full head of hair.[255] However, this doesn't mean that baldness promotes heart disease or that hair protects against heart disease. Nor is it recommended that bald men try to grow hair or buy toupees in order to lessen their disease risk.

Instead, further research indicates that high levels of testosterone may promote both baldness and heart disease. "Confounding factors" can often serve to confuse the interpretation of epidemiologic research.

It is clear that weight is *associated* with increased risk for some diseases, but causation is an entirely different matter. In some cases, the causality may travel in the opposite direction, as in the case of diabetes (to be discussed shortly). Some of the medications intended to treat weight-associated diseases may also encourage weight gain, such as the insulin, sulfonylureas, and thiazolidinediones used to treat diabetes.

Lifestyle habits can also confuse the picture. A sedentary lifestyle, for example, may predispose someone to weight gain *and* make them more vulnerable to many diseases. It is well established that the relationship between activity and longevity is stronger than the relationship between weight and longevity.[256, 257, 258, 259, 260, 261, 262] Consider the research conducted as part of the Aerobics Center Longitudinal Study in Texas, which found that obese men who are classified as "fit" based on a treadmill test have death rates just as low as "fit" lean men.[257] Moreover, the fit obese men had death rates one-half those of the lean but unfit men, indicating that fitness is more important than weight in longevity. Similar results were demonstrated for women.[258]

Larger people may be more likely to have tried dangerous weight-loss methods, which may also be reflected in higher incidence of disease. For instance, in 1970, 8 percent of all U.S. prescriptions were for amphetamines intended to treat obesity[263] that are now known to increase heart disease risk.[264] Heavier people may also have gone through damaging cycles of losing and regaining weight, making them more prone to certain diseases. For instance, even a single cycle of losing and regaining weight may damage blood vessels and increase risk for cardiovascular disease.[265]

Reduced access to health care and poor quality health care may also confuse the picture.[266, 267, 268] Weight bias among health care practitioners is well-documented[269, 270] and life-threatening. As an example, several research studies indicate that fatter women with cancer may not get the appropriate dose of chemotherapy for their weight, which adversely affects survival.[271] Studies also indicate that fat women may delay or avoid seeking health care for fear of discrimination and receiving an unsolicited weight loss lecture.[267, 268]

Also, it is well established that obesity is higher among ethnic minorities and people of lower socioeconomic status,[272] both of which are also highly associated with disease risk. The higher pollution levels in poorer neighborhoods[273] may play a role, and the increased discrimination to which ethnic minorities and people of lower socioeconomic status are subject may be a factor as well.

And of course, stress from the discrimination and widespread hostility directed at larger people may also be a significant contributor to the risks currently blamed on body fat alone. Researchers find larger people experience more cynical mistrust, which is highly associated with inflammation, a major risk for heart disease.[274] There is extensive research documenting the role of chronic stress in conditions conventionally described as obesity-associated, such as hypertension, diabetes and coronary heart disease.[275, 276] Stress itself alters metabolism independent of changes in BMI.[277]

I suspect that it is our attitude about obesity that may also put us at risk. Cross-cultural studies suggest that larger people are not subject to the same diseases in countries where there is less stigma attached to weight.[254] Also, in the United States, there is a stronger relationship between BMI and morbidity (disease) and mortality (early death) among groups more negatively affected by body image concerns (younger people, Caucasians, and women).[278, 279, 280, 281] Even more telling, when researchers looked at a nationally representative group of more than 170,000 U.S. adults, they found the difference between actual weight and perceived ideal weight was a better indicator of mental and physical health than BMI.[282] In other words, *feeling* fat has stronger health effects than *being* fat.

This finding is not surprising given the well established relationship between stigma and stress, which in turn increases disease risk.[276] And of course, weight discrimination is pervasive and severe—so severe that its prevalence now equals or surpasses discrimination based on race or gender.[269, 270, 283]

Take a closer look at the four most common conditions that have been blamed on weight: hypertension, atherosclerosis, type 2 diabetes, and cancer. The data present a very different picture than is commonly portrayed.

Obesity and Hypertension

Hypertension refers to high blood pressure, a condition that is two to three times more common among obese people than lean people.[284] To what extent this is caused by fat, however, is unclear. It may have more to do with the weight cycling that results from trying to control weight than the actual weight itself.[285, 286] One study showed that obese women who had dieted had high blood pressure, while those who had never been on a diet had normal blood pressure.[287] Rat studies also show that obese rats that have weight cycled have very high blood pressures compared to obese rats that have not weight cycled.[288, 289] This finding could also explain the weak association between obesity and hypertension in cultures where dieting is uncommon.[285, 286, 287, 288, 289 290] Since admonitions to lose weight typically result in weight cycling, the proposed "cure" for hypertension may actually be its cause.

Also, it is well documented that obese people with hypertension live significantly longer than thinner people with hypertension[291, 292, 293, 294] and have a lower risk of heart attack, stroke, or early death.[295] Rather than identifying health risk, as it does in thinner people, hypertension in fatter people may simply be a requirement for pumping blood through their larger bodies.

Does weight loss reduce hypertension? Many studies document that blood pressure improves during weight loss in hypertensive people. However, the long-term results are disappointing, even when the weight loss is maintained—including massive amounts of weight loss after bariatric surgery.[286] Studies that demonstrate weight loss through various interventions, such as exercise, sodium reduction, and stress management, show promising short-term effects on blood pressure. However, it is unclear whether the weight loss itself brings about this improvement. For instance, studies document that when weight loss is achieved, the reduction in blood pressure parallels a reduction in dietary sodium, suggesting that dietary change is actually the mitigating factor.[296] The well-known DASH (Dietary Approaches to Stop Hypertension) diet, which is a reduced sodium diet, has been shown to lower blood pressure successfully, even without lowering weight.[297, 298]

It is also interesting to note that the prevalence of high blood pressure dropped by half between 1960 and 2000, declining much more steeply among those deemed overweight and obese than among thinner individuals.[299] (To what extent this is the result of improved medical care or medication is unclear.)

Given this evidence, why is the standard advice given to people with high blood pressure to lose weight?

Obesity and Atherosclerosis

Atherosclerosis refers to the buildup of cholesterol-laden plaque on artery walls that narrows the passage, restricting blood flow. Because atherosclerosis makes the heart work harder, it can damage the heart.

Since obese people have more fat on their bodies, they must have more fat in their arteries, right? Yet research doesn't support this. Five decades of autopsy studies consistently show no relationship between body fat and atherosclerosis.[300, 301, 302, 303, 304] Ultrasound studies corroborate this,[302, 305, 306] and well over half of the angiographic studies conducted between 1976 and 2000 show obesity has no relationship to either the presence of atherosclerosis or its progression over time.[302] The largest, most comprehensive angiographic study examined 4,500 angiograms and concluded that every eleven-pound *increase* in weight was associated with a 10 to 40 percent *lower* chance of atherosclerosis.[307] In other words, fat men and women had the cleanest arteries!

Furthermore, research frequently indicates that overweight and obese adults with atherosclerosis (like those with high blood pressure, as discussed earlier) have a lower risk of heart attack, stroke, or early death, compared with their normal-weight counterparts.[295] The famous Framingham Heart Study followed a cohort of men for more than thirty years and found that the men who had gained weight were less likely to have developed heart disease or to have died from heart disease.[308]

It is interesting to note that the incidence of heart disease has dropped dramatically in the time since obesity rates started to rise and is now occurring much later in life.[299] Heart disease death rates have been falling for more than five decades, including an impressive 22.1 percent drop just between 1993 and 2003. Research indicates that improved medical care is only part of the explanation.

Given the preponderance of evidence, why advise people to lose weight in order to prevent or treat atherosclerosis?

Obesity and Type 2 Diabetes

Type 2 diabetes is a metabolic disorder in which people have a reduced sensitivity to insulin. Insulin helps certain nutrients, such as glucose, get into cells, and when insulin doesn't work effectively, cells don't get the energy they need to work effectively.

Type 2 diabetes is much more common among obese individuals than leaner individuals (80 percent of people with type 2 diabetes are obese),[309, 310] and thus diabetes is commonly blamed on weight. However, it is clear that risk of type 2 diabetes includes a genetic component, and there is strong evidence to support the idea that the genes that play a role in causing diabetes also cause weight gain.[285]

The "thrifty genotype" theory was first proposed in the 1960s and has gained increasing acceptance ever since.[311] The insulin resistance that is characteristic of type 2 diabetes could be viewed as a helpful genetic adaptation to the cycles of famine common in history. Insulin resistance supports efficient storage of fat when food is available and slows energy usage when food is less available, which would have contributed to longevity in earlier times. Our ancestors didn't have fast-food caves on every corner, nor could they dip into their refrigerator/freezers for an always available supply of preserved food.

Research shows that high levels of insulin appear *before* weight gain in future diabetics.[285, 312] The mechanism looks like this: Insulin resistance develops first. Because the cells are partially resistant to the insulin, glucose and other nutrients can't get into most cells, despite the cells' increasing need for the nutrients. The pancreas pumps out even more insulin to try to accommodate the cells' need for energy. The high insulin levels increase insulin resistance and stimulate appetite. Because fat cells are less likely than other cells to develop insulin resistance, the high insulin levels readily allow fat storage, resulting in weight gain. As this cycle continues, the insulin resistance takes on a new name: diabetes. In other words, weight gain is actually an early symptom of type 2 diabetes.

This is not to suggest that body fat is entirely benign in the type 2 diabetes disease process. But the relationship between type 2 diabetes and body fat appears to be self-perpetuating: The high levels of insulin characteristic of type 2 diabetes lead to weight gain, and high levels of abdominal fat increase insulin resistance, worsening type 2 diabetes.

On a short-term basis, weight loss is very effective at improving control of blood glucose. However, this doesn't mean that the diabetes is being cured; even skipping one meal will similarly lower blood glucose. A 1995 review of all of the controlled weight-loss studies for type 2 diabetics showed that the initial improvements were followed by a deterioration back to starting values six to eighteen months after treatment, *even when the weight loss was maintained.*[313]

Surgical studies allow us to see the effects of weight loss without changing other factors like eating or activity habits. Gastric bypass surgery appears to reverse diabetes within days, before significant weight is lost, which suggests that it is not the weight loss that brings about the improvement but some other factor (such as a change in the release of gut hormones).

Liposuction studies provide further support that it is not the weight itself that is problematic. For example, in one study researchers examined obese women, half of whom were diabetic, before and ten to twelve weeks after an average of about twenty pounds of body fat was removed.[314] Despite the weight loss, their metabolic profiles did not improve, including their fasting glucose and insulin levels and their insulin sensitivity.

Though body fat is certainly a contributor to type 2 diabetes— no doubt it's the strongest card the obesity alarmists hold—numerous research studies document that type 2 diabetes can be improved or reversed through changes in nutrition or activity habits, *even when little or no weight is lost.*[65, 315, 316, 317, 318] Eating better and becoming more active are much more effective for curing, preventing, or controlling diabetes than shedding pounds.

It is also interesting to note that obese persons with type 2 diabetes live longer than thinner people with the condition, suggesting that diabetes, like hypertension, may actually be less problematic in a larger body.[319]

Given this evidence, why is the first suggestion to people with diabetes that they lose weight? Why not encourage improving lifestyle habits—a strategy which has actually proven effective?

Obesity and Cancer

What about the headlines proclaiming that fat gives you cancer? One report, from the American Institute for Cancer Research (AICR), was all over the media claiming that overweight and obesity increases risk for six cancers: pancreas, kidney, endometrium, breast, colorectum, and esophagus.[320] All that was lacking in this very comprehensive, 517-page report was convincing evidence to support these claims!

Take a look at the evidence they present for pancreatic cancer. Their researchers found that of the twenty-three cohort studies* they deemed well-designed, only four showed a statistically significant association between obesity and pancreatic cancer. I had the opportunity to discuss this with a representative of the AICR on the BBC World Report radio program,[321] and when I asked him to explain how this data justified their claims, his defense was that they also examined case-control studies.[321] He's right. Here's what his researchers found: Of the fifteen case-control studies†, only one showed a statistically significant increased risk—and one showed a statistically significant *decreased* risk.

Breast cancer? Of the twenty-six cohort studies discussed in the report, only three showed a significant association, while two showed a *decreased* risk of breast cancer for the obese!

For esophageal cancer, risk was indicated for those who are morbidly obese, but not for those who are moderately obese.

---

*In cohort studies, a group ("cohort") of people is followed over time. During the follow-up period, some individuals will be diagnosed with cancer and comparisons are made between those who are diagnosed with cancer and those who are not.

†In case-control studies, individuals with a particular type of cancer ("cases") are compared with otherwise similar people who have not been diagnosed with cancer.

Based on the evidence the report presents, do you share their conclusions? Or is this just more fearmongering from the "experts"?

Investigation by the Centers for Disease Control and Prevention also contradicts the obesity-cancer link.[322] In the words of the CDC epidemiologists, there is "little or no association of excess all-cancer mortality with any of the BMI categories."[322] While there are some associations between specific types of cancer and obesity as well as mechanisms through which fat tissue affects cancer, it is clear that obesity has been greatly misrepresented and exaggerated as a cancer risk.

"Obesity costs us millions of dollars in healthcare expenditures."[323]

So say some pundits in another well-publicized report. How did they arrive at this figure? They calculated the expenses associated with treating a host of conditions, including type 2 diabetes, coronary heart disease, hypertension, gallbladder disease, and cancer, assuming that susceptibility to all of those is caused by fat. Nowhere did they account for mitigating factors that might cause these conditions, such as genetics, activity habits, or diet—nor did they account for the fact that thin people are subject to these conditions as well.

Get Fat: It's Good for You?

Less well publicized is the idea that body fat may actually protect us from many diseases. There is a long list of conditions less common in heavy people than their thinner counterparts, among them lung

Good Fat/Bad Fat?

There are two different types of body fat, which in part explains the ambiguity of the effects of body fat: One is more apt to give us benefits, and one more likely presents us with health risks, though the picture is not as clear-cut or as well understood as we'd like to believe. The two types are differentiated by their location. So-called "bad body fat" is known to scientists as visceral fat and is located around abdominal organs, in particular the liver. It is more metabolically active in terms of both storing and releasing fat, which can be dangerous in two ways: First, because the fat it releases can end up clogging your arteries, and second, much of the released fat can go directly to the liver, impairing its ability to carry out other functions. Women are not as susceptible to high levels of "bad body fat" as men are.

So-called "good body fat" is known to scientists as subcutaneous fat. The cells have high levels of an enzyme (lipoprotein lipase) which cause them to store fat easily and hold on to it more tightly. This means that the fat stays in the fat cells where we believe it has a positive effect on health.

Our body shape tells us a lot about how our fat is distributed. If you have an "apple-shaped" body distribution—fat around the belly rather than below the waist—you are more likely to have a high level of visceral body fat, the stuff more highly associated with risk. If instead you have a "pear-shaped" body distribution—fat on your thighs and hips (much more typical for women), you probably get more benefits from your fat.

cancer, chronic bronchitis, tuberculosis, mitral valve prolapse, anemia, type 1 diabetes, premature menopause, and osteoporosis.[302]

Obesity is also associated with improved survival in several diseases. For example, obese persons with type 2 diabetes,[319] hypertension,[291, 324] cardiovascular disease,[295] and chronic kidney disease[325] all have greater longevity than thinner people with these conditions.[283, 326, 327] And obese people who have had heart attacks, coronary bypass,[328] angioplasty,[329] or hemodialysis[330] live longer than thinner people with these histories.[327] Also, obese senior citizens live longer than thinner senior citizens![331]

3. The "Obesity Epidemic" Myth

No doubt Americans have gained weight over the last few decades. But if we are so concerned about an epidemic, why aren't we celebrating its apparent end? The incidence of obesity is no longer increasing.[332, 333, 334] According to government statistics, obesity rates for women have leveled off and stayed steady since 1999,[333, 334] sufficient time to consider it a plateau. They also have leveled off for men, having been stable since 2003.[333, 334] Same is true for kids: The prevalence of obesity for children and teens is no different today than it was in 1999.[335] It may just be that we've reached our metabolic limit; our bodies have adjusted to our current lifestyle habits and environmental conditions and are now kicking in to maintain us at a new setpoint, albeit a higher one than our ancestors, who experienced different conditions.

In addition to having gained weight over the last few decades, we're also growing taller. American men are over an inch taller than they were in the 1960s[336] and nearly three inches taller than they were 100 years ago! Why isn't that subject to the same media attention and concern? It may be that both the height and weight increase are the result of *improved* nutritional status and health.

What's even more important to notice than our weight gain is that there is no evidence this weight gain is a crisis. As mentioned earlier, life expectancy has increased dramatically during the time period in which weight rose.[249] The very diseases that are linked to obesity, like heart disease, are the ones that are declining.

We are simply not seeing the catastrophic consequences predicted to result from the "obesity epidemic."

4. The "Lose Weight, Get Healthy" Myth

The idea that health will necessarily improve with weight loss is dubious at best.[302] *No one has ever proved that losing weight prolongs life.* There is great controversy as to whether weight loss is necessary or even desirable for improved health. While it is clear that research indicates a short-term improvement in health risk factors with weight loss, no randomized clinical studies have observed the long-term effects of weight loss, and the observational research (epidemiological studies) has typically found weight loss to be associated with dying younger.

For example, well-respected physiologist Glenn Gaesser examined the research and found fifteen studies published between 1983 and 1993 that show that weight loss actually *increases* the risk of dying early.[337] Only two studies published during that same period showed weight loss reducing the risk of dying early, and one of these only showed an eleven-hour increase in longevity for each pound of weight loss![337] Even when subjects with unintentional weight loss (such as might occur with cancer or AIDS) are excluded, the research is ambiguous at best.[338, 339, 340, 341, 342, 343]

When the National Institutes of Health convened a conference to review the evidence about dieting, they concluded: "Most studies, and the strongest science, shows weight loss . . . is actually strongly associated with increased risks of death—by as much as several hundred percent."[344]

Note, of course, that just because the research indicates an association between weight loss and decreased longevity doesn't mean that weight loss *causes* early death. I suspect the explanation for this association lies in the unhealthy methods people use to achieve weight loss, as well as the difficulty in separating weight loss from weight gain.[345] Many people who do achieve weight loss go through cycles of weight loss and gain before finally stabilizing at a lower weight, damaging their health in the process.

Also, when people lose weight through dieting, particularly the more extreme diets, they shed lean tissue (from muscle and organs) in addition to fat. There may be a cost associated with losing lean tissue that offsets any possible benefits of shedding the fat. (Weight loss that results from increased activity may present a different picture, as exercise helps to preserve or increase lean mass, at least when sufficient calories are consumed.)

Nonetheless, extensive evidence documents that attempts at dieting typically result in weight cycling, not maintained weight loss. Weight fluctuation is strongly associated with increased risk for diabetes, hypertension, and cardiovascular diseases, independent of body weight.[346] In other words, the recommendation to diet may be causing the very diseases it is purported to prevent!

In contrast, whether the concern is type 2 diabetes, atherosclerosis, hypertension, cancer, or a host of other conditions, the evidence is clear: An abundance of studies indicate improvement through nutrition or activity habits, independent of weight loss.[285, 345, 347, 348, 349] We're on much firmer ground when we promote lifestyle change. Lifestyle improvements may also result in weight loss, but this is not a given.

5. The "You Control Your Weight" Myth

Many genes interact to determine whether the food you eat gets stored as fat or burned for energy—whether that dash to catch the bus will get its fuel by lightening your fat stores or by emptying your carbohydrate stores and driving you to eat more. It's a biological fact that identical eating and activity habits can result in thinness in one person and chubbiness in another.

Studies of adoptees provide good data on the degree to which your weight is inherited. After all, if there is a strong genetic component, you would expect a child's weight to be similar to his or her biological parents regardless of how he or she was raised. The research supports this. For example, one study, published in the *New England Journal of Medicine*, looked at 540 adults who had been adopted when young: 55 percent in their first month and almost 90 percent within their first year.[350] The study found that adoptees were similar in size to their biological parents, and their size had *no* relation to their adoptive parents.

A similar study, published in *JAMA*, compared twins who were reared apart to twins reared together, and had similar findings.[351] The identical twins in this study had nearly identical BMIs regardless of whether they were brought up together or in different environments. There was a little more variation among the fraternal twins, who share some but not all genes. The researchers concluded that 70 percent of weight variation can be accounted for by genetics—making the heritability of obesity[351, 352, 353] greater than that of almost any other condition, including breast cancer, schizophrenia, and heart disease![5]

Thin people may think they stay thin because they are morally superior. The data suggests it is more likely that they're genetically lucky (in this time when thinness is valued). The most direct route to thinness is to choose your parents well.

Your Genes Determine the Result of the Habits You "Choose"

Think again of two people with similar eating and activity habits, one of whom may be lean and the other heavy, one of whom may lose weight from consuming the same foods that result in creeping weight gain in another. In the past, experts believed this discrepancy was explained by a lack of honesty in reporting, rarely believing the fat person who claimed to eat like a bird. But today, that blame-laying is on shaky ground. Now experts recognize that the way in which people respond to diet and exercise is genetically determined.

Morgan Spurlock's *Super Size Me* experiment is currently being replicated, this time under scientific conditions.[354, 355] Research volunteers are eating double their normal calorie intake in the form of "junk food" and avoiding physical activity. Preliminary results confirm that a certain type and number of excess calories don't result in the same across-the-board weight increase. There is huge variability in their weight gain (and in health risk factors).

This is not surprising when one is acquainted with the research conducted on twins on the effects of diet and exercise. An example:

Researchers put twenty-eight pairs of identical twins on a six-week high-fat/low-carbohydrate diet, followed by a six-week low-fat/high-carbohydrate diet.[356] In each pair, one twin ran an average of thirty miles per week more than the other. Consistent with other studies, when the men were compared to men who weren't their twins, there were large differences in weight change. However, despite the extreme difference in physical activity, each twin had very similar changes in weight. Getting more exercise didn't result in a weight difference! The men's bodies so strongly wanted to maintain a certain weight that they somehow found a way to compensate for the increased energy expenditure.

In other experiments, identical male twins exercised on stationary bicycles twice a day, nine out of every ten days, over either twenty-two days[357] or one hundred days.[358] Diets were consistent, and the exercise caused them to use an extra 1,000 calories a day. Just as the previously mentioned study revealed, these experiments showed that each man's weight loss was similar to that of his twin, although there was large variability when the sets of twins were compared.

There are plenty of thin people among McDonald's regular customers. There are also plenty of people who are fat despite birdlike eating habits and active lifestyles. Making assumptions about someone's habits by looking at their body size will lead you astray.

As discussed earlier, research shows no differences in the eating habits of the heavy and the lean.[126] Being thin or fat largely reflects how well your body is genetically predisposed to store fat.

6. The "Everyone Can Lose Weight" Myth

We believe that if we eat a wholesome diet, exercise regularly, and take care of ourselves in other ways, we can lose weight. We believe that fat people just don't take care of themselves or lack willpower or self-respect. Though these beliefs are accepted as if they are common sense, they are not supported by the evidence. The little data gathered on what happens post–weight loss shows that the vast majority of people regain whatever weight they lose.[344, 347, 359] As noted in one review, "It is only the rate of weight regain, not the fact of weight regain, that appears open to debate."[360]

So can you actually lose weight and keep it off? First, remember that your setpoint is not a firm number, but a range, possibly from ten to twenty pounds. This fact means that for many people, a ten-to-twenty-pound weight loss may not meet with biological resistance. Since how you live your life does influence setpoint mechanisms, it may also be true that many Americans could lose *some* weight by improving the quality of their lifestyle choices.

However, even if everyone in America exercised regularly, meditated daily, and ate nothing but brown rice, broccoli, and tofu, many people would still be fat, and most bodies would be heavier than the ones glorified in our culture.

Yes, there are individuals who beat the odds and maintain large weight losses over time. Some researchers were so determined to "counter the belief that no one succeeds at long-term weight loss" that they actually designed a registry, called the National Weight Control Registry (NWCR), to track those successful losers.[361]

The Few, the Proud, the Losers

At a recent family reunion, a large crowd gathered around a distant cousin of mine. He was sixty pounds lighter than many of us remembered and had maintained his weight loss for several years. With religious zeal, he waxed poetic about his new diet and exercise habits and how he lost the weight. The crowd was entranced, everyone anxious to learn the winning formula.

If you have witnessed a scene like this, you are not alone. We all know someone who has actually lost weight and kept it off. It is possible, though uncommon. It keeps our hopes up. We believe that if they can do it, we should be able to as well. So we listen closely to every story, anxious to learn the secret.

The commercial diet industry is savvy to our desperation and the opportunity this creates. We are easily exploited. Every advertisement draws us in with an inspiring testimonial or before and after pictures. The message is clear: I did it and so can you. (What goes unsaid: If you can't, it's your own damn fault!)

No doubt the NWCR has located some of the small minority of people who do indeed maintain weight loss long term. And small minority it is indeed. One review compares a conservative estimate of the number of people dieting to the population estimate and calculates that the NWCR researchers "demonstrate a 'success rate' of .001 percent, which is not even close to the dismal 5 percent estimate cited in the scientific literature."[362]

Their results don't inspire optimism. First, the data they gathered is hardly long term: It includes individuals who have maintained a thirty-pound weight loss for one year or more. Studies show that two-thirds of weight regain happens within two years, and at five years all the weight has been regained.[344] So some of the individuals in the NWCR registry haven't even made it past these danger points. And even among this elite group, 72 percent are regaining![362]

To maintain her weight loss, the average woman in NWCR follows strict eating rules, consumes 1,306 kcals,[363] and gets sixty to ninety minutes of moderate to high-intensity exercise daily. Do these behaviors raise a red flag for an eating disorder?

Clearly, the people in the NWCR are the anomalies. Just because your office-mate maintained her weight loss doesn't mean that the majority of people can. A few individuals can also touch their nose to their toes, but the majority of us will never achieve this, even if we commit to daily stretching.

Despite the overwhelming odds against any one person maintaining weight loss, the fact that some do allows us to believe that we could be them, perpetuating the belief that there is something wrong with us when we can't. Weight loss just may not be physiologically possible for many people, or at least not to the degree that we believe it is.

7. The "Thinner Is More Attractive" Myth

From an early age we are taught to despise fat. Our culture tells us that the size of our body defines our merits as a person and barrages us with images of ideal body shapes that we can never achieve. While this may have begun as a women's issue, it has been increasingly extended to include men. The emotional toll on all of us cannot be calculated. Few people are at peace in their bodies.

Every culture has its own standards of beauty, which change over the course of time. This is true of all traits that we consider beautiful, including our weight standards. Beauty standards reflect the political and economic interests of the times.

Historically, more often than not, a larger body was considered more desirable. It was a sign of beauty, health, opulence, sex appeal, and fertility. This current historical moment, during which flesh *isn't* appreciated, is a rare anomaly.

For example, historians have found numerous depictions of the Venus of Willendorf (dating back to 24,000-22,000 BCE), a stone female figure and a symbol of female beauty. She had a beautiful rounded stomach, big hips, and huge breasts. Artwork from the ancient Greeks and Romans also show beautiful large women, such as Aphrodite and Venus, both of whom would be considered fat by today's standards. In the seventeenth century, Peter Paul Rubens painted voluptuous women deemed beautiful in his time.

It wasn't until the 1830s that thinness first came into vogue in North America, though only for a relatively brief period of time. By the turn of the century, we had reverted to a larger ideal. Lillian Russell, the leading sex symbol during this time, weighed more than 200 pounds.

In the early 1900s, thin women were sold pills, creams, and potions to help them get fatter. False breasts, thighs, and hips that had natural dimples (which we now call cellulite) were also sold to help women project a more attractive look. Doctors advocated for more flesh, as a heavier body fought disease better. Insurance companies even screened out thinner applicants.

The 1920s and 1930s brought changes, and thinness was once again in vogue for a short period, though the ideal body size was much more substantial than the one currently accepted. This standard of perfection didn't last very long, however. By the 1940s, fashion magazines were again running articles on how *not* to be thin and larger models were again popular.

After World War II, the cultural climate shifted again rather suddenly. 1951 is often marked as the beginning of the war on fat, a war that has gained momentum over time. Currently, the average model is hardly a healthy role model: She is 5 feet 9½ inches tall, weighs 123 pounds, and often has too little body fat to menstruate.

To understand the implications of this history, consider standards of beauty other than weight. Other traits that are considered beautiful in women show similar variations across different cultures and in different time periods. For instance, in other parts of the world, the following are considered beautiful:

■ Decorative scars on the face
■ Stacked rings to elongate the neck
■ Jewels placed in holes drilled in the teeth
■ The maiming of women's feet to make them smaller

Even in the United States, standards of beauty vary. For example, some consider the following beautiful, although they aren't as universally agreed upon as weight standards:

■ Decorated faces (make-up)
■ Shaped eyebrows, curled eyelashes
■ Tattoos
■ Nose, tongue, nipple, and belly piercings
■ Shaved heads
■ Shaved armpit hair/leg hair

Notice that none of the traits in the above lists is natural. These are all ways that people manipulate their bodies in order to appear attractive and conform to cultural beauty standards. The point here is that what you and others find attractive is not objective. Some of these standards may seem unattractive or barbaric to you, but perhaps if you were raised in a different cultural environment you would feel differently. Similarly, people from other cultures may view your standards as unattractive or barbaric.

Why did these cultural standards evolve, and whose interests do they serve? Certainly not our own; our tacit acceptance of these standards is not in our best interest.

Consider conditions for women. Clearly, women's rights have advanced tremendously in recent times. We now have choices that our mothers and grandmothers couldn't even conceive of, such as reproductive options, higher education, and careers in most any trade, profession, or sport we could desire. Whether you exercise these options or instead prefer a more traditional role personally, the changing cultural landscape presents women with a greater sense of freedom and choice.

Despite these advances, and regardless of the choices we make, few women truly feel free. We share a feeling that we aren't good enough. We are ashamed of our physical appearance and ashamed that it matters so much to us.

I believe that there is a connection between women's increasing personal and professional power and our increasing disappointment in our physical selves. We are much worse off than women of previous generations regarding how we feel about ourselves physically, and I don't think this is an accident. Instead, I am concerned that we are in the midst of a backlash against women's advancement. This backlash is particularly insidious as it is being enacted psychically rather than politically. More so than ever before, our identity is premised upon our attractiveness (as opposed to men's identity, which is more firmly rooted in their accomplishments). We are no longer as limited by laws, but instead by our (and others') internalization of social beliefs about attractiveness and our failure to measure up.

This isn't a conspiracy enacted by men to keep women oppressed; all of us, male and female, participate in reinforcing these social beliefs and standards of beauty, and all of us are damaged by it. Though the damage to women is obvious, we're less apt to talk about how it also harms the "oppressor." Think of the loneliness of heterosexual men with their "trophy" wives. Choosing women based on their looks doesn't allow them true intimacy in relationships.

There are huge industries heavily invested in our acceptance of these cultural standards, and they have a big stake in convincing us to conform. The fashion, cosmetics, and diet industries survive by telling us that we are ugly and unacceptable as we are, but if we buy their products we can become beautiful. In other words, they get us to participate in our own oppression! And it seems as if advertisers have recently realized that they were so busy exploiting women's insecurities that they'd forgotten half the population. So now they're doing their best to make men feel equally horrible about themselves.

In fact, being a man these days seems, well, an awful lot like being a woman. For men, more than ever, looks count. Check out the magazines where modern-day Adonises sell everything from cars to cologne. Manly men used to be burly and soft, but now it's all about a pumped-up low-fat physique.

Men eye the washboard abdominals in the ads and think that maybe, with enough dieting and time in the gym, they too could trim the fat and get "buff." The average guy, of course, can no more shape his torso into the media image than the average gal can. But the fantasy is very captivating.

This turning of the tables is not without consequences. Men are catching up with women in body dissatisfaction, acquiring problems formerly associated with women: eating disorders, body obsessions, low physical self-esteem. In fact, Cornell researchers recently found that men and women are similarly dissatisfied with their weight (though women are more likely to want to lose weight and men have more mixed desires, including the desire for increased muscle definition).[364] This sure isn't what I have in mind when I advocate for gender equity!

There is nothing objectively attractive about thinness. Our cultural beauty standards are a reflection of political and economic interests. When you buy into them, you support commercial interests and the status quo and undermine the health and well-being of all of us as individuals. Chapter 8 helps you opt out.

8. The "You Can Trust the Experts" Myth

When solid scientific evidence is considered, the ideas in this book are not particularly heretical, nor even new. Why do they differ so much from what is more commonly promoted by health "experts"? Why is it that these views have not found their way into the beliefs of the public or even to a significant portion of the scientific community? Why are so many intelligent and compassionate people invested in reifying an old paradigm that not only doesn't work, but exacerbates people's difficulty with weight regulation and wreaks havoc with their self-esteem?

I suspect it is because our views have been shaped by our own personal experiences of managing our weight within a cultural context marked by an obsession with thinness and a belief that success can be achieved through that thinness. No individual can escape the influence of culture. Scientists and health care practitioners are subject to the same bias against fat and are exposed to the same unrealistic images of bodies and relentless pressure to "purchase beauty" that we all experience in our culture. They are also subject to intense pressure from people desperate for solutions and may feel a strong need to cling to something, even if it's baseless, rather than acknowledge that they just don't have an answer.

The weight-loss industry, of course, has a multibillion-dollar interest in promoting the view that "overweight" is dangerous and unattractive and that weight can be controlled by dietary manipulation, drugs, or other consciously applied techniques, and we can't ignore the tremendous influence they have had in fueling our cultural hysteria about weight. Body-conscious Americans spent over $58 billion last year to lose weight, and that number is expected to continue to balloon.[365]

We wouldn't be spending that kind of money if we thought we had such limited ability to lose weight. Clearly, it pays for the weight-loss industry to have us believe that losing weight is, with a little help from them, not all that hard. Weight-loss advertisements give the impression that losing fat and keeping it off is easy. The people in these ads are having fun and look great, especially compared to the way they used to look before they signed up for the program, or ordered the "natural" herbal weight-loss pills, or bought the diet book.

It also pays for the weight-loss industry to have us believe that weight has negative health consequences, as is evident from the enormous resources that the pharmaceutical industry has put behind research that exaggerates the health risks associated with weight. Knoll Pharmaceuticals, for example, offers funding to those who "advance the understanding of obesity as a major health problem,"[285] as they explicitly state in a call for proposals. After mobilizing concern about obesity, they can profit by selling the cure.

Exaggerated claims regarding the dangers of obesity are in fact at the cornerstone of efforts to get Food and Drug Administration approval for long-term use of weight-loss drugs known to be hazardous. When defending themselves against lawsuits, the pharmaceutical companies justify sales with the argument that obesity is so dangerous that it overshadows the dangers of their drugs.

Exaggeration of obesity's dangers similarly benefits physicians, for whom there is a tremendous market in promoting various weight-loss methods, particularly surgery. It mobilizes patients to use their services—and helps secure insurance coverage. Health practitioners are among the most insidious players in this fat-hating drama, as they have legitimized the cultural mandate for thinness by reframing it as a health concern. Bariatric surgery poses a particularly egregious example. Ironically, as Eric Oliver astutely points out, bariatric surgeons actually *create* disease, by damaging a healthy organ, and justify this practice by asserting an imaginary disease, obesity.[366]

The government has played a particularly potent role in propagating this cultural hysteria. It was unlikely a mere coincidence that the article[234] wrongly attributing 400,000 deaths to overweight and obesity appeared in *JAMA* just days before Julie Gerberding, the director of the CDC, was to appear before Congress to request increased funding. The report was prepared not by the CDC's top experts on the subject but by Gerberding herself, who holds no particular expertise in obesity, and other researchers attached to her office. Gerberding, of course, cited the paper in her testimony.

The *Wall Street Journal* and *Science* magazine both noted that anonymous sources within the CDC were concerned that the report had been influenced by political pressure to make the results consistent with CDC's public health policy.[367] The report was so blatantly problematic that even conventional obesity researchers questioned its methodology and conclusions, suggesting that a political agenda to exaggerate the risk of obesity had trumped scientific concerns. A host of reasons were expressed, among them that the authors added an arbitrary number of deaths from poor nutrition to the obesity category. The following *JAMA* issue featured several contentious letters. The criticism prompted an internal review and the CDC was eventually forced by a Freedom of Information Act request to post the results of this review on its Web site. The updated information was eventually published in *JAMA* and, as discussed earlier, reduced the estimate for excess deaths a whopping 94 percent.[235]

Lest people actually allow the data to inform practice, the CDC's next step was to issue a disclaimer to state health agencies stating that "despite the recent controversy in the media about how many deaths are related to obesity in the United States, the simple fact remains: obesity can be deadly." Apparently the CDC doesn't want the evidence to distract us from continuing to impose baseless policy.

Also problematic is that those who determine public policy and federal grant funding are almost always simultaneously on the payrolls of weight-loss and/or pharmaceutical companies, thus presenting a conflict of interest. Government panels favor economic interests over health interests whenever they identify obesity as a major public health threat, define obesity at low standards, promote unsuccessful treatments, or minimize the dangers of various treatments.

For instance, at least seven of the nine members on the National Institute of Health's (NIH) Obesity Task Force were directors of weight-loss clinics,[368] and most had multiple financial relationships with private industry.[369] Thanks to this task force, one magical night in June of 1998 twenty-nine million Americans went to bed with average figures and woke up fat. They woke up with a presumed increased risk of type 2 diabetes, hypertension, and atherosclerosis and a government prescription for weight loss. Of course, nobody gained a pound. The task force had simply lowered obesity standards,[370] a change which was obviously favorable for private industry.

The research presented in their report did not support the value of lowering the standards.[371] Indeed, the only relevant peer-reviewed research they cited in their report, a review of studies on the association between BMI and mortality,[372] suggested that *raising* the standards would be a more astute application of the science. The review didn't find a statistically significant relationship between BMI and mortality until BMIs in excess of 40 (yet they set the cutoff for overweight at 25 and for obesity at 30)!

The Politics of "Evidence-Based Science"

I was a PhD candidate at the time the BMI standards were lowered. My mentor was a member of the NIH Obesity Task Force. When I expressed my surprise at the standards being lowered, she encouraged me, as an academic exercise, to conduct a review and make recommendations as if I were sitting in her place on the task force.

A careful review confirmed my suspicions: There was significant evidence in support of *raising* the standards, not lowering them. I presented my review to my mentor, who laughed and congratulated me on my insightful analysis.

I asked the obvious question of why the NIH Obesity Task Force recommended lowering the standards in the absence of supporting data. I paraphrase her response: "We were pressured to make the standards conform to those already accepted by the World Health Organization."[373]

In other words, this decision was made for political reasons, not because it was supported by science or for the betterment of public health.

Trace the origins back further and it becomes even more disturbing. The World Health Organization report that helped to establish a BMI of 25 as the cutoff for overweight was predominately drafted by the International Obesity Task Force (IOTF).[374] On the surface, IOTF appears to be a scientific organization. However, probe a little and you find that IOTF receives much of its funding from Hoffman-La Roche (makers of the weight-loss drug Xenical) and Abbott Laboratories (makers of the weight-loss drug Meridia). Their primary mission is to lobby governments and advance an agenda that is consistent with the platform of the pharmaceutical industry. Indeed, many outsiders describe them as no more than a front group for the pharmaceutical industry.[366]

In other words, private industry is writing public health policy.

Over the years I've been privy to rumors of a lot of dirty secrets among obesity researchers. There are way too many stories circulating about research results being suppressed when they are unfavorable to industry, industry writing papers under the name of prominent academics, bogus numbers being reported by researchers and government agencies, "scientific organizations" that front for private industry. . . .

Knowing many of the players and the pressure many of us feel from our universities to make ourselves known and bring in grant money, and given my own personal experiences of being tempted by potential conflicts of interest, it doesn't take a leap of faith to believe those rumors are true. Indeed, evidence is accumulating, and many exposés have already been written.[263, 366, 375, 376, 377]

Examine the key players in the two major organizations for obesity researchers, The Obesity Society and the American Obesity Association (which recently folded), and you will not find a single officeholder who does not have some financial tie to a pharmaceutical or weight-loss company. Indeed, I cannot think of one obesity researcher, other than myself and the government researchers that are prohibited from these relationships, with a policy of refusing industry money.

Eric Oliver calls this a "health-industrial complex," built on a "symbiotic relationship between health researchers, government bureaucrats, and drug companies,"[366] and he and health writer Thomas Moore describe the interlocking relationships.[366, 378] Drug companies sponsor the research that defines health issues and fund the researchers who sit on government panels; government agencies rely on researchers to provide the data to support their funding requests; and drug companies rely on health advisories issued by government agencies to promote and justify their products. Everyone benefits from reinforcing the same (fearmongering) message.

While the very nature of these relationships is problematic and true corruption exists to some extent, I also believe that it is unlikely many of the people promoting the obesity myths are acting consciously to mislead us, and I am not suggesting all of those holding conflicts of interest are dishonest or part of a conspiracy. Indeed, I believe that most are well-intentioned. Rather, the myths about obesity are so much a part of our culture, and the penalty for questioning them so high, that assumptions are not even recognized, let alone challenged. Many obesity warmongerers are sincere in their belief that fat leads to death and disease. And for those concerned about Americans' health, the "obesity epidemic" is a convenient, attention-getting way to highlight problems with nutrition or activity habits.

Indeed, my concern is that obesity researchers are highly vulnerable to accepting cultural assumptions—even more so than the general public—because their status, reputation, and livelihood are in large part determined by how well they promote the diet and pharmaceutical industries. Career opportunities are limited if they choose not to participate, resulting in little incentive to question the status quo. The result is that cultural bias plays a role in every aspect of research, including our underlying assumptions, what research we choose to undertake, what gets published, and how we interpret and report scientific data.

Public/private conflicts of interest, combined with the extraordinary financial clout of the weight-loss industry, is not conducive to being open-minded about new ideas or making sure important research gets conducted or reported, or that the best information directs public policy and gets out to the general public.

Take-Away Message

Fearmongering about weight is worth billions to the health care system, government agencies, scientists, and the media. And it ties in seamlessly with cultural values. The result is that weight myths have become unquestioned assumptions, so strongly a part of our cultural landscape that we regard them as self-evident.

Yes, Americans have been gaining weight, though the degree to which this is true has been blown out of proportion. No doubt our weight gain is symptomatic of changing environmental conditions, and our eating and activity habits are part of those conditions. There is, however, little evidence to suggest that the symptom—weight—is a problem in and of itself. The epidemic exists only because we have defined it to exist. The epidemic will vanish as soon as we stop pathologizing weight and relegating people into baseless and arbitrary categories like overweight and obese. While I am not arguing that we encourage weight gain in order to improve health or that body weight is irrelevant to health, it is clear that the threat posed by our weight and the benefits of weight loss have been misinterpreted and exaggerated. At both extremes—high and low—body weight adversely affects health. But the vast majority of Americans fall closer to the middle of the body fat bell curve, where weight is little more than a benign marker of an individual's genetic predisposition to carry it.

I hope you're coming to the end of this chapter feeling a sense of relief. Being fat is not a death sentence, nor does it doom people—your family, friends, patients, or clients, or yourself—to a life of disability. Fat or thin, you don't need to feel anxious about your weight.

Encouraging weight loss as our first line of defense or attack is just bad science. Weight loss is not effective for prolonging life or managing many diseases. Furthermore, we don't have effective methods for maintenance of weight loss, and health may worsen as people lose and regain weight repeatedly. Ironically, the admonition to lose weight may actually have contributed to the very diseases it is prescribed to cure.

Though a heavy weight may be the result of imprudent lifestyle habits or underlying disease in some individuals, there are also many large people who eat sensibly, exercise regularly, and have excellent health readings—and many thin people who don't. Regardless, a low weight—or healthy lifestyle habits—shouldn't be a requisite for respect.

Size is a sloppy and unscientific way to judge someone's health or character, and the social and medical imperative for a thin body is not only misguided, it has caused much damage. *"Normal weight" is neither normal (most people exceed it) nor ideal in terms of health.* All that can be determined by judging people based on their weight is one's own level of prejudice.[379]

Let's switch our emphasis to encouraging health-promoting behaviors for all, and let the fat fall where it may. Everyone, fat and thin, can reduce their risk for health problems by making good lifestyle choices. It's time for a new peace movement: one that supports people in developing healthy lifestyle habits, regardless of their size. It's called Health at Every Size.

PART TWO
Health at Every Size

SEVEN

The Story Behind the Health at Every Size Program

B y now you understand that your body *wants* to be at its naturally healthy weight (chapter 1); that you can trust your hunger
drive and rejoice in the pleasure of eating (chapter 2); that certain lifestyle habits support you in maintaining the weight that is
right for you (chapters 3 and 4); that the food industry—even the
government—is working hard to undermine your efforts to eat
healthfully and maintain your natural weight (chapter 5); and that
much of what you've been taught about your weight just doesn't
hold, well, *weight* (chapter 6).

Right about now you've probably figured it out: You've been set
up. Your struggle with weight is an inevitable result of our modern
culture and lifestyle, not your own shortcomings or lack of
willpower.

But there's hope! There is an easy way to win the war against fat
and reclaim your pleasure in eating: Just give up. Yes, give up. Stop
fighting. Instead, turn to science. Specifically, the scientifically proven

Health at Every Size (HAES) program.[1, 2, 3] (The concept of HAES has a long history that predates my research. The term "HAES" is widely used and does not refer to my program exclusively.) Another investigative team has since conducted an additional HAES study which also demonstrates remarkably positive results.[380]

The rest of this book focuses on the program itself, providing step-by-step advice for incorporating all the information you've learned so far into actionable, realistic steps. A program guaranteed to help you enjoy your food again . . . *and* maintain a healthy weight.

The Evidence

I wish I could just give you a magic pill and tell you to take two a day with a full glass of water and you'd never have to worry about your weight or nutrition again. But you know as well as I that nothing is that easy.

Instead, I'm going to give you a set of guidelines to live by, tools that have stood the twin tests of both time and science.

First, the evidence. When I put together this program, I knew each component was based on solid science. And, as you can tell from the first six chapters, I'm big on science. What I didn't know, however, was how the whole thing would work in the real world, with real people. As a scientist, of course, I knew just how to find out. I set up an experiment.

I wanted to see not only if HAES worked on its own, but how it measured up to the gold standard that was currently recommended, i.e., dieting to lose weight.

To make sure my own bias didn't affect the results, I teamed up with one of the most well-respected diet researchers in the world, Judith S. Stern, RD, ScD. I'd known her for years—she was my PhD advisor when I started this research and had more than thirty-five years of experience and a very well-established reputation.

Her résumé still awes me. She's a distinguished professor in the departments of nutrition and internal medicine at University of California, Davis; has served as an invited member on prestigious government panels, including one that established criteria for the definition of obesity and overweight and another that set the criteria for judging weight-loss programs; has published several hundred research articles; and has received a long list of awards, including the Secretary's Honor Award, the most esteemed award the U.S. Department of Agriculture presents, in the category of "Improving the Nation's Nutrition and Health." She is also a member of the prestigious National Academy of Sciences' Institute of Medicine.

I teamed up with her not only for her expertise and the respect she receives in the field, but because I knew she believed strongly in dieting and weight loss and would supervise the study carefully to ensure fair testing of the conventional model. Together we analyzed the research that had already been conducted on dieting and chose what appeared to be the best diet program to compare to HAES.

I didn't stop with Dr. Stern. I also asked two top-notch obesity researchers from the United States Department of Agriculture (USDA) to collaborate and oversee the research, both of whom fell somewhere between Dr. Stern and me in their biases about weight. Nancy Keim, RD, PhD, is a research chemist with the USDA, and Marta Van Loan, PhD, a research physiologist. Both also have awesome résumés and are well published and extremely well respected in the field.

Not only were my three collaborators extremely knowledgeable, but they came with the added advantage of access to money and resources that would support our research. But in the final analysis, I must confess: I also chose the three of them because they are wonderful people who are great fun to work with.

Now I should acknowledge up front that Dr. Stern was hesitant about conducting this research. She worried that if we didn't encourage the women in our study to diet and lose weight, we might be harming them. In fact, she was so skeptical about the HAES program that she required that we test the women's progress after three months, including surveys, blood samples, and weight. If we saw either the weight-loss or HAES group getting *worse,* she said, we had to stop the study immediately. I agreed with her condition.

Money Matters

The weight-loss industry is a $59 billion industry, composed of a wide range of companies, from Weight Watchers and supplement makers, to pharmaceutical companies, food manufacturers, physicians, and publishers. When you read a study that shows the importance of weight loss to your health, I want you to do one thing: Ask who is funding it. Quite often, you'll find that the money for the study came from a company with a stake in the outcome. Why does this matter? Because statistics clearly show that when industry funds research, the published results are much more likely to show beneficial effects than research conducted without industry funding.[207]

I'm quite concerned about this conflict of interest, which is why I follow a strict policy of never accepting research money from private industry. Not that private industry would have been interested in funding this research anyway—I mean, there's no profit to be made if we show people getting healthier with lifestyle change, without worrying about weight loss, or if we show that weight isn't the be-all and end-all when it comes to health.

Consequently, I'm limited to public funding, which is a very small pool. Plus, as with anything else in life (and the government), the decision on who receives funding depends not just on the quality of the project, but on the politics involved in the topic. Given that Congress shares the general perception that Americans need to lose weight, that's where much of the nutrition money goes these days. Plus, many (all?) researchers who sit on the panels that review the grant requests are on industry's payroll themselves. In fact, some in my field jokingly refer to a group of researchers from the Universities of Colorado and Pittsburgh and Columbia University as the "obesity mafia," given their control over National Institutes of Health funding.

With my HAES study, I managed to wrangle a relatively small grant out of the NIH—about $100,000. My co-investigators generously dipped into other odds-and-ends funding to pull us through, and much of the time we spent on this project was voluntary—or least not funded with grant money.

I'd like to believe we got the grant because of the outstanding proposal. But I'm not that naïve. The reality, I think, is that I took my name off the proposal as the primary investigator and substituted Dr. Stern's, who is better connected to the mafiosi.

Time to Recruit

Now we were ready to recruit women to our study. We needed at least seventy non-smoking, Caucasian women between the ages of thirty and forty-five who wore at least a size 16. Why seventy? Because that's how many women were predicted to be required to ensure our results would be statistically significant. We also needed our participants to be similar in terms of gender and ethnicity and thought we'd have a better chance at recruitment if we chose Caucasians.

We put the word out in typical fashion, distributing press releases to newspapers, radio and TV stations; contacting local churches and community groups; and putting up flyers on campus and around the city of Davis, California.

At the same time, I started giving press interviews about the study. While we never explicitly promoted it as a weight-loss program—we left the description of HAES decidedly ambiguous—it seemed everyone assumed it *was* a weight-loss study. After all, what else would you do with large women in a health improvement study?

We were flooded with women begging to be admitted to the study. One after another, they told us their stories of endless attempts to lose weight, desperate to be enrolled in a scientific study at a respected university. When I told one forty-six-year-old woman that she couldn't participate because she was too old, she broke down in tears, telling me we were her last hope. Her physician, nutritionist, and social worker called me the next day to pressure me into bending the rules. (I still couldn't let her in!)

Eighty-two women who met the initial criteria attended an informational meeting, where we explained the program and answered questions. Every one signed the consent form.

We then weighed and measured them to ensure their size met the medical definition of obese (BMI greater than 30) but didn't surpass the arbitrary upper limit of a BMI of 45. The women also completed questionnaires about their health status.

When we checked identification, we were surprised to find that several women had lied about their age! There were other signs of these women's desperation: One participant was willing to undergo a two-hour commute each way to participate. Their stories of how their weight affected their lives pained me. One woman told me her boss was threatening to fire her from her job as a receptionist if she didn't lose weight. Another was about to lose her job in a fitness center, while one woman's husband was threatening her with divorce if she didn't lose weight.

I heard story after story about how painful it was to live in a large body. And yet every woman had tried numerous diet and exercise programs. By now, they felt beaten up by the process and were plagued by an overwhelming sense of failure.

The seventy-eight women who met our criteria were enrolled in the study, and a computer randomly assigned them to either the HAES group or the conventional diet program group.

Each group was then broken into four smaller sections of nine or ten women who met weekly for six months, providing individualized attention and small group support. During the second six months of the program, which we called the follow-up period, the groups met monthly.

The women in the diet group received conventional messages about dieting and attitudes toward their bodies. They learned to moderately restrict their fat and calorie intake, and were encouraged to monitor their diet with a food diary and to weigh themselves weekly. They were also encouraged to walk or participate in other exercise. They learned how to count fat grams, understand food labels, and shop for food. They were taught the benefits of exercise and behavioral strategies for success. They were also encouraged to lose the weight slowly.

The women in the HAES group received an early draft of this book and support in implementing the HAES program. Initial meetings focused on enhancing body acceptance and self-acceptance and on leading as full a life as possible, regardless of weight. The goal here was to first help the women disconnect their feelings of self-worth from their weight before we jumped into talking about food, activity, or other lifestyle choices.

An experienced registered dietician led the diet group while I led the HAES group. Each group gave us equally high marks in terms of enthusiasm, knowledge, and leadership ability, suggesting that the qualities of the group leader didn't affect the research results.

The Final Results

And the results? (Drum roll please. . . .)

The HAES program won hands down, showing phenomenally better results than the conventional diet. Among the many great outcomes, these women no longer struggled with food issues. They'd moved from dieting (restrained eating) to intuitive eating (unrestrained eating), free to eat what they wanted, when they wanted.

The dieters? They remained restrained eaters. Which, of course, is just what diets teach us to do.

But what about the health effects?

The dieters didn't fare very well. Although they showed some initial weight loss and health improvements, they didn't sustain those health benefits—or the weight loss. Yup, back to the same size. A year of deprivation and watching themselves for nothing.

Unlike the dieters, however, the HAES women were flying high. They showed significant declines in levels of so-called "bad" LDL cholesterol and blood pressure. They almost quadrupled the amount of energy they spent being active and told us they felt more vital and enjoyed their bodies more.

Our HAES participants also showed noteworthy improvements in their body image and self-esteem. Here's what some HAES partici-pants told us:

> *Food sure tastes good now! I remember before I started the program: Thinking about what to eat terrified me and was always on my mind. Now it's simple and fun.*

Every morning I used to get on the scale. Whether I was up or down, it didn't matter—the number always told me I wasn't good enough. While in the program, I took the advice to change my scale, putting affirmations where the numbers once were. Now, the scale tells me I'm "perfect," "sexy," or "looking good!" And seeing that actually helps me eat better!

Who would have thought that I'd ever have broccoli cravings? And chocolate tastes better than ever now that I eat it guilt-free!

I never thought I'd ever enjoy exercising. But now a group of us meet at the basketball courts every Thursday night. Sure, it's probably more socializing and laughing than playing basketball, but I look forward to it every time. And when I come home, I sure am tired.

I use to blame the fact that I had a four-year-old on my lack of time to exercise. But now the two of us blast the music and dance wildly—I don't know which of us enjoys it more!

There's a bathroom just a few doors down from my office. But now I make it a practice to take the stairs to a bathroom a few flights away. I actually look forward to the time walking there—my time—and I always come back to work feeling more energized. Sure it takes a few more minutes, but I'm also sure I more than make up for it in increased productivity.

My boss and I have walking meetings now. It's so much more fun than hanging out in our offices. And I feel like I know her so much better now. It's as if doing something together creates intimacy.

I went for a checkup recently and got the typical weight-loss lecture. When I interrupted to tell my doctor how proud I was of my glucose and LDL improving, he said,

"All well and good, but what are we going to do about your weight?" "We're going to fire you, Doc, that's what we're going to do!" I can't believe how freeing it felt to say that!

Sadly, all these variables that improved in the HAES group (blood pressure, LDL, activity level, depression . . .) either stayed the same or worsened in the dieting group.

Even more important: Almost half the dieters dropped out of the study (compared to less than 8 percent of the HAES women)—proof again that no one wants to stay on a diet.

And here's the final nail in the dieting coffin: The dieters' self-esteem plummeted while the HAES women grew more empowered. It didn't surprise me: Happier, healthier people feel more empowered and make better choices.

We could see this coming. At the midpoint of the intervention, in response to the statement "The program has helped me feel better about myself," 93 percent of the HAES group indicated "agree" or "strongly agree" compared with only 51 percent of the diet group.

The Weight-Loss Disclaimer

I can hear you now: *But did the HAES women lose weight?* The answer is no—at least not enough to be considered scientifically significant. But neither did the dieting women. Well, they did at first, but then they gained it all back. Which makes them less well off in the long run than if they'd never lost the weight in the first place! Plus, of course, these women's existing feelings of failure and self-blame simply got worse.

But, you're probably thinking, *why bother if the HAES group didn't lose weight?* Because what's really important here, as I've tried to show you throughout this book, isn't some nebulous number on the scale; it's coming to the same conclusions the HAES women arrived at: that weight loss just isn't as important as they thought.

These women discovered that their focus on weight loss had hidden their real quest: a desire to feel better about themselves, to have more vitality and good health, to feel attractive *for themselves,* not for anyone else. Once they dropped the weight-loss focus, that's exactly what they got.

I'm sure it's crossed your mind: If the women were eating better and exercising more, shouldn't they have lost weight? Isn't this the "magic formula" for weight loss? If you still think that, go back and reread chapter 1. Our bodies are invested in maintaining fat (weight) for "lean" times. They are just not very good at giving up that weight.

So even though some people can do pretty well at short-term weight loss by reducing their calories relative to the amount of energy they spend, maintaining that weight loss over the long term is the tricky part. Ergo, the dismal statistics on long-term weight loss, even when people persist in their diet and exercise programs, as discussed earlier. Even the most optimistic scientists acknowledge that the majority of dieters will regain the weight. Remember leptin's double role? That it's much more aggressive at preventing weight loss, but fairly laid back as your weight ratchets up? That's why these women, for all their healthier habits, still didn't lose weight.

Of course, they *might* lose weight over the long term as the work they did in HAES becomes more ingrained in their lives. We just don't know, given the difficulty and expense of conducting that type of long-term study. In my opinion, what's most important is that these women got healthier and felt better about themselves and their lives.

If you want a weight-loss book, take this book back to the bookstore and get your money back. This isn't it. But if you want a plan that helps you feel better about yourself, physically and emotionally, improves your overall health, and provides you with the tools you need to maintain the weight that is right for your body, then you've come to the right place.

The next chapters will provide you with the Health at Every Size program.

Chapter 8 helps you enjoy your body.

You'll learn how to look in the mirror and love, really love, what you see there, hips, stomach, thighs, and all. You'll learn to accept yourself *as you are,* regardless of what your family, friends, or society say you *should be*. Just imagine how this kind of thinking can change your life.

Chapter 8 also gives you some survival tips to challenge the self-acceptance-damaging and setpoint-raising environment of our current culture that tries to undermine your efforts to live a healthy life without focusing on weight.

Chapter 9 helps you listen to your body, supporting you in eating for pleasure and nourishment.

At my son's birthday party, a mom asked me for advice that would help her seven-year-old son, a binge eater, develop healthier eating habits. Moments later, her son joined us.

"I want another piece of cake," he said. This request came shortly after eating a large meal and while he was still finishing up the remnants of his first piece.

"Why do you think you want it?" I asked.

He looked at me, surprised. "What do you mean? Because it tastes so good!"

"How did you feel when you ate the first piece?" I pushed.

Again, the confused stare. "I felt good, I felt happy."

"So what you *really* want is to feel happy?" I asked.

"Is this a trick? Are you trying to say I can't have another piece?"

"Nope, it's all yours if you want it," I said, cutting a piece to show I really meant it. "I'm just trying to help you figure out if you really want it."

He looked pensive for a moment and then said, in a rather surprised voice, "Maybe I'd rather play on the trampoline."

Fully engaged in play the rest of the afternoon, I'm not sure he thought about food.

It's that simple. When you take care of yourself and give yourself what you really want, the need to overeat dissolves.

In this chapter, you will learn how to recognize your eating triggers. You'll understand why food doesn't fix feelings and explore the links between emotion, hunger, and eating as you learn how to recognize and short-circuit those connections. Once you learn how to take better care of yourself, you will lose interest in eating when you're not hungry.

When you're only eating when food appeals to you, you no longer have to try to control every bite that goes into your mouth.

Eating is simple. You eat what you want, and you get pleasure from satisfying yourself.

Chapter 10 helps you decide *what* to eat and *how* to live well.

You'll learn which habits are wholesome and how to become naturally drawn to these wholesome habits rather than consciously having to choose them and fight other desires. What if being vibrant and active was a core part of your identity and you didn't feel the burden of needing to "work out"?

Chapter 11 helps you change your tastes.

What if your mouth watered at the smell of roasting beets? If you craved an apple, fennel, and watercress salad drizzled with balsamic vinegar? This chapter uses the latest in "taste science" to show you how to retrain your taste buds and reinvent your eating patterns. For instance, did you know that your taste buds have a three-week lifespan? After three weeks of eating foods with less salt, you won't even notice that the high sodium of yore is missing.

Enjoy your journey into Health at Every Size.

EIGHT
Respect Yourself, Body and Soul

No matter how closely we resemble the ideal seen on television, in magazines and advertising, most of us—particularly women—feel shame about our bodies. We don't create this shame out of thin air: Our culture constantly sends us messages that who we are and how we look is definitely *not* okay.

Just think about how many times you've heard the following:

- "You have such a pretty face; if only you'd lose some weight."
- "It's your fault you're single. If you'd lose weight, others would notice you."
- "Lose weight, girl! Don't you have any self-respect?"
- "If you really loved me, you'd lose weight."

People think they're being kind when they tell you, "It's what's on the inside that matters." The unspoken assumption, of course, is that your outside is unappealing—which is really an insult, thinly veiled as support.

We also heap the shame on ourselves. One participant in our study encouraged her family to snort like a pig every time she moved her fork to her mouth. She thought the shame and disgust it inspired would help her stay on her diet. The result? She exhibited tremendous self-control during family meals, but the binge during cleanup more than offset the saved calories . . . and she dreaded family meals.

Even if you'd never go to such extremes, and regardless of your weight, you might still feel like a "pig" inside, certain that neither you nor anyone else can like you until you're thin enough to measure up to cultural standards. That's because our culture accepts dieting and body hatred as normal. We unconsciously absorb these disturbed messages. So instead of uncovering and confronting our disturbed attitudes about our bodies or food, we focus on trying to change our weight. Our unsuccessful efforts at losing weight or maintaining weight loss just reinforce our feelings of personal failure and disgust.

To break out of this cycle and heal, you need to recognize the value of your body and understand that you—and only you—own it and live in it. This chapter provides you with the tools you need, enabling you to reclaim your body and your sense of self no matter what size jeans you wear. Most importantly, it will help you develop compassion for your body, enabling you to trust yourself with food and make better, more enjoyable choices.

Shame Backfires

If you're hesitant about reading this chapter, you're not alone. Many people are concerned that if they accept their bodies they may become complacent and remain "stuck" forever with a body they've grown to loathe. They believe that hating their body is an essential motivation for change, so they resist letting go of that self-hatred.

These fears are not only unfounded, but also stand in the way of your ability to make changes. Change comes from valuing and caring about yourself enough to want to improve your life. By first learning to have a positive relationship with your body, even if that body is not "perfect," you strengthen your ability to make change.

Think about it. When you feel better about yourself, you make better choices, whether it's how you eat, how often you exercise, if you'll quit smoking, start walking, etc. But when you're down on yourself and your body, you're much more likely to act self-destructively. If you exercise as "punishment" for weighing too much, how can you learn to enjoy being active? If you eat salads only as a way to change the body you hate, how will you enjoy the wonderful tastes of fresh vegetables?

Besides, if hating one's body effectively motivated change, do you really think there would be many heavy people in the world?

Accepting yourself as you are today doesn't mean giving up. It means learning to live in the present with the body you have. It means facing and acknowledging reality.

Change the Question

It's way too easy to believe that a thin body will right everything wrong in your world. It won't. Moving toward increased self-acceptance and taking power away from your weight will do much more to improve your life.

Think about what you have believed you will gain from being thinner. Fill in the blank with your fantasies: When I'm thin, _____.

These were some responses from the research participants:

- When I'm thin, I'll be more attractive to others.
- When I'm thin, someone special will love me.
- When I'm thin, I'll have a sex drive.
- When I'm thin, my sex life will get hot.
- When I'm thin, I'll get the job I've always wanted.
- When I'm thin, my dad will be proud to be seen with me.
- When I'm thin, I'll be more outgoing and charming, have more friends.
- When I'm thin, I can go to my high school reunion and show them how successful I've become.
- When I'm thin, I'll order what I *really* want at a restaurant.
- When I'm thin, I won't have diabetes.
- When I'm thin, I won't feel guilty about having diabetes.
- When I'm thin, I'll be more athletic.
- When I'm thin, I'll be more adventurous.
- When I'm thin, I'll be a rock star.

Once you consider the extent of the magical thinking that tends to be tied in to the fantasy of thinness, you can understand how threatening it is to consider the idea that you may never get the thin body you crave. It means that you never get to become the person you want to be. Wow! No wonder it's so painful to let go of the drive to lose weight! Accepting your body is not just about physicality, it's about accepting *who you are*, not continuing to wait until you become the person you imagine being.

The truth is, fat or thin, you may never be a rock star. You may never get the job you want or feel your father's pride. You may never get the attention you want from someone unwilling to give it. It's not because of your weight . . . it's because you're you and others are who they are. When you're invested in your thin fantasies, you avoid the opportunity to face who you really are and to try to become who you really want to be. It's the hope that your life will automatically improve when you're thin that stops you from taking steps to improve your life right now.

Your anger gets directed at yourself for not fitting in, as opposed to a prejudicial culture that values certain bodies over others. After all, thinner people often *do* get better treatment and more respect in this culture. But rather than directing the brunt of our anger where it belongs, many of us feel ashamed of ourselves. Instead of trying to erase the stigma, we try to fight the fat. Think about it: Would you encourage people who face prejudice due to their dark skin to try to lighten their skin? Or would you support them in appreciating this aspect of themselves and fighting the prejudice?

If there is one message to take away from this book, it's this: Start living life fully now, in your present body, because waiting until you lose weight is a big old waste of time. Your fantasies are available to you, right now. The thin person inside you can come out, though he or she may just reside in a fat body. As you become more legitimately accepting of yourself, you'll find that you will make better choices that support a healthy body. Others will react differently to you as you hold yourself with more pride, and even more so as others do the same.

It's a big leap of faith to move on from the "when I'm thin" fantasies. But when you change the question to reflect what you're really looking for, your fantasies become more achievable.

Instead of asking "How can I get thin?" ask yourself, "What can I do to [fill in the blanks with your response, such as . . . be happier, get others' respect and attention]?" Go after those directly, instead of believing you need to first lose weight. Everyone has a right to respect and happiness in their life, regardless of what they weigh. Trying to achieve them through weight loss provides a hollow and tenuous victory, not the core satisfaction that you are really seeking.

As you learned in earlier chapters, your weight is not necessarily in your control. The way you live your life *is*.

What Are Your Myths?

In earlier chapters, you learned to identify the "obesity myths" so prevalent in our culture. Myths that say you must lose weight if you want to be healthy, and losing weight is just a matter of control and discipline.

Learning the truth about these myths will help destroy the power they have over you now. That's why the first half of this book is so important. In fact, you might want to go back and reread the early chapters. Remember learning in chapter 3 that diets don't work? The message in chapter 6 was that you can be healthy even if your weight is still in the "overweight" or "obese" range? That biology, not discipline, controls our weight?

Start by acknowledging the cultural and societal voices you've unconsciously absorbed and believed throughout your life. These are the voices that say things like:

■ Fat people are lazy.
■ Fat people have no self-control.
■ Thin is best.
■ How you look is what's most important.
■ No one will love you if you're fat.

Now take this quiz to learn how much you've internalized these hurtful cultural messages.

Answer each question with either "never," "occasionally," "regularly," or "often."

How often do you . . .

1. Talk negatively about your own weight?
2. Choose clothes based on your perception of whether or not they make you look fat?
3. Assume that someone wants to lose weight?
4. Assume that someone should lose weight?
5. Make negative comments about someone else's weight?
6. Encourage someone to lose weight?
7. Admire someone for having lost weight?
8. Admire someone's ability to control his or her eating?
9. Admire someone for burning calories through exercise?
10. Assume someone is doing well because he or she lost weight?
11. Admire someone's slenderness?
12. Assume that being fat is bad?
13. Disapprove of someone because of what he or she weighs?
14. Make comments to a heavy person about losing weight?
15. Smile or laugh at fat jokes?
16. Compliment a fat person on his or her appearance?
17. Compliment a fat person on his or her personality traits?
18. Actively oppose anti-fat comments?
19. Challenge someone who conveys a myth about body fat?

Questions 1 to 15 are cultural messages that are harmful, never helpful, while questions 16 to 19 show support for living proud, regardless of appearance.

How did you do? Don't blame yourself if you found you've internalized and transmitted these negative cultural myths. They're hard to avoid.

Instead, use this exercise to become more aware of them within your own thinking. Reason through them so you're clear on why they're harmful. Use the information in the first part of the book to counter those voices in your head and other people's arguments and hurtful comments about weight, diet, and appearance, even if those "other people" are just an article in a magazine or another anorexic actress on TV.

Next, consider how you can respond differently when you hear these hurtful messages. For instance, if those negative voices in your head and in your life insist "You'd look so much better *if you'd only lose weight*," try one of the following snappy responses:[381]

- Oh, no. A heart as loving as mine wouldn't fit in a diminutive body!
- Heaven forbid! There's not enough of me to go around as it is!
- Bite your tongue! A personality this huge would starve in anything smaller.
- Why would I want to lose weight, when I'm so damn gorgeous right now?

Or my personal favorite:

- And make less of me to love?

Practice saying the ones you like—or develop your own responses. Then the next time you hear that demeaning comment, whether it's inside your head or from your best friend, you'll have the perfect answer.

If it feels too intimidating to challenge hurtful comments, try arming yourself with written information you can pass on. The HAES Manifesto in the appendix, for example, is a great tool to help you challenge weight myths. So is the How You Can Best Support Me in Good Health letter, also in the appendix, which my clients find helpful for getting families and friends off their backs.

Shape Your Own Values Around Weight

Since our culture has such a strong voice in defining thin as the only acceptable body shape and size, it's difficult to appreciate your own size if you don't create your own value system separate from society's. Until you do this, you will never learn to accept yourself.

Creating your own values around appearance means deciding for yourself what's important to you and what beauty looks like *to you*. It also means being able to separate your own needs from social expectations. Compare that to how most people behave these days: determining their self-worth based on how well they meet society's expectations.

Those Dreaded Doctor Visits

Many large people recount horror stories of physician visits. Indeed, health care practitioners are among the worst offenders of weight bias,[382] and surveys show that most heavy people have felt shamed by their physicians. The result? Many larger people delay or avoid medical care.

Don't. People deserve the same treatment, regardless of size. You do not deserve to be flippantly told that your problems are due to your weight or will be solved if you only lose weight. You have the right to competent, unprejudiced, and sensitive care.

To help ensure that your visit doesn't end with a weight-loss lecture, ask your friends for referrals or interview prospective health care practitioners about their attitudes toward weight before scheduling an appointment. You can also write a letter to the prospective doctor, introducing yourself and explaining your needs so you can learn up front whether or not you'll get the care you want. Or supply your physician with the cover letter provided in the appendix, along with the HAES Manifesto.

And remember, you're in charge of your body and health. If you don't see the relevance of stepping on a scale in your physician's office, you have the right to skip it! Or hop on backward if you feel the information is valuable to your physician, but may just trigger bad stuff for you. While it may feel scary to stand up to your health care practitioner, when you're armed with the knowledge that your weight shouldn't change the way your doctor treats you, it's much easier to assert yourself.

Claim your independence from "them." You know who "they" are . . . they're the people who dictate what we wear ("*they* say capris are in style this season"), what we eat ("*they* say that soy milk is best"), what we listen to ("*they* say this is a great band").

Pay attention to how *you* feel about things, whether it's what you wear, eat, or say.

Here's an example. Before she started the Health at Every Size program, Sarah associated ice cream with weight gain and ill health—the voices of the "fat police" that she had internalized. Though she loved the taste of ice cream, it was difficult to have a healthy attitude toward eating it and to fully enjoy it. After the HAES program, Sarah noted that those voices had disappeared. She could hear her own inner messages of satisfaction. She found she could naturally stop eating ice cream after a moderate amount, which was in sharp contrast to her pre-HAES days when ice cream meant guilt and no amount ever felt satisfying.

So in claiming your independence, you need to first understand what's important to *you*. Determining what's right for you is challenging, given the strength of cultural attitudes and our concern with others' judgment. So give yourself a break when you feel comparisons coming on or a nagging sense of inadequacy. Deep inside your psyche, you know that *you're* the only one who can determine if you're okay. Remind yourself whenever necessary.

Surviving in a Social World

It is hard to accept your body and new lifestyle habits when you are constantly bombarded with messages that you need to change. You will always be surrounded by people who are dieting and obsessed with their weight and by people—ostensibly with your best interest in mind—who encourage you to do the same. It is a sad fact of life that women often bond over commiserating about their flawed bodies or failed diets. To stop participating in this ritual may require large and difficult changes in your social relationships.

How do you confront these cultural attitudes that might otherwise undermine your journey? No one should have to hurt and to rally their defenses against a hostile world, yet we all do. The most potent response is to fortify your own defenses. The more you cultivate your internal resources, the more you recognize your beauty and your value—and the higher your self-esteem—the less others can infiltrate your world.

Next, recognize that you didn't get to your openness to kicking the diet habit and becoming more accepting of your body weight—if you are even there now—overnight. It probably took a long time for you to be open to reading this book, to accepting the futility of dieting, and to knowing there is a better alternative, and you yourself may be somewhere along that journey, still not totally convinced. We can't expect others to be magically transported there. It takes time for anyone to make this journey, and we need to be patient with others' process as well.

Everyone has received the same false messages about dieting and weight that we have, and it's not surprising that others want to prescribe weight loss and their pet diet—and that many are doing so because they sincerely want to help.

Acknowledging that drive to help is the best place to begin. Your friends and family—your doctor—probably don't want to hurt you and are not likely to be aware of the pain they are causing. Once they become aware of the destructiveness of their comments or advice, they may be willing to act differently. Let them know that you understand that they care and want to support you. Then teach them how they can best accomplish that.

What's clear from the research is that social support is extremely helpful. Friends and family keep us afloat. If they give you a hard time, your process will be that much more difficult. But if you can bring them along, all of you are likely to benefit greatly.

Painful as it may be, your friends and family may not come around to support you. You do not have the power to change someone's mind or to make people see the world on your terms. There may not be the perfect argument that will catalyze open-mindedness. All you can do is present your truth. And then you can make choices about whom you want to surround yourself with. You are worthy of love. There are people who will enjoy you as you are, who will love and support you, even if you haven't met them yet. Make it a priority to find them.

Understand Your Internal Motivation

In exploring your feelings about weight and appearance vis-à-vis society's messages, I want you to ask yourself a question: Do you *want* to be fat? Some large people unconsciously do. When I first present this idea, most people think I'm crazy. No one can even remotely consider that they might prefer to be fat in this fat-phobic culture. But suspend your disbelief for a moment as you try the following exercise:

Picture yourself at a party at your current weight. Pay attention to your clothes, how you feel in your body, how you interact with others. Now replay the party, this time visualizing yourself at what you view as your "ideal weight."

When I asked my study participants to do this, the results were surprising. Even though they are the same person in each scenario, they report that their weight played a dramatic role in how they felt and the quality of their participation and interaction with others. Many reported that their fat afforded them some "protection"—it allowed them to recede into the background and hide. It helped them avoid being marketed, judged, viewed as a sexual object or in competition with others.

It's not surprising that so many of us feel this ambivalence about our body size, that we revile ourselves for being fat, but we value the protection it affords. This experience derives from our social context. For some of us (certainly not all), overeating and getting fat is an unconscious rebellion against the social expectations placed on us.

Listen to what my study participants found.

Several women said they felt that while others at the party were judging the other women there, their fat enabled them to escape the pressure of evaluation based on appearance. It was as if their fat was saying, "Take me for who I am, not for who I am supposed to be." The result? Relief that they weren't being "checked out" by others.

Several women in my study connected their weight gain to motherhood. Once they became mothers, it meant that everyone else's needs came first. So they learned to take care of others, but not to acknowledge or make space for their own needs. They viewed their fat as a physical representation of their role as nurturers and caretakers and a sign they had abdicated their role as sexual beings, which they felt was an important part of being mothers.

The benefit of this exercise wasn't limited to women. When I asked a man I was counseling to try this exercise, he recalled being sexually molested as a child. His weight gain began soon after. It was as if he were trying to make himself unappealing so his abuser wouldn't approach him anymore. He acknowledged that his current weight still provided the same protection; as long as he's "overweight," others are less likely to pay attention to him. When a woman flirted with him at work, it made him very uncomfortable and he started to binge.

Another client described his fat as allowing him to look (and be) substantial. It's as if by taking up more space, he could be noticed and taken more seriously.

If you recognize yourself in any of these stories, it's time you explored the benefits of being fat and the ways in which you rely on your fat to protect you. Otherwise, you may continue to sabotage yourself when it comes to developing healthier habits. If you feel stuck, it may be because you continue to address your weight as an eating/exercise problem you need to control, rather than understanding it as a protective device you've created to help you get through your days.

But be careful before you jump to this conclusion. Some of us may assign it to ourselves because we've heard it over and over—you know, the "fat people are fat because they're scared of intimacy" stereotype. We generalize the legitimate problems of the minority onto the majority of larger people. Contrary to popular belief, however, studies indicate that larger people are not significantly different than thinner individuals with respect to sexual satisfaction.[383]

Try this exercise to help answer the "do-I-need-my-fat" question.

Picture yourself in various social settings—parties, family gatherings, sporting events, time alone with your partner, a first date, being sexual—at various weights. Focus on the *positive* elements of your weight and, in each scenario, ask yourself the following questions:

- What are the advantages of being fat?
- What parts of my personality does my fat express?

- How could I express these parts of myself if I were thinner?
- Are there any negatives to being my "ideal" size?
- Are there any fears associated with being my "ideal" size?
- What aspects of my personality do I currently suppress because of my size?
- How might I express these aspects if I weren't worried about my weight?

As you start to acknowledge the ways in which your weight benefits and protects you, you can move toward taking conscious responsibility of these benefits and protection, instead of allowing your fat to do it for you.

For instance, if this exercise shows that you use your fat as an excuse not to be sexually active, you need to examine your fears about sex. You then have the option to decide you don't want to be sexually active and own that choice instead of using your body as an excuse not to have sex. Or you can decide that you want to become more sexually active and move beyond the limits you've set for yourself.

Other steps to take:

- Brainstorm other solutions for every problem you think weight loss will solve. For instance, if you think losing weight is the only way you'll ever get a promotion, meet someone special, or be able to go to the beach, brainstorm other ways you can reach these goals.
- Wean yourself off the scale. Don't give some stupid machine the power to weigh your self-esteem.
- Acknowledge and appreciate what your body can do. Isn't it amazing that your legs can hold you up, that they can help you walk, run, or dance?
- Get rid of clothes that don't fit. No need to have the constant reminder of what *could* be, or what *used* to be; instead, you want to live in the here and now.

Live your life for *today*, not ten pounds from now!

Accept Yourself and the Rest Will Naturally Follow

Now you're ready to move to the next step: accepting yourself, regardless of how much you weigh, how you look, or what others say.

Start with this thought: Your body doesn't represent your core self. You are many more important things beyond your body: Perhaps you are compassionate, intelligent, articulate, and/or creative. Don't give your body more power than it deserves; it can't define you. Instead, cultivate a value system that puts appearance in its place and honors bodies for more than their packaging. Your body is valuable because it houses you.

Next, reflect back on the information from chapter 6 in which you learned about the culturally defined beauty standards that so many of us buy in to. Become more aware of the ways in which you have internalized these cultural messages (as with the exercises above) and accepted these standards of beauty.

Then recognize that you have a choice. You can choose your own standard of beauty, one that is realistic and respectful, or you can choose society's hurtful standards. Just remember: You only have one body and despite how well you live your life, it may never change. Can you afford to hate yourself for the rest of your life?

Bring this new thinking to how you view your body. Experts call this vision *kinesthesia*, which simply means how you sense and feel about your body. Kinesthesia is a product of your imagination, much more influenced by your self-esteem than by others' perception of you. Only you have the power to alter it.

Most people try to change their bodies to fit their minds' perception of what their bodies should look like, i.e., starving themselves to lose weight. Moving toward a healthy body image requires just the opposite: changing your mind to appreciate your actual body.

The following exercise will start you on the track to changing your body image.

To start, walk in a public place, perhaps along a busy street or in a store. Consider how you feel about your body *in this moment*. How are you holding yourself? Are your shoulders slumped or erect? Eyes down or level? Are you making eye contact with anyone? What expression is on your face? Are you smiling or frowning? Don't look at yourself in a mirror when you're doing this; just look at yourself in your mind.

Later, sit alone in a quiet place and reflect on these questions:

- What does my body language tell others?
- What kind of response do I expect from others based on my body language?

For instance, if you walk with slumped shoulders, head down, you're conveying the image that you are not worthy of approaching, that you don't even respect yourself, and that you're trying to hide from the rest of the world. But if you maintain a straight, proud posture, smile, and look people in the eye, you're sending the message that you are a person worth knowing, one who feels comfortable within his or her own skin.

Next, remind yourself that you are more than your body. Make a list of everything you like about yourself. Don't leave anything out. If you like the fact that you have wavy hair, write it down. Then list the successes you've achieved throughout your life. Make sure you're listing things *you* feel were successful, not things society deems successful. For instance, if you graduated from college in four years with no debt, write it down. If you landed a career you love, write it down. And don't forget the little successes. How about the time you painted the living room yourself or turned a weedy lot into a lush garden?

Now take that list and laminate it. Once a day, sit down with the list in front of you and make a new list: successes you had *today*, and new things you found to like about yourself *today*. Even if you only add one or two items a day, this exercise will remind you of your strengths and help you support yourself as you move toward self-acceptance.

Once you can believe in your strengths beyond your weight, try the walking-around part of this exercise. This time, walk like the person you really *are*—that wonderful, warm, creative person with talents that have nothing to do with weight. How are you holding yourself now?

Protect Against Negative Self-Talk

The corollary to this exercise is to protect yourself against negative self-talk. Your brain picks up on what you think and imprints these thoughts into your memory. Eventually, they become self-fulfilling prophecies, which is why sports psychologists train athletes to envision themselves sinking a putt, crossing a finish line, or winning a meet. Seeing themselves succeed over and over in their minds strengthens the mental muscle to turn the vision into reality. The same is true of negative thoughts.

If you do have negative thoughts about yourself while you're making your list, or even throughout the day, envision yourself wrapping them up in tissue and tossing them into the trash to make room for more positive thoughts.

Reframe Your Thoughts

Another helpful strategy is to reframe your negative thoughts so you can view your life in new terms. For instance, if one of your negative thoughts is "I hate exercise," try reframing that thought. Instead of thinking about your forty-five-minute walk as exercise, think about it as a gift you're giving your body so it can become and remain healthy, and so you can continue to live an independent life free of pain. Don't view it as a way to lose weight; that's playing right back into the negative thought mode.

Sometimes, however, no matter how much you talk to yourself and will yourself to change, you just can't make any progress. If this happens, don't give up. Just *pretend* that you've succeeded. Imagine that you have the qualities or the body that you desire. Live your life "as if" you are already where you one day hope to be. The more you do this, the more you realize that it is your attitude that limits you. If you act as if you are something, you learn that you can be that something. You can have the life you want in the body you have now. Some day it'll click for you and you'll realize it's not pretend anymore.

Love Your Scale!

Here's another reframing trick that proved to be very powerful for Health at Every Size study participants. Artist, author, and activist Marilyn Wann supplied us with a "Yay! Scale," on which she had replaced the numbers with compliments. Step on, let the dial spin, and be informed that you are "gorgeous." Try again tomorrow and you may just register as "hot." I promise you: A compliment will help you face the day with far more confidence than the numbers you find on a conventional scale!

Seize the Present

Instead of promising yourself new clothes when you lose weight, go out *now* and buy clothes you feel good wearing, no matter what you weigh. How about that vacation you keep promising yourself if you lose weight? Life is short! Call that travel agent *now*.

Taking these actions now allows you to live in the moment, in the body you have today, which is the kind of "presentness" many spiritual disciplines such as meditation, yoga, and martial arts espouse. You want to live in the present moment with full awareness, an essential component of truly inhabiting your body. This ability is particularly important to you right now. If you accept the present reality of your body, you can focus on how you feel and what you want for yourself, and move forward in your life.

Find Support: Internally *and* Externally

The next step in transforming your attitude and behavior around weight and appearance and becoming more self-accepting is to find support. This book is one form of support. Congratulate yourself for buying it! Now find other avenues of support by talking to others who are experiencing similar explorations, educating the people in your life so they can be supportive, and reading more on the subject. (Check the resource bibliography in the Appendix.)

Consider therapy or a support group with like-minded individuals (there are some great online support resources) or even a reading club. There is safety in numbers and comfort in connecting with others.

Open Your Mind to Others

Just as you want others to accept you, it's important that you accept others. While you may be discriminated against because of your body size, others are discriminated against based on their skin color, ethnic background, sexual orientation, or many other characteristics. Developing open-mindedness and empathy toward others who are discriminated against enables you to support and feel empathy for your own position. Being fat, like being Hispanic or a lesbian, is not bad; it's just different.

Our diversity is what makes the world such an exciting place! We can celebrate size diversity in much the same way we are learning to celebrate cultural diversity.

Change the Culture

Repeat after me: "My weight is not a problem. Society's problem about weight is the problem." The true heroes among us are not those who have lost weight. They are the people who move on with their lives, who live proud regardless of their weight.

The single most powerful act available to you is to own your body—to walk proud and let others see you enjoying your body. Self-love is a revolutionary act! A person who is content in his or her body—fat or thin—disempowers the industries that prey on us, telling us we are unacceptable and need their products to gain acceptance.

You can also take another step that will both help you to solidify your new identity and make the path easier for others. Challenge the myths about weight whenever you hear them. Join activist organizations committed to size acceptance. Write letters, make phone calls, SPEAK UP.

You *Can* Live Proud . . . in Whatever Body You Have

In today's world, it *is* difficult to live proud in any body, let alone to live large and proud. There simply isn't enough social support or role models for larger people. When the HAES participants started out, they were sure this was something they'd never be able to do. Although it is a difficult path for people of all sizes, the further we are from the cultural ideal, the more overt the cultural messages that undermine us.

I'm not going to tell you that your size is irrelevant in the world. Even as you move toward greater appreciation of your body, many of you will continue to struggle against cultural images, and friends and family who continue to tell you that "No, you *aren't* okay." Trust me here when I say it *can* be done. My research proves it. And you *can* teach those who love you to see you differently and to treat your body with respect. If you can't, you have to ask yourself if they're worth a leading role in your life.

Eventually, as more people learn to live large and proud and stop accepting the hatred and discrimination society has toward large people, the culture will shift to accommodate. Don't believe me? Consider the parallels with other social change movements. Would you encourage African-Americans to lighten their skin to become better accepted? Or gay men to date women so they'll "appear normal"? Of course not. I firmly believe that in the not-too-distant future, we won't expect heavier people to lose weight before we view them as part of the beautiful spectrum of human diversity.

I already see this occurring. Just look around you. People of all sizes are living full, happy, fulfilled lives, and are in satisfying relationships. With the help of this chapter, and this book, I know you can be one of them!

NINE
Take Care of
Your Hungers

Dieting. It's so seductive. It gives us hope, the promise of weight loss and happiness. But by now you know it doesn't deliver. So acknowledge that. Repeat after me: *Diets. Don't. Work.* Bottom line: Any plan that has you giving over control to someone else's idea of what you *should* eat is doomed to fail.

Every time I think of diets, I think of some women I once saw standing near a buffet filled with food. One looked at the display and said, "Oh, I really shouldn't." Another commiserated, saying, "It really is tempting, isn't it?" They all looked on sadly.

Who wants to feel like they constantly have to fight their desires? Yet that's exactly the message of diets: "Do what we tell you, not what you want." "Control yourself." Any system that emphasizes external processes to determine what to eat is fragile and ineffective and promotes discontent and periodic rebellion and binging.

The good news is that you don't need a diet to achieve happiness, health, or whatever else underlies your quest for weight loss. Just go after them directly!

There's more good news: You are innately capable of making satisfying food choices that improve your health and take you to a healthy weight, without following any diet. Trust yourself and you will find that you are far more effective at managing your weight than any diet can be.

Yet more good news: Indulging your desires will actually *help* you achieve and maintain a healthy weight. Why? Because you already have everything you need inside you directing you to make good food choices. I know that's a difficult concept to accept, given the years you've spent hearing how inadequate you are because of your weight and that you need to subscribe to this or that theory or diet plan to "save" you.

No one profits from internal trust, except of course the individual. Perhaps that's why it's such an unfamiliar concept.

But now you're ready to take a leap of faith and trust yourself. Trust that your body knows what it wants and will guide you to eat what's right for you. Now you understand that no one else but *you* can provide this knowledge. Your body doesn't know the diet language of good or bad: It just knows what it wants and needs in the moment. The less such knowledge is mediated by our culture, the better off you are.

We can all resist a piece of chocolate cake or a slice of meat-lover's pizza on occasion, just as we resist buying a surround sound home theater system when we've just lost a job. It's called willpower and control. But it's a short-term answer to a long-term issue. Instead of closing your eyes and repeating to yourself, "I won't eat that ice cream; I won't eat that ice cream," this chapter teaches you to hear a different message from your body: "As good as I know that pizza tastes, it's just not appealing to me right now. I'm not hungry."

You'll not only learn how that inner voice works, but how to listen to it. When you learn how to listen, you can determine what you really want—whether it's food or something else. And as you learn how to better take care of those non-physical needs, you become less interested in eating when you're not hungry. If you're only eating when food appeals to you, you no longer have to try to control every bite that goes into your mouth.

Guideline 1: Eat Delicious Food

Hard to believe this is part of the prescription for maintaining a healthy weight, isn't it? But it's the key to making this work. Sensual pleasure is our biological reward for taking care of ourselves.

When you eat what you want and allow yourself to truly experience the pleasure, you feel satisfaction and contentment, which allows you to stop eating when you feel full. I'm not just saying this to make you feel good; numerous studies support this: Eating pleasurable food when you have a physical drive to eat won't trigger consistent overeating *in intuitive eaters*. Also, if you are consumed with guilt, you don't enjoy (or even experience) the food.

Unfortunately, however, the opposite is true for people with a dieting mentality. If you avoid eating food you truly desire, you'll often wind up eating more in a never-ending quest for satisfaction.[384] The next time you want those French fries, go for it! Eat them attentively and notice if they satisfy you. That is much better than substituting a baked potato, which typically results in an ongoing grazing binge in search of satisfaction. Commit to choosing food you love.

Concerned that your tastes may not be conducive to good health—or to choosing foods that register on your internal weight meter? Not to worry. Future chapters help you identify—and love—the foods that nurture you best.

Guideline 2: Pay Attention When You Eat

In a very interesting study, researchers monitored the digestive processes of twenty-four healthy college students while they ate.[385] They monitored them while eating before a film and then when they ate during a film. When they ate while watching the movie, activity in their digestive tract was reduced and their digestion was less effective overall.

This result wasn't too surprising. Research consistently finds that as much as 30 to 40 percent of your total physical response to a meal occurs during the "cephalic phase of digestion," which is just a fancy term for the time you spend seeing, smelling, and tasting your meal.[386] This process initiates a wide range of digestive activities, including releasing saliva and digestive enzymes, sending blood to the digestive organs, and contracting the stomach and intestinal muscles.

But as the above study shows, if you're not paying attention to the food itself, this process doesn't work as well. You don't metabolize your food nearly as effectively and your body doesn't get all the nutrients it needs, nor does it get the full range of chemical messages it needs to trigger stop-eating cues. You're still getting the calories, however.

Here's another study to ponder if you're not convinced of the value of attentiveness. Study participants first consumed a mineral drink under relaxing conditions.[387] They completely absorbed two of those minerals, sodium and chloride. The same individuals were then exposed to stressful conditions—two people simultaneously talking to them, one in each ear—while consuming the drink. Their bodies *completely* shut down to assimilating the minerals. From 100 percent absorption to 0 percent! The simple act of inattention dramatically altered their ability to assimilate those nutrients.

How often do you eat while watching television, driving, reading, etc.? How are you ever going to feel satiety sensations or get the full range of nutrients contained in your food, if you're chomping on that hamburger while negotiating a left turn in your car?

So from now on, aim to be fully present for your meals. Eat with awareness. Turn off the TV, put away the newspaper, put on some soft music, set a nice table, and sit down to enjoy the food—even if it's just a peanut butter and jelly sandwich!

Guideline 3: Satisfy Your Hunger

Even though you can't always get your hands on a just-picked piece of fruit, you can still learn to savor every bite. Start by eating when you're hungry—not when you *think* you should eat, or when you're eating to assuage some uncomfortable feeling. When you're hungry, your senses are sharper, primed for the smells, taste, and feel of good food.[388]

Try this exercise. Eat a piece of chocolate just after dinner. Write down how it tastes, what you feel, and all the related sensations that you're aware of. Now eat a piece of chocolate *before* dinner. Take the same notes. Which piece of chocolate tasted richer?

Your appreciation of tasty food doesn't just support you in eating when you're hungry; it can also support you in moderating amounts. Try another exercise, a favorite of the HAES study participants. This time get a chocolate truffle—a super-rich dark chocolate truffle. Take a small nibble. Hold the piece of chocolate in your mouth and close your eyes as you experience the sweet/bitter taste melting on your tongue. When that small piece is entirely gone, take another bite, and another, eating slowly and staying attentive to the experience.

HAES group participants observed that after the first few bites, the truffle was progressively less delicious. It still tasted good, just not quite as good. In scientific jargon, they experienced negative alliesthesia[389]: your taste buds toning down on repeated exposure, nature's way of prompting you to eat less once your calorie needs are met.

In other words, if you commit to eating foods when they're maximally pleasurable, you feel satisfied with a lot less. (You also have more stable moods and healthier blood sugar regulation.)

But if you've spent years ignoring your body's hunger/fullness signals, how do you learn to recognize them again? It's not as if you can look at a picture!

First, forget about how *other* people define hunger or fullness. Many say they're hungry when their stomach starts growling. By the time I reach that point, I'm ravenous; my body is in panic mode, geared to force me into overeating so it can pack extra food away as fat to protect against future deprivation. Such desperation won't allow me to make good food choices. Better to catch hunger in an earlier stage.

At the same time, how do you know when you've had enough? Hint: "Full" occurs long before you feel bloated and have to unbuckle your belt.

To help give you a sense of how someone might perceive the range of hunger and fullness, check out the following scale, a composite of my experiences and those of the HAES research participants. We all feel hunger and fullness differently, so it may not jive with your experience. Use it as a starting point as you explore how hunger and fullness manifest for you.

Sample Hunger/Fullness Scale	
1	Can't think straight and feel crazed. I think I should eat, but feel incapable of making a decision about what to eat and how to take care of myself. Just want to lie down and do nothing.
2	Very low energy, irritable, cranky, and anxious. Snapping at people. Shaky. Difficulty concentrating. My stomach is rumbling and feels empty.
3	May be preoccupied with thinking about food. Energy starting to lag. Mild concentration lapses. A little anxious. May have a slight empty feeling in my stomach, but not uncomfortable.
4	Starting to think about food. Light in my body. Energized.
5	Comfortable. Energized.
6	Feel a little heaviness in my stomach. A little tired.
7	Feel a little stuffed and heavy in my body. Lethargic, want to nap. Generally low energy.
8	Stuffed and heavy in my body. Lethargic and very low energy.
9	Uncomfortable, bloated. Tired. Want to sleep.
10	Whoops, it really hurts. Stuffed to the gills. Want to lie down.

Now it's your turn to explore these feelings in yourself. HAES group participants found journaling, and the other exercises in this chapter, to be helpful. By the end of the study, testing showed that their "interoceptive awareness" had increased dramatically, which is scientific jargon for their having become more sensitized to body sensations. In simpler terms, they were more adept at recognizing hunger and fullness.

Eating Journal

A journal can help you recognize hunger and fullness and identify patterns between eating and your physical state, emotions, thoughts, and moods. These patterns can eventually reveal how hunger and satisfaction manifest in your body.

In case the thought of a food journal conjures up bad feelings, let me alleviate your fears. This log is not a food journal like so many diet programs use to help you control the quantity and quality of food you eat, with the typical result being beating yourself up. Instead, your task is to be a nonjudgmental fact-finder. The goal is to explore whether the timing, quantity, and quality of foods you eat are truly satisfying and to figure out how to make your eating habits more enjoyable.

How to Chart in the Eating Journal

The Hunger/Fullness journal is provided on page 195. I recommend you make a copy of the chart and carry one with you when you leave the house and leave one in the kitchen.

Before you eat, put an X in the pre-eating box that describes how hungry you are. Also note your mood, thoughts, physical sensations, and emotions. Jot down anything that stands out in your mind that might be related to your degree of hunger or your appetite. What is your energy level? Notice any physical sensations in your body? Is your mind focused or wandering? Are you happy, sad? If you cannot identify your emotions or mood, is there something particular that you are thinking about? If you are not sure if some of these are related to hunger or appetite, write them anyway.

After you eat, rate how full you feel by putting an X in the post-eating rating box, again describing your mood, thoughts, and physical sensations. Draw a line connecting the Xs so you can see how much your hunger level changed before and after eating.

Are you resistant to trying this out? Study participants sure were! But trust me on this one: it's a really valuable learning experience. You never know what will come up if you just let it flow, and writing stream-of-consciousness is often a great strategy to get around your inner censor.

Journaling can help you note common feelings that are your personal experience of hunger. Without journaling, you might not notice that certain sensations reappear consistently. For instance, one woman noticed a few mentions of being particularly tempted by the smells of restaurants as she drove by. These observations always appeared several hours after she had last eaten. She realized that a strong aspect of her hunger signal was that her senses, particularly smell, were heightened. From then on, she relied on her nose to tell her when it was time to eat!

Eating and Its Relation to Moods, Thoughts, Body Sensations, and Emotions: A Journal

Date/Time	Food	Hunger/Fullness Scale										Feelings/Moods/Thoughts/ Body Sensations Before Eating	Feelings/Moods/Thoughts/ Body Sensations After Eating Additional Comments
		1	2	3	4	5	6	7	8	9	10		

Analyzing Your Eating Journal

Only you can determine when and how much to eat. The purpose of this journal is to figure out what is most satisfying for you. Your task is to look for the patterns to help you to respond to these questions:

1. What does hunger feel like to you and how does it progress?
2. What does fullness feel like to you and how does it progress?
3. What degree of hunger do you feel best responding to? Does the context matter?
4. At what level of fullness do you feel most content? Does the context matter?

Some patterns you may identify are listed below. See where you are.

I never seemed to get hungry.

There are two common reasons for this. Maybe you don't allow yourself to get hungry because you eat before you're hungry. In my study, one participant told me she thought that if she waited until she "felt" hungry, she'd eat until she exploded. It makes sense she would feel this way after believing for so long that she couldn't trust her body. But recognize that there is nothing magical about getting hungry. Your body needs fuel, and hunger sensations are its way of asking for it. It will also feel satisfied, and it will let you know that as well. If you don't give in and let yourself feel hungry, you never learn to satisfy yourself.

The only way to learn that you can handle your hunger is to prove it to yourself. Wait longer between meals or snacks instead of eating for "future hunger." If you're a creature of habit, delay eating at the usual times. So, for instance, if you typically eat breakfast as soon as you wake up, delay eating for an hour and see how it feels.

Another possibility is that you *are* getting hungry, but psychological barriers prevent you from feeling that hunger. For example, you may be afraid that your needs are too big to handle, so you deny them. Or you may feel that you don't deserve to have your needs met. Or—very common—you may so strongly connect food and weight gain that you don't allow yourself to feel hungry.

One woman in my study noticed that a croissant first thing in the morning led to a nine on the hunger/fullness scale. She realized it was unlikely that she was this full from a single croissant and figured that she *imagined* the croissant would make her fat. Dropping the judgment allowed her to check in with her body. She was able to learn that a single croissant was a comfortably satisfying snack—not overfilling—to get her through a couple of hours. In other words, *giving yourself permission to eat the foods you want when you're hungry enables you to enjoy your favorite foods in moderation.* She also discovered that it wasn't sufficiently filling to get her through to her lunch break. The croissant became less appealing as a breakfast on a typical workday because she knew it wouldn't satisfy her.

I felt dizzy, sensitive to cold, tired, moody or had a headache or difficulty sleeping or concentrating before I ate.

If this described you, then you were letting yourself get *too* hungry. These symptoms are better described as starvation than hunger. Try to be more attentive to your physical sensations throughout the day, particularly three to four hours after eating.

I bounced back and forth between extreme hunger and overeating.

This is a familiar pattern: getting extremely hungry (1–3 on the Hunger/Fullness scale) followed by overeating (9–10 on the scale). That's because it's a response to a biologic phenomenon. When your blood sugar levels drop because you've gone too long without food, eating triggers your body to secrete large amounts of insulin so your starved cells can gobble up the energy from your meal. Chemical signals encourage you to eat tremendous amounts to replenish your body, with fullness sensors suppressed.

However, since you're not using this energy at a faster rate, much of it ends up in storage. Also, you're likely to be so desperate for quick energy that you crave foods high in sugar (which gets into your bloodstream quickly) and calories (like fat). You are unlikely to be tempted by more wholesome foods. When your blood sugar is low, you may also get moody and mean and feel generally lousy.

Remember all those times you felt so self-righteous because you felt hungry but didn't eat, picturing the pounds tumbling off? Now you know this strategy backfires. It's ironic that eating can actually help you maintain a lower weight, often doing a better job than not eating!

I never felt full, no matter how much I ate.

Eating should alleviate hunger. If it doesn't, then you may be eating because of emotional rather than physical hunger, and food isn't addressing your "real" hunger. Later in the chapter I'll discuss some strategies to tackle emotional eating.

You might also be "eating without eating," allowing yourself to become so distracted while eating that you don't pay attention to fullness signals. Remember what I said earlier: You must be present and taste your food. Eating in front of the television or while driving won't allow you to be fully sensitive to your food. Nor should you be eating while participating in a stressful meeting at work or while squabbling with your family at home. Food has to satisfy you on numerous levels to fully activate your satiety sensors.

It may also be that you are eating foods that don't register on your fullness meter and not getting enough of the foods that readily contribute to fullness. Chapter 4 identified some of the culprits, and upcoming chapters will help support you in changing your tastes toward the more nutritious and filling stuff.

I consistently overate and felt stuffed.

This is a very common problem. For many people, overeating is driven by emotional eating. Let's save that for later in the chapter.

For others, it's because there's a time lag between when our stomachs are full and when that fullness message reaches our brains. Too many of us never slow down enough to get that signal until it's too late. The typical American meal doesn't even last the twenty minutes it takes an average meal to register. (Some foods might take quite a bit longer, perhaps up to an hour.)

Your past experiences can play an important role in helping you anticipate how the food will affect your satiety level beyond the moment. For instance, history tells me that a typical San Francisco burrito goes down easily, at least in the moment. Thirty minutes later though, I feel lousy—overstuffed and uncomfortable. This teaches me a lesson. Next time I eat a burrito, I stop after finishing three-fourths of it, even if I don't feel particularly full at the time. A half hour later, I'm perfect!

So check in while you're eating, and find ways to reduce the amount you're eating until the fullness signal has a chance to get to your brain. Try out these ideas if they speak to your issues:

- **Be present.** Appreciate all the taste sensations. I like to start with a pre-meal moment of silence to bring my awareness to the table.
- **Choose satisfying foods.** Foods with higher fiber, protein, and water content do a pretty good job of filling up your stomach and more readily activating fullness sensors.
- **Eat slowly.** Put down the fork between bites, sip some water, chew your food well.
- **Take smaller portions initially** (and keep the food away from the table, giving yourself permission to come back). Then, if you're still hungry, get up and walk over to get more food. This interim provides a time to "check in" with yourself.
- **Leave the dining area** or clear your plate from the table after a meal instead of lingering over the food. This will lessen the "mindless eating."

Here are some other tricks I've found to be helpful. Though they sound very diet-like, remember the context. These tricks are intended to support you in feeling fullness and stopping when you're satisfied, which gets you to a very different place than trying to reduce your calories.

Eat off smaller plates. I didn't think I could be fooled by this, but when my partner changed our dinner plates, we ate smaller portions and were just as satisfied. This suggestion fits with numerous studies finding that when we're given food in large containers or servings, we're more likely to eat it all than if we're given food in smaller containers.[390, 391, 392, 393]

In one experiment, movie-goers were given free popcorn. Some received medium containers and others large ones.[392] Even though the popcorn was five days old, people ate it anyway, and interestingly, those with the large containers ate an average of 50 percent more than those with the medium containers. More interesting still, those with the large containers said that the container size didn't affect the amount they ate. But it did. They didn't eat the popcorn because it tasted good (it was stale!), they ate it because of the external cue: the container size.

Choose high-volume foods. Dozens of studies show that you eat the same volume of food at a meal, as opposed to the same number of calories.[394, 395] Makes sense: A full belly is a simple but sure sign that the body has taken in energy as food. Also, nerves sensitive to stomach distension trigger appetite-reducing mechanisms.

In one study, researchers served participants who were used to eating a half-pound hamburger a quarter-pound burger instead.[394] After eating, the participants said they were still hungry. However, when researchers added lettuce and tomato to the burger, and used a fluffy bun, the participants ate it and said they were full. Why? The researchers suspect that was because they received a visual signal of an amount of food they thought would make them feel full.

Eating fewer calories at individual meals is not ultimately successful as a weight-control technique, as people tend to compensate at future meals. But you're not doing this to lose weight, remember? The point here is that eating high-volume foods may be valuable for you if you have trouble stopping without a full-belly feeling.

You can increase the volume of food without significantly increasing calories by concentrating on foods with high water content, like vegetables, fruits, soups, casseroles, and stews, as opposed to more energy-dense foods like candies, cookies, and chips.

Bringing It All Together

Now that you've explored what hunger and fullness feel like to you, it's time to throw out the sample scale and make your own. Fill in the blanks using your own experience!

Hunger and Fullness Scale	
1	
2	
3	
4	
5	
6	
7	
8	
9	
10	

Choosing Foods and Amounts

How do you know what's the best level of hunger to respond to? Only you can determine what's comfortable. For me, on a normal workday, that's about a 4. Dipping into a 3 is also fairly common for me, but I try to catch myself before I fully settle there. Sometimes I can't always recognize stage 3 before I get there, particularly if I'm distracted. That's why I always keep snack items around so I have food immediately available before moodiness sets in. Having snacks around also helps ensure that I get the food I want. If I get too hungry, I'm more likely to eat whatever is around. And in our culture, if you're not prepared, that usually means your options won't be very nutritious or satisfying.

And what is the best level of fullness? Again, only you can determine that. For me, it's very context-dependent. I notice that during the workweek, I'm most energized and productive if I don't get beyond a 5. So I fall into the routine of eating small meals spread frequently throughout the day and have a fairly small range of hunger/fullness. I couldn't function well on the frequently recommended pattern of three meals a day. Eating enough to carry me through long meal intervals leaves me lethargic.

WARNING!

If you're accustomed to a diet mentality, you may be tempted to morph this into another diet—one in which you follow a "must be physically hungry" rule. Resist the temptation. Use the information in this chapter to help you identify your body's needs and what else you might be hungry for.

There's no reason to be rigid. Occasionally eating for reasons other than hunger is a normal and healthy aspect of being human. That your choices are conscious is more important.

Guideline 4: Tackle Emotional Eating

What many people view as an eating problem they need to control is, as discussed in chapter 2, actually an emotional problem. The larger issue that underlies this drive to eat is related to caretaking. If you can get your emotional needs met in appropriate ways, your drive to eat for emotional hunger disappears. Here's my six-step plan to help you get there. Be patient and gentle with yourself as you move through them.

1. Thank your appetite.

For decades now, you've been eating for reasons other than hunger. Take a moment to show your appreciation for the help you've received from that drive to eat. Acknowledge the importance of taking care of yourself and that without food or another similar technique, life might have become so overwhelming you might have fallen apart. Recognize that your drive to eat has been a good thing. It alerted you to the fact that you had needs that weren't being met and led you to where you are today—a place where you can finally take care of yourself.

2. Question yourself before you eat.

Before you tear open that bag of cookies, ask yourself: "What am I really looking for here?" and "What would it take to satisfy this need?" So, for instance, if the answer to that question is that you really need to tell your mother that you're angry with her, how else could you meet that need besides eating? Maybe writing her a letter (even if you never intend to give it to her)? Would walking briskly around the block help? How about taking your anger out on a punching bag?

Say you're about to unwrap a candy bar because you're bored and frustrated having to wait for an appointment. Maybe you could catch up on paying the bills in your purse? Or call a friend and chat (quietly) while waiting? Or read a book? Maybe you could simply tell the person you're waiting for that your time is valuable, and you're not going to wait more than another five minutes.

3. Sit quietly.

Next time you find yourself reaching for food in the absence of hunger, go into another room and sit quietly. Let the feelings you're experiencing wash over you. Try to name the feeling you're having. Can't put it into words? Pick from the following list:

Happy	Angry	Sad	Hurt	Afraid	Miscellaneous
Content	Annoyed	Depressed	Lonely	Uncertain	Lonely
Peaceful	Bitter	Distraught	Embarrassed	Worried	Jealous
Relaxed	Irritated	Despairing	Shameful	Frightened	Bored
Cheerful	Disgusted	Melancholy	Guilty	Nervous	
Joyful	Frustrated	Hopeless	Foolish	Scared	
Excited	Furious	Miserable	Humiliated	Terrified	
Satisfied				Overwhelmed	

Note one word that is conspicuously absent: "fat." Fat is not a feeling! Also absent are "good" and "bad." These are all judgments about feelings, but feelings just *are*. If these words come to mind, back up and try to get at the feeling behind the judgment.

Pay attention to how you feel physically and where in your body the emotions reside. Don't try to change the feeling, just feel it. Does it evoke any memories or associations? Particular conversations? Try to tolerate the feeling for as long as you can, even if only for a minute, and see what you can learn. Many times simply acknowledging feelings removes some of their intensity.

Be sure to take *all* your emotions seriously, treating boredom with the same curiosity you would sadness. Even feeling bored can provide important information about who you are.

Check out this life-changing experience of one HAES study participant. She was a data entry operator, sitting all day entering information into computer programs. While she worked, at lunch, and when she got home, she ate and ate. But she didn't know why. When I asked her to sit quietly and feel the emotion that led her to the refrigerator, she realized she was eating to distract herself from the boredom in her life and job. When she actually *felt* the boredom, she realized it was intolerable. With this understanding, she quit her job, returned to school, and is training for a more fulfilling career.

When you experience your emotions, rather than numbing them with food, you can realize that you have a choice. You can continue with what is familiar and boring or you can make a change, perhaps by returning to school or looking for a new job. If you don't experience the boredom, you resign yourself to a vague dissatisfaction that may stay with you forever—and the continual drive to binge.

It may be that you can't quite figure out what's going on for you. That's okay. Be patient and try to stay with the feeling that washes over you anyway. Sometimes just allowing yourself to feel is enough.

4. Feel those emotions.

If you've identified the emotion(s) in your mind, try to experience them rather than drowning them in food the next time they hit. Some things I recommend include:

■ Writing in a journal
■ Talking with friends
■ Releasing your emotions physically, such as punching a pillow, running, crying, or screaming
■ Talking to a psychotherapist

Having unsettling feelings doesn't mean that you need to do something. You may just need to sit with them until you can figure out how to resolve them. An important part of the healing is being able to tolerate the discomfort, rather than distracting yourself from it with food.

5. Take care of the most important person in your life: you.

Pick at least one activity from the following list and *do it*:

■ Take a bath, or sit in the sauna or hot tub.
■ Play with your pet.
■ Buy yourself presents (retail therapy!).
■ Pick up some fresh flowers.
■ Spritz yourself with perfume or burn some incense.
■ Garden.
■ Curl up with a blanket and a good book or your journal.
■ Build a fire and sit before it, watching the flames dance and thinking about how warm and protected fires make you feel.
■ Get a manicure or pedicure.
■ Watch reruns of your favorite sitcom.
■ Read a trashy magazine or novel.
■ Work on a crossword puzzle, jigsaw puzzle, or sudoku.
■ Play a computer game.
■ Take yourself to the movies.
■ Rent and watch a favorite movie.
■ Call a friend.
■ Take a drive.
■ Clean out a closet or drawer (amazingly invigorating!).
■ Take a nap.
■ Listen to relaxing music.
■ Breathe/meditate.

▪ Play a game with a friend or your kids.

▪ Go for a walk or bike ride.

▪ Put on some great music and dance around the living room.

▪ Go for a massage.

▪ Enjoy a hobby: knitting, scrapbooking, and needlepoint are examples of fun options.

We get lazy about finding pleasure as we get older. This realization became clear to me during a party I recently attended. Adults and kids alike were indulging in ice cream. Ice cream is high on the list of my son's favorite foods. But when his friend arrived and invited him into the pool, my son forgot about his half-eaten ice cream and jumped in. The food was no longer interesting because he had another source of pleasure. The adults, on the other hand, vied for his half-eaten leftovers.

Food is a wonderful source of pleasure—but it will get you into trouble if it's the *only* source of pleasure you have in your life. Finding enjoyment elsewhere allows food to fulfill its primary role as a source of nourishment, while still providing you with joy and fun.

6. Show compassion toward yourself.

The corollary to this is to stop blaming yourself when you *do* overeat. It's going to happen. Sometimes you may also eat to cope with that emotion. *Doing so doesn't make you a bad person!* It makes you someone who has made a conscious decision about the way you want to manage this feeling. Note I said "conscious." If you've identified the emotion and *chosen* eating to cope with it this time, you're making progress. Note whether eating is effective and, if it is effective, how long that benefit lasts. If it doesn't work, that knowledge will help you to choose a different option another time.

Stop judging yourself. Enough already with the weight! Despair you feel about your body and your weight is counterproductive. It makes you feel that something is wrong with you; that you're not entitled to the food you want, and that you need to deprive yourself as punishment for being "overweight." All this causes a powerful retaliatory appetite and puts up a big barrier to becoming an intuitive eater.

Moving On . . .

Once you complete all the exercises and steps in this chapter, you'll be one step closer to trusting yourself to eat well. When you indulge yourself, making sure that eating is a pleasurable experience, you'll find the satisfaction you are looking for. Trust in pleasure, trust in yourself, and you'll find your own ability to make choices that nurture you.

Here's some more good news: HAES study participants reported that as they let go of the prescriptive aspects of weight-loss regimens and learned to trust themselves, these lessons spilled over into other aspects of their lives. They made better health choices overall and felt more fulfilled throughout their lives.

In the next chapter, I'll share with you some of those other adjustments, including *what* to eat, how to manage stress, and how to live an active, healthy life.

TEN

Live Well

This book is not a weight-loss book, but a book about living a life that will make you healthier, no matter what your size. Although the focus in this chapter is on health, not weight, suggestions are consistent with maintaining a healthy weight.

Developing a Healthy Lifestyle

We live in a tough world. Although we're pressured to lead a more wholesome life and to be thin, the American lifestyle supports poor health habits, some of which may result in a high weight. The bottom line is that although many people would like healthier (and thinner) bodies, we're just not willing to change our lifestyles.

And although health care practitioners suggest that exercise and nutrition are simply a matter of personal choice, I know that's not entirely true. Not only is there a biological component that underlies our choices, but our lives occur within a cultural context that supports a sedentary lifestyle and eating low-nutrient foods. To choose to live differently takes so much more effort than passively living the lifestyle most of us are accustomed to. Social inequities make this particularly challenging for people with lower incomes.

Throughout this book, I have emphasized following your body's lead, eating what you want, when you want, and being attentive to the full experience of eating. I've told you how important it is to move when you want to, because it feels good, not because you have to. Many experts, however, are concerned that this is tantamount to "giving up" and will result in indiscriminate eating, inactivity, and more weight gain.

As you know, however, my research found this concern to be unfounded. We clearly documented that dumping the obsession with food and weight, along with the self-hatred and shame about your body, and following your body's lead can result in marked health improvements.[1, 2, 3]

In this chapter, my goal is to help you identify the type of life you want and take responsibility for your choices in achieving it.

Maybe your main goal in the past was to be thin. Having this goal undermined your ability to eat a nutritious, delicious, and satisfying diet. It also undermined your ability to enjoy moving your body, since you probably viewed exercise as your penance for weighing too much. And imagine the toll that stress is taking on you!

Hopefully by now you've changed your mindset and decided you want a new focus in your life. Instead of thinking thin, you're thinking happy and healthy. In this chapter, I'll show you how to integrate physical movement, nutrition, and stress reduction techniques to achieve that goal. What I *won't* show you is how to use things to lose weight. I do, however, promise that these strategies will help you achieve and maintain the weight that's right for you.

Let's start with physical activity.

Move It for Fun!

There's no doubt that physical activity tops the list of lifestyle habits that influence your health. Physical activity or, to put it more simply, *movement,* triggers tremendous changes in the hormones and neurotransmitters involved in weight regulation and health. Activity even helps you become more sensitive to hunger and satiety signals.

However, if you think hitting the gym or sprinting around the block is required, I've got some good news: Vacuuming the living room can be as, or more, beneficial than strenuous aerobic exercise for some people.[396, 397, 398, 399, 400, 401]

This is part of a new model for exercise called "active living." Active living refers to moving more as part of your everyday life. It means taking the stairs instead of the elevator, raking the leaves yourself instead of recruiting a neighborhood child to do it or using a leaf blower, or parking at a distant spot instead of circling the parking lot looking for the closest space.

Studies find that it's easier to stick to activity in short bouts of physical movement throughout the day instead of one long episode of continuous activity, like running, taking an aerobics class, or lifting weights.[402, 403] So far there's evidence that individuals are maintaining these activity patterns for up to two years or more,[3, 400, 404] which is in direct contrast to the short-lived attempts of people who jump on the gym bandwagon.

So forget about carving time out for your workout, if that's not appealing to you. Instead, just find ways to integrate more movement into your daily life. To be most successful, keep it simple and don't ask or expect too much of yourself. Instead, think of creative ways you can move more without making major alterations to your schedule. Try these on for size:

- Wear or have comfortable walking shoes with you at all times. Any time you have to wait or have a few minutes to spare, take a walk.
- Park far from your destination and walk to it.
- Walk to a different floor or neighboring building to use the restroom.
- Deliver things personally instead of using interoffice mail or e-mail.
- Take the stairs, not the elevator.
- Stand, stretch, and move every hour.
- Walk around when talking on the phone.
- Hold walking meetings instead of sitting in an office.
- Set challenges for yourself: How quickly can you get from your office to the lunchroom?
- Walk to the store instead of driving.

- Get off the bus or subway at an earlier stop.
- Park at the far end of the mall and window shop until you reach your destination.
- Houseclean with extra vigor. Pump the music up and rock to the beat while folding clothes. Master those dance steps with your vacuum as your partner.
- Play games with your kids. The little ones will love to dance and get silly with you!
- Throw away the television remote control.
- Stand while reading on the computer and march in place (easier in the privacy of your own home!).
- Walk with your friends and colleagues instead of the usual coffee break.
- Use an old-fashioned push mower for lawn work.

Challenge yourself with these small bouts. If you climb four flights of stairs one day, add an extra one the next. But don't feel the pressure to push yourself. Even a little bit has big payback.

The beauty of this approach is that you can forget about any fitness plan, weight loss, target heart rate, number of calories burned, etc. Instead, just move. An added bonus? Just a single short bout of activity will release endorphins, feel-good chemicals that pick up your mood immediately. It also makes muscle cells more responsive to insulin, even when you're not moving, dramatically reducing your risk of diabetes and other concerns.

As you move more and find yourself getting stronger, consider getting involved in structured activities like hiking, running, cycling, golf, tennis, skiing, dancing, kayaking, swimming, basketball, or horseback riding, either alone or with a friend or family member.

Whatever you do, be creative. One of my favorite activities is playing fetch with my dog. I'm not sure I totally understand the rules, but this is how it usually goes: I throw the stick, she chases it, then she teases me until I chase her. Then we both run until I collapse on the ground laughing, her signal to start kissing me. She scores extra points if she can make me run through the mud. I'm not sure which of us looks forward to this game more, but I know both of us are getting a great workout in addition to the fun!

Build your socializing and work around active ventures. For instance, instead of meeting a friend at a café, meet at the neighborhood basketball court and catch up on the week while trying to sink baskets and steal the ball from each other. The longer it's been since you both played, the more you'll both laugh! One of the HAES participants reports that Thursday night with her best buddy and a basketball is the highlight of her week.

At work, hold your one-on-one meetings while walking, or walk to the coffee shop four blocks away instead of hitting the stale brew in the kitchenette.

Of course, you can also join a gym and participate in classes such as aerobics, spinning, dance, boxing, etc. A few gyms are getting more progressive and making it more fun for people of all sizes to participate, although many still cultivate an environment unkind to larger people or to non-jocks.

Don't forget walking, which can be one of life's greatest pleasures. If you don't typically enjoy walking, concentrate on your surroundings instead of letting your mind wander. Smell the air, notice the landscape, check out the details of the architecture. As you tune in to your surroundings you'll find plenty to keep you interested and engaged. My dad's currently trumping my mom in their contest to find the tackiest garden displays in the neighborhood, and I enjoy their weekly reports. Apparently, pink flamingos are all the rage in Florida.

You may also find that walking is an enjoyable escape from daily demands, and a relaxing way to spend time with someone else. For me, the key to enjoying walks is making sure I actually show up. What do I mean by this? If I'm distracted, thinking about what I should or could be doing instead, walking becomes a chore. But when I allow myself to just be present, to let go of other thoughts and responsibilities, it's a great relief. I feel a real sense of lightness, which may just show up as a bounce in my step. With this attitude, walking becomes a welcome respite during my day. I'm also a better listener and friend if I've got company.

Swimming and other pool activities are other great ways to appreciate movement. Being in water has the added advantage of providing a very different way of experiencing your weight. It's particularly beneficial for people who experience joint pain or have limited mobility.

Active living is accessible to people along the full range of mobility, though it may take a little more creativity for some. For those in wheelchairs, I highly recommend chair-dancing, having recently had a great time rocking out with some friends.

The key is to stop associating exercise with "working out" or with weight loss. Notice, instead, how good it makes you feel. You may find that exercise is not only enjoyable, but a reward for the hard work you do in the rest of your life.

Why I Love to Move

I'm generally active, including riding my bike all over town. Here's what being active gives me:

■ Time for myself. When I exercise, I can let go of the overwhelmed feeling I often have.
■ Improved mood and energy.
■ A feeling of total freedom. I can let go and forget about everything else but the experience of moving.
■ A sense of wholeness. Exercise reminds me that I am more than just my brain.
■ Awe at what my body can do. Exercising takes my focus away from how my body looks to how it functions. I love feeling myself get stronger and better at different activities.
■ Challenges. I love setting challenges for myself and working toward them, as well as feeling pride and accomplishment.
■ Adventure. For instance, I've biked from San Francisco to Los Angeles, climbed tall mountains, rafted turbulent rivers, and rappelled down high cliffs.

- Outdoor time. I love feeling connected to the environment.
- Social connections. I love the social aspect of team sports. Playing on a team helps me feel connected to people in a way nothing else can.
- Spontaneity. I can chase my dog because I'm in the mood, quickly run and get something I need.
- More restful sleep.

What does exercise mean to you? What can you do to expand the possible roles that exercise plays in your life?

Ten Ideas to Support You in Becoming More Physically Active

1. Find activities that are *fun* for you, that you can look forward to.
2. Take risks and try new activities and different types of movement.
3. Lighten up! You don't have to reach a particular heart rate or exertion level for exercise to be beneficial.
4. Enter the flow of movement. When your body and mind are in sync, you are in the moment, and all other concerns are forgotten.
5. Connect to the environment. When you're outside, try to become more involved in your surroundings. Smell the flowers and notice the scenery.
6. Ditch the self-limiting attitude and challenge the cultural myths about exercise and movement that you've internalized. For instance, don't allow your size, age, or ability to limit your participation.
7. Be confident in your right to exercise. Stand up to people who ridicule you and let them know that *they* are the ones with the problem. For additional support, try to exercise with people similar in size or ability.

8. Make your exercise social. Involve your family, friends, and pets and try to meet new people through your activities.
9. Be patient. It takes time for your body to adapt to new movements. As you become used to a particular activity, it will become more fun.
10. Set goals. Exercise may not always be fun for you. But, if you're working toward a goal, like participating in a 5K walk for breast cancer, or being less winded when you run after your kids or try to catch the bus, you may be more motivated.

Address the Resistance

This "just do it" attitude may not work for everyone. We all differ in our attitudes toward physical activity. While some people find movement fun, others find it work. Some want to move and others have to push themselves. There are biologic reasons behind this; for instance, some people produce more endorphins and get more of a feel-good response from physical activity than others. If you don't get such a strong reward signal, then it's harder to find the joy in exercise.

What can you do to make exercise more natural and appealing, something you look forward to and crave?

Consider some of your reasons for not liking exercise. The most common ones relate to social stigma.

Fear of humiliation. Maybe you still remember the humiliation of being picked last for sports teams or being teased about your weight in gym class. Most of us have horror stories from our childhood; kids can be especially cruel in this way. Many of us also associate exercise with punishment for our weight.

To overcome this fear, first accept that you deserve a healthy, strong body. Recognize that neither your size nor your physical ability can determine your right to move. And remind yourself: You no longer have to wait to be chosen to play; as an adult, you can choose yourself!

Fear of ridicule. Some thinner people feel they have the right to yell insults at larger people who exercise in public. Even if people don't actually comment, you may still fear they're thinking bad thoughts and judging you. Larger people also often get treated poorly in organized sports or in fitness clubs, with exercise instructors and coaches making disparaging comments about their weight in order to "motivate" them to move or assigning inappropriate exercises.

To move beyond this type of judgment, let me repeat again: You *deserve* a healthy, strong, capable body to facilitate your movement. You have as much right to move your body and feel good about it as anyone. The prejudiced have the "weight problem"—not you!

Fear of looking awkward or ugly. Do you compare yourself to others and feel you don't measure up? Do you find exercise clothing too revealing? Do you despise the "jiggle and bounce" you see when you move?

It takes courage to challenge the cultural bias that says you're unattractive or that you shouldn't be physically active because of your weight. The best way to get over this fear is to find a safe environment in which to work out. Maybe that's an exercise DVD in your living room or an exercise class with three of your friends.

Find some comfortable clothes. Exercise clothing designed specifically for larger people is less easily accessible, but you can find a guide to accessing retailers in the resource guide.

Fear that you won't be able to keep up. You're scared that you won't be able to walk around the block or ride a bike because of your weight.

Exercise builds endurance over time. Maybe one day you can only walk for ten minutes. The next day, however, you might be able to walk for twelve minutes. Within a few months, you're walking for forty-five minutes a day and your stride is getting faster. You are not competing against anyone except, if you want, yourself.

Fear of injury. You're worried that you'll hurt yourself exercising. To get over this fear, take it slow! Build some warm-up and cool-down into any structured workout. Make sure you have proper equipment, such as a good pair of walking shoes. If you feel any strain or pain, take a day off, or cut back a little. Some muscle soreness is to be expected; it's a sign your body is getting stronger. Significant pain, however, is not to be expected. And know that you run a greater risk of physical problems by *not* moving than you do by moving.

Physical limitations. If weight-bearing activities are uncomfortable or impossible for you, you just have to get more creative: Check out what you can do in a pool, on a stationary bike, or even in a bed or chair. There's an exercise routine that can accommodate any specific body challenge. Wheelchair aerobics, in particular, can be way fun! And many larger people find that weight limitations melt away when you have water to support you.

Summing Up

Your body is your physical connection to the world. Becoming active can help you chip away at any bad feelings you may have had for your body, enabling you to appreciate its functionality, de-emphasize its looks, and revel in your strength and capabilities. So now it's time to put this book down and go play!

Nutrition

When it comes to nutrition, you do have to employ a modest amount of direction to support good health and maintain a healthy setpoint. In the past, when the only options available were nutritious ones, people may have easily selected a nutritious diet when left to their own devices. But modern food processing has done a pretty good job of stripping nutrients from the tastes we're programmed to love.

Nor will you get cravings for all the little stuff you need. When you are low on zinc, for instance, it is unlikely that you'll crave zinc-rich foods. The biological drive for variety is probably nature's way of ensuring you get the range of nutrients you need.

Chapter 4 also alerted us to the fact that many low-nutrient foods don't trigger your weight-regulation system, making the rules of nutritious eating consistent with healthy weight regulation.

Since your food cravings won't ensure nutritional adequacy, *some* conscious effort has to go into choosing foods that ensure you get the nutrients you need to support good health. So here is state-of-the-art nutrition advice—Linda Bacon's eight magical words to eat by: Enjoy a variety of real food, primarily plants.

Easier than counting your servings of each food group, isn't it?

But really, it's that straightforward. This one-sentence rule will help naturally regulate your blood sugar and enable you to get all the nutrients you need. Be sure to combine it with chapter 9's information about *how* to eat and chapter 8's attitude adjustment advice. Prioritize meat from animals raised under more natural conditions; these will be much more nutritious—and will also more actively stoke your weight regulation system.

Let me flesh out a few more details:

Enjoy what you eat. Really. Eat with gusto. It's so much more satisfying.

Eat real food. Real food comes from nature, not a box, can, or bag. Processed foods are typically stripped of vital nutrients and laden with excessive amounts of salt, sugar, fat, and synthetic chemicals. The less food is messed with and the quicker it gets from farm to table, the more nutritious it is, and as discussed in chapter 4, the more likely it is to kick your weight-regulation system into gear.

Be sure to maintain perspective when incorporating this advice rather than get stuck in black and white thinking: Not all of your choices need to be nutrient-dense whole foods! Think big picture and give yourself permission to eat a range of foods. Put your focus on eating whole foods and you'll naturally find a little less room for the processed stuff.

Eat mostly plants. Plants are densely packed with nutrients that nourish you. Meat and dairy provide valuable nutrients, but they work better in moderation—as a side dish rather than a habitual main course. The more plant-based foods you eat, the fewer animal-based foods you eat, which is overall much healthier for you. This simple fact is likely the reason populations that eat diets high in meat have higher rates of "diseases of affluence" like diabetes and heart disease than those that follow diets high in fruits, vegetables, and whole grains. In the United States during World War II, when meat and dairy products were strictly rationed and people ate more plant-based foods, the rate of heart disease temporarily plummeted.

Again, perspective is recommended. Wholesome eating doesn't require that you become a vegetarian or vegan. Humans are omnivores, meaning that we have the ability to eat and obtain nutrients from a wide range of foods. We have evolved to have choice: We can survive with animal foods as part of our diets or as vegans, and a well-chosen diet in either of these categories can supply us with all of the nutrients we need. Moderation regarding animal foods, not avoidance, is key.

Get variety. Foods of the same type, and with the same colors, textures, and taste, tend to concentrate the same nutrients. Eating a variety of foods ensures that you get a wider range of nutrients. Aim for foods with vibrant colors and strong aromas, as these often parallel nutrient density. You get more nutrients for your caloric buck, so to speak.

The menu's not limited to unprocessed plant foods. Just use them to form the base of your diet and complement them with other foods you love.

My advice may seem simplistic, especially given daily nutrition hype in the news, unending talk about super-foods, and excruciating debates over high-carb vs. low-carb eating, good carbs and bad, low-fat and non-fat diets. Remember that fearmongering and confusion serve the weight-loss industry. The same is true for the food industry.

When it comes down to it, food is just food. Individual foods rarely have the ability to significantly transform your health or overall well-being. You're much better off paying attention to your overall dietary patterns rather than individual foods. So cut yourself some slack. There's plenty of room for Twinkies in the context of an overall nutritious diet. Subscribe to this basic eight-word mantra (enjoy a variety of real food, primarily plants) and other aspects of the diet matter much less.

Advice given in the previous chapters bears repeating here. Choose foods that help you to feel good. Use your nutrition knowledge to support you. For example, do you find yourself straining on the toilet? Increasing your fiber is likely to help you feel more comfortable. Do you have inconsistent energy throughout the day? Consider changing the types and amounts of foods you eat to stabilize your blood sugar.

You can trust your body to guide you in making good nutrition choices. After all, you are the best nutritionist you know!

Action Tips . . .

Take the Pledge . . . today and every day. To help you commit, there's a copy in the appendix, suitable for photocopying and with a place for a signature.

Live Well Pledge

Today, I will try to feed myself when I am hungry.
Today, I will try to be attentive to how foods taste and make me feel.
Today, I will try to choose foods that I like and that make me feel good.
Today, I will try to honor my body's signals of fullness.
Today, I will try to find an enjoyable way to move my body.
Today, I will try to look kindly at my body and to treat it with love and respect.

Relaxation and Sleep

As we discussed in chapter 3, your mental health and sleep habits have a major influence on many of the neurotransmitters and hormones involved in weight regulation and health. When you're stressed, you pump out the hormone cortisol. Cortisol kicks up your appetite, prompting you to want to eat large amounts of foods, high in sugar for quick energy. How do you get enough sleep and learn to manage stress?

Getting Sufficient Sleep

The best strategy to ensure you're getting enough sleep is to let your body guide you. If you need an alarm clock to get you out of bed instead of waking up to your body's natural rhythms, especially if that alarm pulls you out of a deep sleep, then you're not getting enough sleep.

Conversely, if you feel really sluggish after sleeping, you might be getting too much sleep. Studies find most people need between six and eight hours a night.

If you're not sure if you're getting enough rest, try going to sleep fifteen minutes earlier each night to see if you wake more rested.

Every night, go to bed another fifteen minutes earlier until you reach the right amount of sleep, i.e., waking up on your own and feeling rested. If you're like most Americans, you're trying to burn the candle at both ends, so don't be surprised if you find yourself going to bed an hour or two earlier than normal in order to wake rested.

If you have trouble falling asleep or staying asleep, pay careful attention to the next section on managing your stress. You may also want to check in with a trusted health professional.

Managing Your Stress

Everyone in our society talks about being stressed. But stress is not necessarily a bad thing. For instance, when you get a promotion, buy a new home, or have a baby, you're stressed, but in a *good* way. There is no way you're going to get rid of the stress in your life, nor should you want to. That would make for a very boring life! Instead, you can learn to manage the stress in your life so it has the least negative impact on your physical and mental health. One of the best ways I know is meditation, also known as mindfulness.

First, if you have preconceptions that meditation is reserved for New Agers, drop them. Meditation is just a simple practice geared to helping you experience the present moment. You don't need to burn incense, nor do you need to sit cross-legged. It's becoming quite accepted in the medical mainstream, thanks to studies showing significant benefits for a variety of medical conditions. It can reduce blood pressure, improve sleep, reduce the perception of pain, and increase your self-awareness. It also changes the point at which a traffic jam sets your blood boiling.

There are dozens of meditative flavors that can help you revise your stress response, including breathing exercises, yoga, relaxation training, mental imagery, and martial arts like t'ai chi. But the basic strategy is the same.

Here's one helpful approach. Find a quiet place with few distractions. Sit or lie comfortably. Try to let go of outside thoughts and focus instead on your breathing, noticing the sensation of air moving in and out of your body. If a thought pops into your mind, simply acknowledge it and then let it go.

It is that simple. All you are doing is bringing your awareness to the present. The more you practice meditation as a discrete exercise, the better you'll be able to bring mindfulness into your everyday life. This practice will help you in immeasurable ways, increasing your sensitivity to your body's signals; allowing you to more fully taste and enjoy food; and helping you live in and appreciate the body you have. Meditation will support you in your quest to stop chasing the elusive goals of weight loss and the fantasy that thinness equals happiness. It will help you appreciate who you are and what you are doing in the moment.

Particularly in the beginning, the practice of meditation is difficult. Your mind wanders; one thought leads to the next, which leads to the next, and much time goes by before you remember to come back to the present. This experience itself can be quite instructive. It tells you that you don't need to take each individual thought so seriously. It's just a momentary thought and your mind will be wandering on to something else soon. Think about that the next time you feel driven to finish off that quart of ice cream. If you can just "sit" with the thought for a few moments, experiencing it in a nonjudgmental way, the drive may just dissipate—a clear sign that you weren't really physically hungry.

Help Your Kids Establish Nourishing Eating Habits, Too

Your kids also need support in developing a healthy lifestyle and feeling good about their bodies. Establishing good habits while they're young will help them grow up trusting themselves and without the self-hatred and weight obsession many of us learned early on.

Children learn most by mimicking what they see around them. Don't fall into the trap of thinking that taking care of yourself is selfish. The Health at Every Size changes *you* make will have huge payback for your kids' health and well-being.

Research finds that sharing responsibility with your child about what and how much he or she eats is the most effective approach, from infancy through adolescence.[405] It's your job to provide enjoyable food and cultivate an atmosphere that supports pleasure in eating. It's your child's job to decide whether he or she wants to eat and how much. Since you will have less and less control over your child's exposure to foods over time, your best bet is to support him in honoring his body, learning how to make good choices, and taking care of himself.

Though kids have slightly different nutritional needs than adults, the same advice that works for you will also support healthy growth in your kids: *Enjoy a variety of real food, mostly plants.*

Protein Myths

Did you know that many green vegetables get more than 50 percent of their energy from protein, packing in more protein per calorie than meat and dairy? That even a low-protein vegetable food like a potato gets 10 percent of its energy from protein? That a low-protein processed grain like white bread gets 12 percent?

The dietary recommendations for kids are based on body weight, but approximately translate to 12 to 15 percent of total energy, so even these low-protein sources contribute a considerable protein punch. Assuming overall dietary variety (not just sugar!), when kids get enough calories they get more than enough protein to meet their growth needs.

Don't let the protein-pushers fool you. Americans err on the side of getting too much protein, rarely too little. Don't start your kids on that path. While growing bodies need proportionately more protein than adult bodies, nearly all unprocessed plant foods, including vegetables, beans, grains, nuts, and seeds, contain adequate protein to support healthy growth. Meat and dairy can certainly be a part of a nutritious diet, but it's no more necessary for children than for adults.

Children—often even more so than adults—are easily seduced by the intense flavorings found in processed foods. When their diets are centered on processed foods, it dulls their ability to sense and appreciate more subtle and wider-ranging flavors, a trait they will carry on into adulthood.

Exposing them to a wide variety of whole foods when they are young will make them less interested in fast foods and processed foods. This isn't to say that they will lack interest in those foods entirely, but that they are more likely to achieve a healthier balance. Provide a variety of foods so they can choose foods they like and develop their own tastes.

There's no need to ban "junk food." Offer foods like candies, cookies, and ice cream—in moderation. Deprivation won't do anything except make "forbidden" foods more enticing.[406]

A vivid example brought this home for me. I was cleaning up after my then six-year-old son and his friend and found an empty cookie bag. My son acknowledged that he had taken the full bag from the cupboard and ate a couple. "But they ruined our play date, Mom. Miguel just wouldn't stop eating them and didn't want to build Legos anymore."

Cookies were taboo in Miguel's home. Apparently, the deprivation he experienced left him without the skills to set appropriate limits. My son, on the other hand, knowing he had access to cookies much of the time, could enjoy them—and stop. He could also enjoy playing and wasn't distracted by the food.

Research indicates that parents who restrict access to certain foods are actually more likely to have heavier kids![407] This fact makes sense: The kids lose their ability to self-regulate as a result of parents' interference.

Promising a child dessert if she eats her vegetables or encouraging a child to clean his plate can also contribute to developing unhealthy eating practices.[408]

What's the best predictor of whether or not your kids eat their fruits and veggies? Whether or not they like them! Put effort into tasty preparation and you'll see the results, though you might need to exercise some patience. Young children are often hesitant to try new things.[409] This wariness is normal. In fact, there's even a scientific name for this: neophobia, or fear of new things. Pressuring your child to eat a new food can backfire.[410] The best strategy is to eat well and wait for your child to follow your lead. He or she might not like mustard greens the first time around, but may be more open after watching you enjoy it over time.

Eating together has many benefits beyond more nutritious eating.[411] Studies show that the more often families eat together, the less likely kids are to smoke, drink, do drugs, get depressed, develop eating disorders, and consider suicide, and the more likely they are to do well in school, delay having sex, and eat their vegetables.[412, 413]

Farm-Fresh Balsamic Braised Beets (Often a Big Winner with Kids!)

Peel beets and slice them into quarter-inch strips. Be sure to get hands and face as stained as possible. Add the beets, some balsamic vinegar, and a little brown sugar (optional) to a large skillet. Bring to a boil and allow the beets to brown lightly, then flip them to brown the other side. Reduce heat to medium and continue simmering, uncovered, until beets are tender. Add balsamic vinegar as necessary to make sure the liquid doesn't get too low. Serve alone or on a bed of sautéed beet greens with the concentrated sauce drizzled on top.

Beets also taste great when cooked in a roasting pan in a 400-degree oven.

Try, too, involving your kids in food preparation. It will heighten their appreciation of what they eat. Consider growing your own food, even if it's just an herb in a windowsill pot; visiting a local farm; or shopping, cooking, and planning meals together. Beets are much more enticing when your child sees one growing in a field, pulls the bulb from the ground, meets the farmer who planted it, and then tries the farmer's recipe for balsamic braised beets. Schools that help students follow food from the garden to the kitchen to the table, doing much of the work themselves, are seeing amazing results.[414]

Keep in mind that children are not just "little adults." Young children need to eat more frequently than adults given their high energy needs and less-developed digestive tracts. Three meals a day just aren't enough for them—at least not without a couple snacks in between. Be sure to have foods accessible between meals.

Structured snack times are more effective than grazing, and also help ensure that your child comes to the table hungry. By late toddlerhood, kids can already develop skills to control mild hunger and wait for a meal to be ready—and you can support them in further developing those skills. If your child is hungry, the food will taste better, and they will be more inclined to enjoy foods beyond their favorites.

Given our cultural fear of fat, you may be tempted to limit or withhold food if you have a pudgy kid. Don't. Kids of all sizes need to learn how to regulate their food intake. Pudgy kids will be feeling plenty of cultural prejudice. They don't need more hassling from you—they need your support. Better to shore up their self-esteem: Reinforce the idea that kids come in a wide range of sizes and that every body is a good body. Teaching them to appreciate, not hate, themselves will support them in making better choices.

Remember, it's about health, not size, even with our kids.

Summing Up

Now that you know how to integrate more healthful habits into your life, let's talk again about food. In the next chapter, I will show you how to reprogram your taste buds so that you are drawn to nutritious foods and, in the process, take another step along the path to Health at Every Size.

ELEVEN
Change Your Tastes

W hat if you craved broccoli in the same way you crave double chocolate Häagen-Dazs? What if a bag of potato chips
appealed to you about as much as a piece of shoe leather?
Sound far-fetched? It's not. Just as the food industry has manipulated
our taste buds into preferring high-fat, high-salt, high-sugar foods
with added flavor chemicals, we can "manipulate" them back,
retraining them to prefer fresh, quality foods like fruits, vegetables,
whole grains, and beans. This chapter helps you revitalize your
palate, based on the latest research in taste science, supporting you
in eating food that tastes truly delicious to you.

The Joy of Eating

Think about eating a just-plucked-from-your-garden strawberry, still
warm from the sun. Even before it reaches your lips, the rich color
and intoxicating perfume have taken over two of your senses. As you
bite into it, the sensations of sweetness with just a hint of acidity
overtake your taste buds. You feel the texture of the seeds mixed
with the soft pulp, the flavors changing and becoming less intense

but no less delicious as you swallow. Mm, mm, good! The next day you return to the garden, eye your strawberry patch, and your mouth waters in pleasant anticipation.

What's going on here is that you're getting your biological reward for nourishing yourself. Ripe fruit looks and smells appealing, titillating your senses and compelling you to try it. Dig in and it unleashes a flood of hormones and neurotransmitters that make you feel good.

And there's more. Experience pleasure and your body releases a hormone called dopamine, which locks onto your brain cells and builds a memory of how that pleasure was derived. Flavors, scents, even sexual experiences are in that memory, making you want to experience them over and over again.

Pleasure. It's a crucial component of the eating experience. Makes sense, doesn't it? The stakes are high: stop eating, die. It's not surprising we come hard-wired with a reward system to encourage us to eat! Some scientists even suggest the reason we naturally produce opiates is to stimulate eating—and the pain relief they provide is only a secondary function.[415]

As an added bonus, pleasure brings an additional reward: You absorb more nutrients when the food is more appealing to you. When researchers fed a traditional Thai meal of rice and vegetables spiked with chili paste, fish sauce, and coconut cream to two groups of women, one Swedish and one Thai,[416] the Thai women, who liked the meal better than the Swedish women, absorbed 50 percent more iron from the same food than the Swedish women.

The presentation is also important: When the meal was blended together and turned into an unfamiliar paste, the Thai women's absorption of iron from the meal decreased by a whopping 70 percent!

More evidence of the importance of pleasure and presentation: When volunteers at the University of Minnesota spent six months on a semi-starvation diet, they developed all kinds of strange rituals around eating. Meals that might ordinarily have been consumed in just a few minutes took hours as the men cut their food into tiny pieces, rearranged the food on their plates, chewed each mouthful two hundred times . . . all behaviors engineered to prolong the enjoyment of their limited food.

The fact that pleasure supports you in getting the nourishment you need—and insufficient pleasure invites neurotic behaviors—reinforces the reality that it's safe to dump the old diet values of deprivation and self-denial. After all, the proof is in the pudding: Eating tasty food actually helps your body grow healthy and strong, strengthening your immune system and bodily defenses. Add a heaping amount of guilt and the food loses some of its benefits.

Scientists have begun tracing some of the other biochemistry that supports these connections. For instance, one chemical called cholecystokinin (CCK) helps metabolize our food, tells us when to stop eating, and makes us feel good about eating. Cholecystokinin is produced in response to protein or fat in a meal, after which it begins stimulating your digestive organs to work. It also travels to your hypothalamus to shut down appetite before activating the pleasure center of your brain. So it's clear that eating—and the pleasure derived from it—is intimately connected to a natural fullness response.

Let's talk a bit more about why you like the food you do.

Your Ancestors' Taste Legacy

Why do some people love Brussels sprouts, yet others find them repulsive? Why do some people find them bitter, others sweet? Genes tell part of the story. No amount of open-mindedness, good parenting, or parental arm-twisting will get some kids (or grown adults) to salivate at their smell as they simmer.

To teach students about the powerful impact of genes on taste, I give them a dried piece of filter paper doused in a chemical called 6-n-propylthiouracil, or PROP for short. I ask the students to place the filter paper on their tongues. Inevitably about one-quarter of students find it nasty (they're mad at me for giving it to them), while another quarter find it tasteless, feeling as if they've licked the paper equivalent of water. The other half note a slight bitterness, nothing too dramatic.

After they argue about what it tastes like, I usually have to distribute a second round of filter paper to reassure the students that I wasn't tricking them—they all got a taste strip doused in the exact same chemical.

PROP is a bitter-tasting substance, but only those with a certain genetic makeup can sense it. Those who perceive a strong bitterness are called "PROP super-tasters" and have a double dose of the gene; those for whom it conveys a mild bitterness are called "PROP tasters" and have one copy of the gene; and those that are insensitive to taste are called "PROP non-tasters." PROP is frequently used in scientific experiments because it is a strong marker not just for bitterness, but for taste sensitivity in general.

You don't need a filter strip to figure out your genetic predilection. Answer these questions:

■ Do you prefer your coffee black (rather than with cream and/or sugar)?
■ Do you like grapefruit?
■ How about cabbage and Brussels sprouts?

If you responded with a resounding yes to each of these questions, you are, in scientific jargon, a "non-taster"—you don't perceive the bitterness or intensity in certain foods that turn others off. Strong cheeses and heavy salad dressings probably go down with no trouble. One advantage to this is that you enjoy a broad range of tastes and it will be easy for you to expand your horizons. You can physiologically enjoy many nutritious foods, such as cruciferous vegetables, even if you haven't developed the hankering. Because you are a little less taste-sensitive, however, you may need more flavor intensity in your foods—making you also drawn to processed foods and sweets.

If you answered a definitive no to those questions, you are a "super-taster" and are very sensitive to flavor. Because a little bit goes a long way, you don't like extremes and are probably a relatively finicky eater. You may need to flood your coffee with creamer and sugar to mask the bitterness you perceive. You can also detect every bit of sweetness in candy and every hint of bitterness in some forms of alcohol—which may curb your appetite. However, you may also snub nutrient-rich vegetables, such as Brussels sprouts and cauli-flower, because you detect their bitterness.

If your answer was yes to some and no to others, you probably have a single "taster" gene, making you flavor-sensitive, though not extreme.

In the old days, being a "taster" or "super-taster" conferred the advantage of helping you to detect and avoid poisonous foods, a trait not nearly as handy in modern times. Nowadays, none of these taste profiles are inherently good or bad. However, knowing your taste style can help you develop a strategic eating plan.

If you are a . . .

- ■ **PROP taster or super-taster**, you may turn away from many vegetables because you sense their bitterness. If this is your plight, your challenge is to be open-minded. Experiment with a wide range of vegetables, rather than writing them all off. You will find that not all have an off-putting flavor; carrots, red bell pepper, beets, sweet potatoes, snow peas, and green beans, for instance, are unlikely to trigger your distaste, and you will probably find their sweetness pleasant.

  You can even love the more bitter vegetables, given the right preparation. For example, cooking cuts bitterness, as does the addition of a sour taste, such as lemon juice. (No one knows why lemon juice is effective, but it is well documented.) Try roasting vegetables. Sprinkle them with salt, then roast in the oven until soft (the timing depends on the veggie). Roasting brings out a vegetable's natural sweetness—even Brussels sprouts.

- ■ **PROP non-taster**, you are more likely to enjoy a wide range of wholesome vegetables, but you're also less discriminatory in general, which may make you more vulnerable to overeating. Paying more attention to recognizing subtle differences in foods and limiting yourself to foods that *really* taste good may help you. Develop your sensitivity to negative alliesthesia. Recall that negative alliesthesia is the decline in our preference for specific tastes as we consume more of them over a short period of time. The chocolate truffle test discussed earlier is one important exercise to help you increase your sensitivity.

Experience Changes Your Tastes

While genes like those that confer sensitivity to PROP play a role in your sensitivity to certain tastes, your tastes preferences aren't hard-wired. In fact, your past experience with food plays an even larger role in directing your desires than your genes.

I wrote a bit about this in chapter 5—that your senses adapt to what they're familiar with. Eat the same flavors over and over and you generate more cells that convey the same receptivity to those flavors while generating fewer cells sensitive to tastes you encounter less often.

The result, also discussed in chapter 5, is that many of us are "hooked" on processed foods. Accustomed to their intense flavoring chemicals, we have lost our ability to appreciate the subtlety and complexity found in "real" food. We're better acquainted with "raspberry flavor" than real raspberries, with "sour cream and onion" flavor than the nuanced taste of the real thing. Too many of us have lost the ability to sense the wonderful range of flavors in whole foods.

That's why trying to get a group of people raised on Chinese food to try a ripe Stilton cheese results in a group of nauseated Chinese people; while getting gourmet cheese lovers to try the Chinese delicacy known as a "Thousand Year Old Egg," a preserved fermented raw duck egg, also sends them running for the bathroom.[417] Each group, trying these tastes for the first time, finds them repulsive. Although both groups had a penchant for strong, adventurous flavors, their taste buds just couldn't immediately accommodate flavors they weren't accustomed to.

But as a species, we have a remarkable ability to learn to love the taste of almost anything given enough time. This ability has allowed us to populate every corner of the globe while most other animals with more restricted diets are limited to locations that provide just the type of food they need. Research suggests that it may take ten to twenty exposures before a child[418] or an adult[419] accepts a new food, so be sure to stay open-minded and be patient.

Craving Sugar

The most common dietary preference is a sweet tooth. There's a good evolutionary reason for this. When food was scarce, it compelled early humans to look for foods that gave instant energy. And the sweet fruits that fit the bill came bundled with lots of other great nutrients. Today, of course, food, particularly sweet food, is more than plentiful—and the sweet tastes we love are often stripped of other beneficial nutrients; that we're genetically predisposed to prefer sweets frequently undermines our efforts to eat more nutritiously.

The evolutionary survival advantage conferred by sugar is one reason why taste buds for sweetness are concentrated front and center on the tongue, where the greatest amount of food tends to land and, bud for bud, are most prevalent. Every time they get activated, they quickly fire off a response to the brain that stimulates feelings of pleasure. Enjoy sweets. But just as your nose gets used to the odor of perfume a few minutes after you sprayed it, your taste buds quickly adjust to the sweetness, losing their sensitivity and requiring more and more to reach that same "reward" level of activation.

This is part of the reasoning behind Guideline 1 in chapter 9: eat delicious food. Nature has you hard-wired to enjoy those first few bites the most. Once you've gotten some initial calories, it tones down the biological reward feedback system. Unfortunately, most people ignore that signal and keep eating, even though they're not receiving the same pleasure from the food. If, on the other hand, you pay attention when you're eating, your body subtly nudges you to stop while you're ahead.

There's another reason many people are drawn to carbohydrate-rich foods like sweets: Carbs increase the ability of the amino acid tryptophan to travel into the brain, where it is converted into serotonin. Serotonin is a powerful hormone that helps stabilize your mood, supports restful sleep, and reduces the risk of depression. Some people theorize that carbohydrate craving may reflect a drive for emotional stability. While tryptophan is found in protein-rich foods—turkey, for instance, is an abundant source—there it competes with other amino acids to get into the brain. Carbohydrates, however, spark the release of insulin, which pushes the other amino acids out of the bloodstream, leaving tryptophan behind. Competition gone, tryptophan can sail into your brain.

A switch to more wholesome carbohydrates (think real food, not processed stuff!) still provides the serotonin benefits, just without the empty calories of excessive sugar or the high-glycemic carbohydrates.

The Allure of Fat

Sugar is on the menu when we need fast calories, but we are also genetically programmed to search out fat, since it provides more calories with less food. Although the research is not conclusive, we probably don't have taste receptors for fat; what draws us in is the texture and "mouth-feel" it brings.

Fats may also act as a mild sedative. There is some indication that calorie-dense foods such as fats trigger the adrenal glands to reduce their release of stress hormones, thus making us feel calmer. If this is true, it's not surprising that many think of ice cream as a comfort food!

Despite the rhetoric, fat is not the monster it's made out to be. Sure, it comes bundled with lots of calories, but it also has a lot of other beneficial traits. For instance, it contributes to the feeling of fullness. That's why low-fat and fat-free, sugar-based snacks leave you hankering for more calories. You also absorb more nutrients from certain foods like vegetables when your meal includes some fat, probably another reason why we're biologically driven to crave fat.

For instance, one research study compared participants who ate a fat-free salad to those eating a salad with half an avocado (rich in monounsaturated fats).[420] The avocado eaters absorbed about ten times the carotenoids (powerful plant chemicals that help protect us from a variety of biological ills) from the salad's greens than the fat-free eaters. Meanwhile, adding avocado to salsa more than quadruples the amount of lycopene you absorb, another important phytochemical that can significantly reduce the risk of heart disease and prostate cancer, among other conditions. Other studies comparing people eating salads with fat-free dressing to those eating salads with traditional dressings find similar results.[421] Fat also confers other qualities onto food, such as carrying flavor molecules. Cook an onion in water and it's much less flavorful than if you sauté it in oil. The oil brings the onion's flavor molecules to the surface, making them more accessible to your senses. Fat also allows you to cook at high temperatures—think deep-frying—providing an appealing crunchy texture to food.

The key to dietary fat, then, is moderation—not avoidance. Don't buy in to the hype behind the low-fat mantra. There is little research to support strong links between dietary fat (including saturated fat and cholesterol) and heart disease, cancer—and even body fat.[422] As researchers from the Harvard School of Public Health, who used to be among the chief recommenders of a low-fat diet, proclaim, "It is now increasingly recognized that the low-fat campaign has been based on little scientific evidence. . . ."[422]

Sugar + Fat = Heaven

Okay, so you've got your predisposition for sugar and your predisposition for fat. Put the two together and the sum is greater than the parts. In fact, research shows that a 50/50 ratio of fat to sugar stimulates the greatest rush of feel-good chemicals called endorphins.[423] Turns out, that's exactly the proportion found in high-quality chocolate. No wonder chocolate remains the single most craved food in the world![424, 425]

It is particularly highly craved by women, and even more so in the days just prior to menstruation. That's because eating a chocolate bar is not unlike a visit to the drugstore. Not only does it contain caffeine and a related energy-inducing compound called theobromine, but it also contains phenylethylamine, which acts like an opiate. Together, the three chemicals can pull a woman out of that premenstrual fatigue/mood swing, back into something approaching normal.

Premenstrual Cravings

Women can often predict the onset of their period just based on the food cravings they experience within the days leading up to the actual bleeding. They're not imagining things. Just before a woman's menstrual period, estrogen levels suddenly drop. This leads to those classic premenstrual symptoms of water retention, irritability, moodiness, and food cravings.

One option? Choose foods to minimize those symptoms. For instance, fatty foods increase estrogen levels while low-fat foods and fiber decrease levels. So, if you typically follow a high-fat/low-fiber diet (like most Americans), you likely have higher estrogen levels throughout the month. When that drop comes, it's more precipitous for you. On the other hand, a lower-fat/higher-fiber diet maintains lower circulating levels of estrogen. Thus, when the premenstrual drop occurs, it's not as severe. The result? Fewer premenstrual symptoms, including food cravings.[426]

Context Matters

How you feel about food also plays a large role in how that food tastes.

Numerous studies find that our preconceptions, ideas, and attitudes, and the context food is consumed in, can actually change the flavor of foods. Chunky green split pea soup may appeal to a blindfolded taster, but taste awry when that same person eyes a bowlful. And research shows that people rate brightly colored foods as tasting better than bland-looking foods, even when the flavor compounds are identical. Food manufacturers know this. Butter is rarely naturally yellow; it's dyed yellow to be more appealing.

One study had participants eat steak and French fries in a room with special lighting. In that setting, the food appeared to be a normal color, but when it was revealed that the steak was blue and the fries green, some participants became ill.[189]

Color can even fool our taste buds into perceiving taste differences where none exist. In one study, researchers changed the sweetness and color of orange juice in various increments, finding participants experienced more difference in taste between the same juice of different colors than between juices with different levels of sweetness.[427]

Of course, brand marketing also makes a difference. Put a carrot in a McDonald's wrapper and kids will tell you it tastes better than carrots served in a plain wrapper.[428]

I expect that it's not too hard to accept that the same food can taste dramatically different when eaten in different circumstances. Just imagine the difference that results from eating an ice cream sundae as part of a birthday celebration compared to one consumed stealthily in the middle of the night. Chianti sipped with your lover on a romantic Tuscany hillside pleases your palate in a way that you'll never reproduce if you're gulping it at the kitchen table while spooning strained peas into your one-year-old's mouth.

Culture and attitude play a large role in our preferences: A delicacy like candied grasshoppers may not be highly valued outside of Mexico, nor would termite cakes be as appreciated as they are in Liberia. And how many Americans relish roast dog, a traditional favorite in Samoa?

Food also tastes different depending on the foods it's paired with. For instance, if you eat a piece of cheese before sipping a glass of wine, the wine tastes smoother because the cheese's fat and protein molecules coat your taste receptor cells so the acidic wine molecules can't connect with them.

The same type of process is at work when you eat artichokes. They contain a chemical called cynarin, which suppresses sour and bitter taste receptors. So any food you eat after the artichoke tastes sweeter.

The flavoring monosodium glutamate (MSG) is highly used because it excites taste receptors, so you need less of a particular taste to fully activate the receptor. In other words, MSG enhances the way food tastes, making it a cheap solution to improve the flavor of low-quality ingredients.

Bottom line: You need to experiment more with your food. Maybe you don't like veggies because they've never been prepared the right way. Maybe you don't like certain foods because of your attitude toward them. Maybe you aren't eating foods with the right accompaniments.

When you change what you eat, eventually your preferences catch up to accommodate your new diet. For instance, the more salty foods you eat, the more salt you need to enjoy the food.[429] This is due in large part to your taste buds adapting to a higher salt content and then needing it for stimulation. But taste buds only have about a three-week lifespan. So if you switch to lower-sodium foods, after three weeks you'll find you stop reaching for the salt shaker during every meal. Then try eating something very salty that you previously enjoyed. You'll find it no longer appeals.[430, 429, 431] Research shows this method also works with sweet and high-fat foods.[432]

Not only can you change your taste buds by revamping your diet, but since consuming lots of high-sugar and high-fat foods alters brain neurochemicals involved in appetite and reward,[201, 202] reducing your consumption of those foods essentially rewires your brain to adapt to your new diet, inducing cravings for this new way of eating.

Be persistent. If you don't like broccoli, don't write it off entirely. Try it different ways: steamed with a bit of butter and nutmeg; sautéed with olive oil and garlic; roasted with Parmesan cheese. As mentioned earlier, research shows that repeated exposure increases people's enjoyment of certain foods. Most people don't like coffee when they first taste it, but many develop a love for it over time.

Putting Meat in Its Place

Suppose you're considering eating less meat. How do you do it? I'm not talking about going vegetarian or vegan, just cutting back a bit. If you're used to the typical American style of eating, you're accustomed to meat at the center of the plate, and it may be difficult to conceive of it otherwise.

The arguments for eating less meat are extensive and well established, whether you are considering your personal health or that of the environment and the world community. It's really not as difficult as many people believe. Rest assured, for example, that there are no physical withdrawal symptoms: No jittery feelings, no headaches, no tiredness. You may get cravings, perhaps, but that's okay. Because remember, there's no need to go all out: You can feed those cravings.

Here's some food for thought on reducing the meat habit:

First, know this up front: The typical concern about getting enough protein is unwarranted. We've been programmed to think of meat as an essential protein source. But it's not. Plants have plenty of protein. In fact, calorie for calorie, many plant foods contain more protein than animal foods. Besides, most Americans get way more protein than is recommended anyway (probably twice as much, according to USDA records). Unless sugary snacks predominate in your diet, protein is not a concern. (And if you are a sugar junkie, expanding your horizons is good general advice; adequate protein is just one of many concerns to consider.) Nor do you have to worry about getting the essential amino acids. It happens naturally with just a little bit of variety, which again, is good general advice. The typical conception that you need to be well-educated to reduce the meat habit (or even dump it entirely) has long been disproven.

Most traditional cultures cook meat as a condiment or an enhancer as opposed to the main deal. In traditional Chinese cooking, for example, bits of meat are added to vegetable stir fries or rice or noodle dishes. In traditional Italian culture, a small piece of meat is served as a second plate, while pasta frequently reigns as the main dish. And when Americans look back to early frontier cooking, bits of bacon or salt pork were used to season beans.

There's no need to jump into alien territory. Just try tweaking the proportions a bit. Bump up the side dishes, reduce the portion of meat. If you're making lasagna, throw in a few more mushrooms, add some zucchini. That stew can get great flavor with added carrots or parsnips. Like chicken teriyaki? That same teriyaki sauce adds wonderful flavor to tofu and vegetables.

Challenge yourself to learn new ways to cook vegetables, grains, and beans. Perhaps you want to make one night a week a no-meat meal? Grab a cookbook and experiment! Call on your friends for help. Host a meatless potluck and see what others come up with. I'm sure everyone has at least one meatless dish they love!

The Addictive Nature of Food

How many times have you heard someone say, "I'm addicted to this chocolate candy . . . or McDonald's hamburgers . . .or my mother's coconut cream pie"? Whether or not food addiction truly exists is a hot topic for scientific debate.

Take sugar, for instance. Several studies in rats find that sugar stimulates the release of opiates,[433, 434] which make you feel good.

Opiates, in turn, stimulate your appetite for more sugar. Give rats enough sugar, and they become addicted, constantly pressing a button to get more of the sweetened solution so they can keep getting that "high." This same mechanism is at work in people (or rats) who get addicted to cocaine. And when you turn off the high sugar or cocaine supply, people (and rats) exhibit anxiety and other signs of withdrawal.[435]

Studies on high-fat foods show a similar opiate response. In addition, researchers at Rockefeller University found that regularly eating fatty foods can quickly reconfigure the body's hormonal system to want more fat. They also found that early exposure to fatty food could influence children's choices so that they would always seek a similar diet.

In another study, scientists puts rats on a cyclic diet of 5 days of standard rat food followed by 2 days of high fat/high sugar processed foods.[436] The rats developed a preference for the processed food. Whenever they went back to the standard rat food, they showed signs of anxiety and reduced pleasure, sometimes refusing to eat. When they were given the processed food, their anxiety calmed, but they ate more than they had before the experiment started. Two months later, the researchers examined the rats' brains. They found increased genetic expression for a brain chemical that resulted in a greater release of cortisol, a stress hormone. This same pattern of brain changes is observed during withdrawal from addictive substances like alcohol. Other research indicates that this type of response triggers cravings.

Does this indicate these foods are addictive? While some individuals may meet the lax psychiatric definition for addiction, I am hesitant to take this seriously. It just illustrates that we have pleasure pathways in our brains designed to reinforce certain survival behaviors. Eating is one of them, sex another. Narcotics use this same brain pathway, usurping the mechanism meant to reward us for eating or attempting to reproduce.

There are of course some other considerations that make use of the term "addiction" problematic. I just can't conjure up the same level of concern when I consider someone eating ice cream compared to their shooting heroin. Nor does taking a kid to a

McDonald's drive-through elicit the same reaction as carting them along while you visit your drug dealer. I also doubt that many murders have been committed to support a Kentucky Fried Chicken habit.

However, there is research that suggests that larger people, on average, have fewer receptors for dopamine, a "feel-good" hormone, which means that the pleasure signal has fewer places in the brain to attach to and work its magic.[437] Maybe, then, these individuals eat a lot to stimulate the pleasure centers that do exist as much as possible, leading to weight gain, in an eternal search for the same satisfied state others take for granted through daily life. If this attribute is genetically rooted, it explains why alcoholism, drug abuse, and compulsive eating tend to run in families: Less ability to experience pleasure makes people vulnerable to anything that provides it.

Of course, there's another possible explanation: Maybe repeated overeating causes the brain to reduce the number of attachment sites.

Regardless of whether the term "addiction" is appropriate, the compulsion to continually seek out certain foods can be extremely painful. Should you avoid this drug-like high that you might get and "just say no" to chocolate? To the contrary, I think we should celebrate that food makes us feel good.

The challenge, then, is to figure out how to enjoy food and eating without constantly being dogged by the need for more. Start by asking yourself: Is your sugar/fat habit causing you harm? Are there other things you can sometimes do that are more effective at giving you the comfort or the high you seek? Cultivate other avenues of pleasure. Instead of relying on chocolate to make you feel good, how about friends, sports, theater, museums, volunteering, family?

In addition to pumping up your self-care skills, you also want to explore alternatives that provide the good stuff. There's nothing wrong with loving particular tastes, but perhaps you can mimic those tastes in a more nutritious way. If you're turned on by sugar, what about a nearly-too-ripe peach, or apples dipped in honey, or the sweetness of caramelized onions? Or spice it up: Allspice, cloves, anise, ginger, cardamom, mace, cinnamon, or nutmeg all provide tasty sweetness and can help expand your taste range. If salty foods are your thing, try savory flavors with bite, such as black pepper, garlic, curry, cumin, dill, basil, ginger, coriander, and onion.

The next issue to explore is whether your food is truly delivering on its promise. Those first few bites may have given you a pleasure high, but if you become more attentive to your experience you may just find that the next few are significantly less rewarding. This knowledge may help tone down your cravings.

Next, I encourage you to pay attention to the whole experience of food rather than just focusing on the in-the-moment pleasure. For example, you may love the Sunday family brunches and consistently overeat. Then you feel too tired and lazy afterward to participate in the fun of throwing around a football. Once you start to make the connection that the food is not as pleasurable an hour after you have eaten, it may also help you to moderate your intake. You do this because it makes you feel better, not because you are trying to restrict your calories and diet—a much more effective strategy in the long run.

Your goal? To re-educate your palate to appreciate a wider range of flavor sensations and tone down the cravings that may be causing you harm.

Is Pleasure Getting You into Trouble?

In the old days, a penchant for sweet drew us to ripe, nutrient-packed raspberries. But now it's much easier to find a raspberry-flavored Snapple than a raspberry. And those supermarket raspberries, having been bred for shelf life, not taste or nutrient value, just don't inspire that same magical pleasure. They are also relatively expensive.

So what do you do if your drive for good-tasting food draws you to the less nutritious processed foods? What if craving cabbage is incomprehensible to you but the distinctive smell of Kentucky Fried Chicken gets your digestive juices flowing?

Hop into the driver's seat. It's time to reclaim your taste for nutritious foods.

The Diet Makeover

It's easy to take on the values of our culture but it takes extra effort to resist. For many people, processed food (including fast food) tastes delicious and seems to be a necessity for the lives we live at such frenzied paces.

If you feel stuck in this rat race, I encourage you to start by considering larger issues than just food. Ask yourself: Is this "fast" lifestyle really delivering on its promises? You may just find that you sleep better at night with a slower lifestyle, where good food and nutrition become more important than the amount of money in your bank account; where pleasure comes from community and nature rather than the size of your flat-screen television and the brand of your car.

Earlier in this book, I encouraged you to consciously choose your value system, as opposed to passively accepting cultural values. Challenging these deep-seated values—and learning more about food—will help you change your taste for food from one that plays to the lowest common denominator of the mass market to one that honors food and pleasure.

I see this all the time in the introductory nutrition courses I teach. When students start the course, they rank the reasons they choose certain foods, often listing "presumed effect on weight" as second to taste, giving less credence to a long list of other food values, such as cost, social justice, animal welfare, and environmental concerns.

In the course, I teach them the same things I'm teaching you—with an added emphasis on the social and environmental effects of our food choices. (If you are interested in learning more about these issues, check out what I've written by visiting my Web site: www.LindaBacon.org.) By the end of the course, my "after" surveys document a dramatic change in their diet and tastes. Students report that they choose more whole foods. Even more importantly, they now prefer them. They eat less meat and enjoy plant foods more. What is most interesting is how they got there: They cite an increased social and environmental consciousness as playing a larger role in their change—not concerns about weight or health.

In other words, once they lessen their preoccupation with weight and increase their knowledge about where their food comes from and its larger impact, their newfound awareness becomes compelling motivation for dietary habit change. Their previous preoccupation with weight was less successful at motivating change. So in case you needed yet another reason to dump the weight focus, there it is.

When you eat processed food, you're digesting the values that go along with it: the idea that food has to be fast, cheap, and easy and that it doesn't matter where food actually comes from. But it does. Your food choices really *do* matter—whether we're talking about personal health and well-being or larger community concerns.

It is difficult to understand the consequences of our food choices when we are so distanced from them in the grocery store or fast-food restaurant. It doesn't occur to us to think about how that ninety-nine-cent burger got on our plate. We tend to not connect supermarket meat and produce to water pollution or global warming. We don't consider the conditions of the pig's life or that of the slaughterhouse worker when we buy our packaged sausage. Nor are we aware of the chronic diseases that may be silently developing in our bodies. The effects are out of sight.

But in fact there's a dramatic story that lurks beneath your food choices. Whether you care about global warming, pollution, animal welfare, food safety, social justice, or a slew of other concerns, the more you learn about it, the less palatable today's fast-food culture becomes. And it turns out that there is a remarkable confluence of values. The same food choices that support good health and healthy weight regulation also support a more compassionate, respectful, and sustainable world. What's good for the planet and our people is good for you!

Of course, animal rights activists, environmental activists, and others have been outspoken about the rampant abuse brought about by the processed food culture. In the past, some activists thrived on employing the "shame and blame" approach to motivate change (and some groups continue in that vein today). But guilt doesn't produce lasting change.

What's different now is that there is a thriving subculture to move toward, one that celebrates pleasure and good food. If you are concerned about the larger issues, it doesn't have to be about feeling guilty and running away from the bad stuff. "Slow food" culture is quite seductive and can easily entice you.

Consider your options. You could spend your morning at your local supermarket, stock up on some produce and packaged convenience foods. The conventionally grown tomatoes will be sturdy and blemish-free, though they lack flavor and nuance. The convenience foods will give you the taste intensity blast you are accustomed to. Each eating experience reinforces a taste for the added flavor chemicals at the same time that it reinforces a disinterest in produce.

Or you could stroll through the local farmers' market, chatting with the farmers and others in your community, sharing tips on the seasonal produce. Along the way, you sample the lovingly cultivated varieties of juicy, vine-ripened heirloom tomatoes, like the tangy Tigerella tomato, with red and gold stripes, or the colorful Green Zebras, bursting with unique flavor, and hear about their folklore. You go home and cook and share the season's bounty with friends and family, savoring the intimacy it fosters. Your Saturday morning doesn't feel "spent" but rather, enjoyed.

In the latter scenario, food is not an enemy to overcome, nor are your eating proclivities a sign of weakness. Instead, eating well is celebrated, an integral part of the fabric of a well-lived life.

If this appeals to you, here are some suggestions to support an attitude shift.

Get connected to the source of your food. Start by buying foods that help you feel connected to their source in places that provide friendly interaction. Farmers' markets are an ideal way to shop, providing a direct sense of where your food comes from. Many farmers' markets also include music and other entertainment. (If you don't know of a farmers' market in your area, the USDA maintains a list of markets online at www.ams.usda.gov/farmersmarkets/map.htm.)

Community Supported Agriculture (CSA) is another great option. Under this model, you "invest" in a local farm through a monthly payment, helping ensure its ability to continue producing healthy, delicious vegetables and other foods. In return, you get regular deliveries of fresh seasonal produce. You get exquisite produce, support farmers with a real commitment to the land, and often wind up paying far below retail prices. Many CSAs also provide great recipes to accompany the produce, helping you to try new seasonal foods in ways in which you may not be familiar. (LocalHarvest has a searchable online database of CSA farms at www.localharvest.org/csa.)

Farmers' markets and CSAs help you get higher quality ingredients. You get fruits and vegetables bred for taste, allowed to ripen in the field, and brought directly to you. No long-distance shipping, no gassing to stimulate the ripening process, no sitting in storage for weeks. The taste difference will knock your socks off.

Learn to enjoy cooking. Too often, preparing "real" food is viewed as drudgery, to be avoided when possible. That's why we so often turn to processed foods. But if you approach cooking with the right attitude, you'll find it's not work at all, but a pleasant way to unwind after a stressful day, to exercise your creativity, to spend some quality time with friends, family—even your kids. Find a couple of cookbooks you like, subscribe to a cooking magazine, take a cooking class, or curl up and get some tips from a television chef. Before you know it, you'll be dicing, slicing, and sautéing like a pro, creating stuff dictated by *your* tastes.

Go for variety. Eating the same thing all the time dulls your senses. Instead, prepare a variety of foods for meals, and when you eat, don't eat all of one thing and then all of another. Mix it up! Try exploring different cultural traditions to expand your horizons.

Enjoy food in a peaceful, loving environment. How you respond to food is strongly influenced by the context in which you eat. And there's no better context for eating than eating with people you love. In fact, sharing a meal is so important to Greeks that they call someone a friend by saying they have shared bread with each other. In the United States, the family dinner is one surefire way to reduce the risk that your kids will engage in risky behavior. So no matter how challenging it is to schedule it around work, sports practices, and other commitments, resolve to share meals with your family or friends. Set a ground rule: No fighting. The dinner table should be a peaceful place where everyone can connect. Conflicts can be resolved in a way that everyone feels respected. If you need some help making that happen, get it. Family should be about love and support.

It's also a good idea to create a ritual around eating. Rituals help provide meaning to everything we do, even the ordinary. In my family, we take a few moments to let go of our day and become present with one another by holding hands and enjoying a moment of silence before eating. We use this time in whatever way we find helpful. Sometimes I do a short meditation to empty my mind, other times I focus on my appreciation for what I have, including my family and lovingly prepared food. To foster shared community, my son then asks a question that we all answer. The typical question is "What made you happy today?" We also acknowledge the food, and whoever cooked that night often talks a bit about the ingredients or preparation.

An added bonus to all this is that talking helps you eat slower, giving your hunger/satiety signals time to kick in. Which brings me to the next suggestion.

Slow down. Eat slowly, allowing the food to mix throughout your mouth. The longer you chew, the more taste cells are exposed. As food becomes liquefied, additional molecules vaporize, increasing the aromas and helping make the flavor more intense and complex. Take a cue from a traditional Japanese tea ceremony, designed to employ all senses: Watch and listen as the tea pours, feel the heat from the cup, smell the aromas of the tea, then, finally, taste the tea.

Pay attention to presentation. It's no secret that how food looks affects our willingness to eat it and our enjoyment. That's why professional chefs spend as much thought and energy on presentation as they do on preparation. So rather than just plunking down the food on plates, arrange it prettily, sit down to a table set with real cutlery and plates, maybe some flowers, and light some candles—even if it's just a typical Tuesday night. Be particularly attentive to aromas: The cat box next to the table isn't going to help your appetite or enjoyment.

Conclusion

The best attitude toward eating is not one of denial and restriction. The best approach is one that cultivates pleasures and honors food and the act of nourishing yourself. By becoming more attentive to and respectful of your food and the eating process, you will be drawn to more wholesome choices, learn to better appreciate the flavorful nuances of nutritious foods, and be able to better hear your body's signals of hunger and fullness. All of which will, in turn, help you in your quest to maintain a healthy weight.

TWELVE
Solving the Weight "Problem"

Identifying the Problem

The path that eventually led to this book began with a simple question: How can I lose weight? The more I examined the science and the deeper I probed, the more I realized how misguided even my most basic assumptions about weight had been. The problem was not that my weight was too high. The problem was the assumptions I had about my weight.

Let's face the facts. *We've lost the war on obesity.* Fighting fat hasn't made the fat go away. And being thinner, even if we knew how to successfully accomplish it, will not necessarily make us healthier or happier.

The war on obesity has taken its toll. Extensive "collateral damage" has resulted: Food and body preoccupation, self-hatred, eating disorders, discrimination, poor health. . . . Few of us are at peace with our bodies, whether because we're fat or because we fear becoming fat.

Health at Every Size is the new peace movement. Very simply, it acknowledges that good health can best be realized independent from considerations of size. It supports people—of all sizes—in addressing health directly by adopting healthy behaviors.

The only way to solve the weight problem is to stop making weight a problem—to stop judging ourselves and others by our size. Weight is not an effective measure of attractiveness, moral character, or health. The real enemy is weight stigma, for it is the stigmatization and fear of fat that causes the damage and deflects attention from true threats to our health and well-being.

The generational increase in weight, like the generational increase in height, results from the complex interaction between our changing environment and our genes. While it's tempting to assume that gluttony or sloth—or lack thereof—determine our weight, the evidence shows that is simply not true. An individual's weight merely reflects his or her particular biological response to these and other lifestyle and environmental factors.

In other words, some people are genetically predisposed to store fat under current lifestyle and environmental conditions while others—the minority—are less efficient at fat storage. While research suggests that those who exercise regularly may average a few pounds less than those who don't, other research suggests that the eating habits of the fat and thin aren't remarkably different.

"Overweight" and "obesity" are misnomers: Many individuals with those labels are neither over an appropriate and healthy weight nor medically at risk. If we simply redefine obesity using the criterion we assign to other disease—defining it instead at the point at which it promotes disease—the epidemic would vanish.

For many individuals, "overweight" or "obesity" is benign, and perhaps even represents an effect of *improved* nutrition. For some, it is a symptom of an underlying metabolic disorder or a result of imprudent lifestyle habits. Many thin people also have an underlying disorder (such as diabetes or cardiovascular disease) or those same imprudent lifestyle habits, but are simply less genetically predisposed to weight gain.

By encouraging positive health behaviors for people of all sizes, we can address real health concerns, giving both fat and thin people the support they deserve, and avoiding stigmatizing people and worsening the problem.

Solutions

How do we shift away from a weight-centered focus and toward embracing Health at Every Size—from fighting fat to fighting stigma and celebrating body diversity?

There are no easy solutions to a problem that is so deeply cultural and institutional.

Part of the solution is to challenge the system that profits from discontent about our weight and to fix the corruption in the scientific process. The convoluted relationships between private industry, academic research, government panels and task forces, and the wider public health establishment need to be more widely acknowledged and disentangled.

Another monumental task is to address the problems posed by the industrialization of our food, which has resulted in an abundance of cheap empty-calorie ingredients (among numerous other woes), encouraging consumption of health-damaging foods. Whenever people in cultures around the world give up their traditional foods and increase their consumption of processed food and industrial meat, there is a predictable rise in "diseases of affluence" such as diabetes, cardiovascular disease, and cancer.

We also need to address the social inequities that make healthy habits, such as access to nutritious food, safe recreation, and the time to enjoy both, particularly challenging for those with lower income.

Next, we need to stop making weight an official concern. Health officials, researchers, physicians, dietitians: Lay off the fat people. It is time for the health-industrial complex to acknowledge that science and reason do not support the value of a weight focus. We need to practice evidence-based medicine and use it as a basis for determining public health policy.

We can support this by adding weight as a protected category under anti-discrimination laws. Fat people deserve full personhood and the right to legal protection when that personhood is denied; the high prevalence of weight-based discrimination and the lack of recourse when it occurs are simply shameful.

As important as it is for industry and government to change their attitudes toward weight and health, we can't look exclusively to them to provide the solution for our weight woes. That profit often motivates action, that the law sometimes prohibits corporations from prioritizing health over profit, that the government has limited ability to regulate, and that context dictates the meaning of lifestyle choices (meaning that the same habits affect us differently in moderation and in excess) requires us as consumers to take responsibility for our choices.

Some of the challenges to positive health behaviors result from modern conveniences, like processed food, television, even cars. In moderation, these are valuable, yet when teamed with one another or in large doses, each makes it harder to stay fit.

As Eric Oliver points out in his smart exposè, *Fat Politics: The Real Story Behind America's Obesity Epidemic*, this is the paradox of progress. Modern life has brought us many advantages that at the same time undermine our needs. We were supposed to be empowered by not having to cultivate our food, cook all our meals, walk to our jobs, or exhaust ourselves in taking care of daily necessities. However, as freeing as our technological advances may be, they also make us vulnerable to health concerns (and at the same time promote weight gain in those genetically predisposed).

Consequently, we have to be a bit more purposeful in maintaining our health. This is particularly challenging in that individual daily decisions may not carry much meaning—an occasional donut will have little impact on my physical health—but it is when these habits become routine or are teamed with others that they become problematic.

We also need to acknowledge that the marketplace is not going to save us. Advertisements try to lure us in with empty promises. The magical pill that will allow us to eat with impunity and be slothful—without health implications—will never materialize. Nor is body mutilation like bariatric surgery proving to be effective for improving health.

Even as we fight the powers that be, individuals concerned about health need to shift our attitudes and make different choices. This is particularly true when considering our attitude toward weight. We have bought in to the myths, internalized fat phobia, and all of us enforce the cultural mandate for thinness: We are oppressors as well as the oppressed. We can all refuse to support this culture of hatred, and we can combat size discrimination, in ourselves and others.

Don't be a sucker for the cultural version of beauty. And don't impose it on yourself or others.

The individual choices we make add up. There is tremendous power in our words, our money, and how we choose to live our lives. Send a message to the powers that be. Walk proud whatever your size. Expose the self-hatred encouraged by advertisements that suggest you need their products to be worthy of respect and love. Expose the self-hatred encouraged by health professionals who demonize fat (for your own good!) and prescribe dangerous and ineffective treatments. Refuse to give your money to those who trumpet the old ideas. Transfer your support to individuals and companies that care.

Barrier to Change: Internalized Oppression

It is difficult to adopt or even consider HAES given the strength of our cultural value system. Many of the ideas discussed as myths in this book are typically unquestioned assumptions. Dissenting views are rarely taken seriously or given air time.

Considering Health at Every Size touches deep emotions. People mired in the conventional approach are threatened by it. I've received my share of hate mail and have been attacked by seminar audience members and callers on radio shows, often in the name of caring. "You can't just tell people to drop their concern about weight. Do you want fat people to die?"

Denial and resistance are understandable. People reach for denial when an intolerable situation has been pointed out to them but the means for change are hard to grasp and the penalties for contributing to that change are high. Myths about weight are so deeply entrenched that it may be difficult to imagine an alternative and to have the courage and means to move toward it.

Conventional thinkers provide a simplistic solution, which is that we can opt out of the oppression merely by losing weight or maintaining a low weight. It's tempting to grab on to weight control as a lifeline rather than confront the overwhelming pain as we acknowledge the damage caused by the weight myths and the major personal, cultural, and institutional shifts required for change.

At the core of the myths are their divisiveness. They ask us to measure ourselves against others or outside standards: "Don't you just hate women who look like that?" One person's body becomes the instrument for criticizing another.

The belief that we can lose weight and opt out of the oppression means that we don't bond with one another about how harmful this message is. It's not surprising that fat people have not had a Stonewall.* People cling to their "temporary status," believing they can escape oppression as "fat" if they try hard enough. They put their energy into escaping rather than fighting cultural prejudice. This accounts for the well-documented anti-fat bias among fat people themselves.

Conventional ideas about weight take away the motivation for self-defense by removing the need for resistance: "Just change yourself and this won't be an issue anymore."

Attitudes toward weight are further complicated by social class. It is said that "You can never be too rich or too thin," and in fact heaviness is much more common among people of lower socioeconomic status. It is common for the privileged class to view weight as a measure of one's character: People are fat because they are too lazy or irresponsible to take care of themselves. Weight carries a moral judgment, allowing the thin (wealthy) to justify their social position. If the poor and minorities are getting fatter, it is even more proof that they are less responsible and less worthy.

---

*The Stonewall rebellion occurred in 1969 when police raided a popular New York City gay, lesbian, bisexual, and transgender (GLBT) nightclub. It was the first time the GLBT community had ever acted together in such large numbers to resist police harassment, and is considered to be both turning point and catalyst for the modern-day GLBT civil rights movement.

Individuals Embracing Solutions

As angry as I may be at the external system that teaches us to hate ourselves, I don't believe that the difficulty of fighting the system is the limiting factor. While I certainly advocate continuing to fight and to chip away at the systemic problems, I think our primary power lies elsewhere.

Because the most powerful force preventing change is our own internalization of the myths. We believe that this cultural value system is real and that there is something wrong with us because we don't measure up. We feel shame. Because we believe there is something wrong with us, we disown our personal experience. When we regain lost weight after a diet, we blame ourselves as opposed to the diet. The culture doesn't have to exert pressure because we do it to ourselves and to each other.

Internalized oppression hurts people across the weight spectrum. The fear of becoming fat can be just as painful as the plight of being fat.

The toughest challenge in adopting HAES is to recognize that change has got to come from inside you. You are trying to define your own beauty and value in an environment that doesn't want you to get away with it. No industry profits from your self-love or from the very simple notion that you've already got the tools for fulfillment right there inside you.

This book's message is that you are the best expert on how to take care of yourself. Think about eating. This message is seriously unprofitable to the food industry, which would like you to believe that eating their income-generating processed products is in your best interest. It's seriously unprofitable to many dietitians, who would be out of their jobs if people didn't need their expert advice. And it's just not interesting to reporters, who can do a much better job of selling a story about the benefits of chocolate than the benefits of self-love.

But this message *is* profitable to you. On the other end of the spectrum is the great relief many people exposed to HAES feel when they realize they can stop fighting themselves, that they can ease up on their vigilance and finally enjoy themselves. I've certainly received much more "Thank you for this very freeing message" mail than I have hate mail.

Over time, I've come to understand that the crucial difference between those in whom the message triggers denial and those in whom it triggers relief has to do with this: the degree to which a person is willing to believe in him- or herself. Because once you trust your experience, HAES just makes sense. Back to that example of dieting: If you trust your own experience, you know it's not effective long term. The science just confirms your experience. If it did work, why would you have to try again?

Self-love may be the most revolutionary act you can engage in. A person who is content in his or her body—fat or thin—disempowers the industries that prey on us and helps rewrite cultural mores.

Your Own Health at Every Size Journey: Your Personal Path

Adopting Health at Every Size is a challenge in this fat-phobic culture. Show some compassion for yourself as you address your pain as a result of your "weight problem." Don't worry if you still feel critical of your body, still judge others, and are confused about how to integrate this new paradigm into your personal life or your work. You haven't failed because you are still struggling. We internalize the culture and it is hard to let it go. Regardless of what you believe intellectually, constantly being told by media, experts, friends, acquaintances, and family that losing weight is paramount to health, beauty, and moral character takes its toll.

Your journey is a long-term process of change. You are unlikely to wake up one day and realize you suddenly love and trust your body. Reading this book has not magically turned you into an unrestrained eater who loves vegetables and whole grains, lives for biking, and feels sexy in spandex, nor will you instinctively know how best to respond in the moment to friends or acquaintances with concerns about your weight or their own.

Focus on a moment-to-moment awareness, rather than worrying about the big picture. You will have tipping points. Some day you will enjoy chocolate pudding without thinking about the calories.

Or you will realize that today, your pleasure comes from the company of good friends and you're less dependent on pizza for that feel-good hit. The pleasure of eating assumes its rightful place alongside the many other ways you obtain pleasure, no longer tainted by your anxiety and neediness.

You will experience on occasion how delicious food can be and how good it feels when you maintain comfortable satiety, choosing the right foods to meet your tastes and needs. You will notice when you are satisfied, when food stops tasting or feeling as good, and how right it feels to stop eating then, knowing you can eat again when you want to. You will, on occasion, spontaneously dance or run, or otherwise experience the sheer joy of embodiment and movement.

Many times throughout the day you can apply healthy-living principles, whether that choice is about what, when, or how to eat; how to take care of yourself; what you see when you look in the mirror; how you feel in your body; or what judgments you make about others. Each time you practice what you have learned, you contribute to a larger cumulative effect on who you are. In time, you will find that you think less about when or how much to eat, since your body will let you know what you need and you will naturally and effortlessly respond. You will be less susceptible to that knee-jerk reaction that says "Where's your self-respect?" when you look in the mirror or see a fat person.

I also want to encourage you to take it to the streets. Re-imagine a more compassionate world, one that supports healthy behaviors and celebrates size diversity. Help make it a reality.

Join a counterculture movement. The "fat acceptance" movement, for example, provides a safe place for people of all sizes to expand the cultural notion of beauty, to celebrate the diversity that fatness adds to our cultural fabric. While the fat acceptance movement poses obvious benefits for fat individuals, I encourage thin people to join the ranks as well. As long as fat is persecuted, thin people will live in fear of becoming fat and will not be free. Fat acceptance benefits people across the size spectrum.

Thin people can also benefit by acknowledging "thin privilege," the ways in which we have benefited from discrimination against fat people. Whether we choose it or not, we receive untold advantages from being thin, from social approval to preferential hiring for jobs. It's hard to feel legitimately worthy if our achievements are based on unearned status in a discriminatory system.

Unearned privilege brings with it responsibility. We can use our privilege to help level the playing field.

Clichéd though it may be, no individual is free until we all are free.

Your Own Health at Every Size Journey: The Professional Path

If you are a health care professional, you may need to confront your own demons while trying to help your clients. You may also need to re-invent your understanding of health itself within an antagonistic establishment.

Know that it's not uncommon for people to feel considerable grief when they first embrace HAES and recognize the hurt they may have unintentionally caused by promoting the weight myths. Show compassion toward yourself: you did the best you could given the information you believed at the time.

When working with clients, keep coming back to the practice of weight neutrality: If a fat person seeks help, ask yourself, "How would I treat a thinner person in this situation?" Show compassion for how difficult it is to live in a culturally stigmatized body. Support your larger clients in handling the unique challenges of their bodies. And challenge the establishment that instructs you otherwise.

Know that HAES principles are equally valuable and effective across the weight spectrum. If an individual's weight is problematic from a health perspective, the best way to address it is to improve health behaviors and let the weight settle where it may.

It may be tempting to jump on the anti-obesity bandwagon. Claims that promote weight loss or obesity prevention attract attention, clients, grants, and money, and refusing to participate in these paradigms limits marketability. Health professionals who might otherwise be drawn to HAES sometimes rationalize their participation in the conventional paradigm by thinking, for example, that they can capitalize on weight concerns to motivate better eating or activity habits. In this way, well-intended health professionals are typically the worst offenders in furthering weight stigmatization and promoting obesity myths.

It is also popular to co-opt the vocabulary of the HAES movement to support a weight-centered focus. Some weight-loss programs promote lifestyle change and increased sensitivity to hunger and fullness, claiming that they're not diets, and then promptly prescribe ways to control your eating or foods that turn off your hunger drive. Also popular are intuitive eating programs (also called non-diet programs) that suggest trusting your body is the best way to lose the weight you want to lose.

Approaching this halfway is undermining and deceptive. Supporting a desire for weight loss or obesity prevention in and of itself promotes weight stigma. It says, "We don't want anyone to be or to become fat," sending a message that there is something wrong with fatness and reinforcing the myth that weight is largely a matter of personal control.

Approaching this halfway is also ineffective. While lifestyle change is valuable, it is rarely maintained when driven by weight-loss goals. Tricks to minimize hunger may result in short-term success but are ultimately challenged by long-term weight-regulation mechanisms. And while certain habits may result in weight loss for some individuals, there are no guarantees. Failed attempts at losing weight make people feel like failures, and even those who succeed feel a never-ending pressure to retain that success that will always limit their ability to feel comfortable around food and in their bodies. By putting an emphasis on weight, we also limit our ability to support thin people in adopting healthy behaviors.

Obesity prevention programs are particularly damaging (and ineffective) when applied to kids. Think about the impact of BMI report cards: The fat kids get stigmatized and put on diets and exercise programs; the thin kids—who may have similar health habits or be maintaining their low weights through damaging diets or obsessive exercise—get ignored; and everyone, fat and thin, is saddled with a fear of fat and a bias against fat people. It's not too difficult to reframe obesity prevention programs as health promotion programs—and health promotion will ultimately be much more successful in instilling healthy habits in kids of all sizes.

Eating disorders and preoccupation with food and weight are in part about trying to avoid being fat, and arise as a side effect of a weight-centered focus. Making the world a safer place for people of all body sizes will go a long way toward preventing these problems.

Perhaps the strongest suggestion I have for health practitioners who struggle with these issues is to find community. Knowing that you are not alone gives you the strength to persevere in unpopular views and supports you in making decisions that you know are right. And though we may not be in the majority, there is a huge community of Health at Every Size practitioners—psychotherapists, dietitians, fitness trainers, physicians, coaches—who have been where you are, can offer support, and can help you define your practice. (Visit www.HAESCommunity.org for resources and to get connected.)

It's worthwhile as well to reconsider the power dynamics in the healing relationship. You can't be as valuable to your patients or clients if you are yet another expert telling them what to do, even if your intent is to encourage HAES. You are more likely to be successful if you exhibit compassion for how difficult it is for all of us to work through our internalized oppression, create a safe environment, and offer education and tools to support the journey.

My Path

Let me end on a more personal note. As I neared the completion of an earlier draft of this book, I noticed that I was drawn to richer foods and needed a greater sense of fullness in order to achieve satisfaction. I was also self-conscious about the rounding to my tummy. I share this to make the point that an urge to overeat is part of a healthy relationship with food and my body. It's a signal from my body that something emotional is going on for me, an opportunity to slow down and consider what is really driving me toward excess eating or body dissatisfaction. We always have a good reason for our feelings and behavior, even if that reason isn't readily apparent. That's the gift of the hunger drive—and even feelings of body discontent. They alert you to your needs.

Food is an ongoing metaphor in our search for nourishment and fulfillment. The drive for nourishment never goes away. My life—all of our lives—is a process in which greater fulfillment is possible. I may never actually reach that final stage of true fulfillment, but I—we—can get closer and closer.

What options did I have? I could recognize that I needed nourishment right then, but that the nourishment I needed was a type that food couldn't provide. By not feeding my appetite physically, by disengaging from the drama of "feeling fat and as if there were something wrong with that," I gave the feelings space to surface. I realized that as I swung into the final stages of writing this book, I suddenly had to face my fears of vulnerability as I exposed my writing to others.

Once I acknowledge my vulnerability, I can make choices. After I finished that earlier draft, I realized that the fear I was experiencing was strong for good reason: The book was not as accessible as it could have been, and needed better editing. So I used this information to improve the book. I asked my friends to review it and give me the support I needed. My vulnerability decreased and my confidence increased, until I knew the book was ready. My hunger gradually dissipated.

Celebrate Your Hunger

Misplaced attention to weight has resulted in many of us losing that precious connection between hunger and nourishing ourselves. We are taught to view hunger as a manifestation of betrayal of our body, a force to be resisted. We're taught to view our weight as a sign of our failure—or to believe that failure is imminent if our resistance to hunger falters. But these ideas stand in the way of change. When you free yourself from the damaging weight myths and the "expert" voices that have infiltrated your mind, when you give yourself permission to feel your hunger, you recognize that hunger is not the enemy, but rather, a friendly, helpful force, alerting you to your needs and inviting you to take care of yourself.

Hunger provides an opportunity to honor your humanity. When you stop suppressing or otherwise denying your hunger, you are able to hear your body needs and know how best to physically nourish yourself. You can recognize that there is much you are hungry for, and not all of it can be satisfied by food. You become more attuned to these other hungers, such as your need for emotional connection and a sense of purpose and meaning in your life.

You have the ability to reclaim that connection between hunger and nourishing yourself. Feeling your hunger—and feeding it, in whatever form, is your power and opportunity for growth. You take back ownership of your body and how that precious body manifests and touches the world.

That's the final encouragement that I'd like to leave you with, the solution for our hungry nation. Free yourself from the limiting cultural biases around eating and weight and challenge them in others. Let go of the rules, the judgments, the "expert" advice. Trust that you know best how to take care of yourself. Respect your hunger and appetite, and let them guide you to better health and fulfillment. Expand that openness to others and celebrate the diversity that makes us human.

Enjoy the Health at Every Size journey.

APPENDIX

CONTENTS

Messages to Assist Specific Groups/People in Shifting Their Paradigm to Health at Every Size

Consider sharing the appropriate cover letter, along with the HAES Manifesto, to support your efforts in educating others.

General Advice to Specific Groups

Follow-Up

Get Involved/Informed

Note: Appendix materials are freely distributable. They are also available for download from the excerpts page on the book's website: www.HAESbook.com.

LIVE WELL PLEDGE

Today, I will try to feed myself when I am hungry.
Today, I will try to be attentive to how foods taste and make me feel.
Today, I will try to choose foods that I like and that make me feel good.
Today, I will try to honor my body's signals of fullness.
Today, I will try to find an enjoyable way to move my body.
Today, I will try to look kindly at my body and to treat it with
love and respect.

Signature: _____ Date: _____

THE HAES MANIFESTO

Health at Every Size: The New Peace Movement

We're losing the war on obesity. Fighting fat has not made the fat go away. However, extensive "collateral damage" has resulted: Food and body preoccupation, self-hatred, eating disorders, weight cycling, weight discrimination, poor health. . . . Few of us are at peace with our bodies, whether because we're fat or because we fear becoming fat. It's time to withdraw the troops. There is a compassionate alternative to the war—Health at Every Size—which has proven to be much more successful at health improvement—and without the unwanted side effects.[1, 2] The scientific research consistently shows that common assumptions underlying the war on obesity just don't stand up to the evidence.

Assumption: "Overweight" and "obese" people die sooner than leaner people.

False! Almost all epidemiologic studies indicate people in the overweight or moderately obese categories live at least as long—or longer—than people in the normal weight category. The most comprehensive review of the research pooled data from 26 studies and found overweight to be associated with greater longevity than normal weight.[3] Analysis of the National Health and Nutrition Examination Surveys I, II, and III, which followed the largest nationally representative cohort of U.S. adults, also determined that the "ideal" weight for longevity was in the "overweight" category.[4]

Assumption: Being "overweight" or "obese" puts people at significant health risk.

False! Epidemiological studies rarely acknowledge factors like fitness, activity, nutrient intake, weight cycling, or socioeconomic status when considering connections between weight and disease. Yet all play a role. When studies *do* control for these factors, increased risk of disease disappears or is significantly reduced.[5] What's likely going on here is that these other factors increase disease risk at the same time they increase the risk of weight gain.

Assumption: Anyone who is determined can lose weight and keep it off.

False! The vast majority of people who try to lose weight regain it, regardless of whether they maintain their diet or exercise program.[6, 7] This occurs in all studies, no matter how many calories or what proportions of fat, protein or carbohydrates are used in the diet, or what types of exercise programs are pursued. Many studies also show that dieting is a strong predictor of future weight gain.[8-14]

Assumption: Weight loss will prolong life.

False! No one has ever shown that losing weight prolongs life. Some studies actually indicate that intentional weight loss increases the risk of dying early from certain diseases.[15-20]

Assumption: The only way for "overweight" people to improve health is to lose weight.

False! Most health indicators can be improved through changing health behaviors, regardless of whether weight is lost.[5] For example, lifestyle changes can reduce blood pressure, largely or completely independent of changes in body weight.[1, 21, 22] The same can be said for blood lipids.[1, 23, 24] Improvements in insulin sensitivity and blood lipids as a result of aerobic exercise training have been documented even in persons who actually *gained* body fat while participating in the intervention.[24, 25]

Assumption: Health is declining as a result of an "obesity epidemic."

False! While it's true that we're moderately fatter than we used to be, life expectancy has increased dramatically during the same time period in which our weight rose (from 70.8 years in 1970 to 77.8 years in 2005).[26] That's right, government statistics predict that the average kid can now expect to live almost eight years longer than his or her parents! Not only are we living longer than ever before, but we're healthier than ever and chronic disease is appearing much later in life.[26] Death rates attributed to heart disease have steadily declined throughout the entire spike in obesity.[27] Both the World Health Organization and the Social Security Administration project life expectancy to continue to rise in coming decades.[28, 29] We are simply not seeing the catastrophic consequences predicted to result from the "obesity epidemic."

Blame Economics

Why do these faulty assumptions continue to proliferate and why isn't the reality more widely known? There can only be one explanation when science so blatantly contradicts popular thought: economics.

There is a huge industry that benefits from widening the boundaries of what is considered a problematic weight, including weight loss centers, supplement makers, drug companies, physicians, and purveyors of diet books, foods and programs. Even scientists benefit by getting research grants and serving as consultants, or by running weight loss centers at universities. Convincing us of a crisis can also aid government agencies in obtaining congressional funding. And expert panels that create public policy and determine research funding are populated by individuals with financial conflicts of interests.

That said, I do not believe that those engaging in this damaging paradigm are part of a widespread conspiracy. We are all raised with the assumption that fat is bad and permanent weight loss can be achieved through dietary change and exercise. These assumptions are so strongly a part of our cultural landscape that they are regarded as self-evident, and few even consider questioning them. As a result, many well-intentioned, caring people unknowingly collude and transmit this cultural bias. Also, there is little reward for questioning these assumptions, other than peace of mind. Indeed, for a professional to challenge these ideas is tantamount to career suicide; this is in stark contrast to the large financial/status incentive for supporting the old paradigm.

What Can You Do?

Refuse to fight in an unjust war. Join the new peace movement: "Health at Every Size" (HAES). HAES acknowledges that well-being and healthy habits are more important than any number on the scale. Participating is simple:

1. **Accept your size.** Love and appreciate the body you have. Self-acceptance empowers you to move on and make positive changes.

2. **Trust yourself.** We all have internal systems designed to keep us healthy—and at a healthy weight. Support your body in naturally finding its appropriate weight by honoring its signals of hunger, fullness, and appetite.

3. Adopt healthy lifestyle habits.
Develop and nurture connections with others and look for purpose and meaning in your life. Fulfilling your social, emotional, and spiritual needs restores food to its rightful place as a source of nourishment and pleasure.

- Find the joy in moving your body and becoming more physically vital in your everyday life.
- Eat when you're hungry, stop when you're full, and seek out pleasurable and satisfying foods.
- Tailor your tastes so that you enjoy more nutritious foods, staying mindful that there is plenty of room for less nutritious choices in the context of an overall healthy diet and lifestyle.

4. Embrace size diversity. Humans come in a variety of sizes and shapes. Open to the beauty found across the spectrum and support others in recognizing their unique attractiveness.

References

1. Bacon, L., et al., *Size acceptance and intuitive eating improve health for obese, female chronic dieters.* Journal of the American Dietetic Association, 2005. **105**: p. 929-36.
2. Provencher, V., et al., *Health-at-every-size and eating behaviors: 1-year follow-up results of a size acceptance intervention.* J Am Diet Assoc, 2009. **109**(11): p. 1854-61.
3. McGee, D.L., *Body mass index and mortality: a meta-analysis based on person-level data from twenty-six observational studies.* Annals of Epidemiology, 2005. **15**(2): p. 87-97.
4. Flegal, K.M., et al., *Excess deaths associated with underweight, overweight, and obesity.* Journal of the American Medical Association, 2005. **293**(15): p. 1861-7.

5. Campos, P., et al., *The epidemiology of overweight and obesity: public health crisis or moral panic?* International Journal of Epidemiology, 2005.

6. Miller, W.C., *How effective are traditional dietary and exercise interventions for weight loss?* Medicine and Science in Sports and Exercise, 1999. **31**(8): p. 1129-1134.

7. Mann, T., et al., *Medicare's Search for Effective Obesity Treatments: Diets Are Not the Answer.* American Psychologist, 2007. **62**(3): p. 220-33.

8. Stice, E., et al., *Naturalistic weight-reduction efforts prospectively predict growth in relative weight and onset of obesity among female adolescents.* Journal of Consulting and Clinical Psychology, 1999. **67**: p. 967-974.

9. Stice, E., K. Presnell, and H. Shaw, *Psychological and Behavioral Risk Factors for Obesity Onset in Adolescent Girls: A Prospective Study.* Journal of Consulting and Clinical Psychology, 2005. **73**(2): p. 195-202.

10. Coakley, E.H., et al., *Predictors of weight change in men: Results from the Health Professionals Follow-Up Study.* International Journal of Obesity and Related Metabolic Disorders, 1998. **22**: p. 89-96.

11. Bild, D.E., et al., *Correlates and predictors of weight loss in young adults: The CARDIA study.* International Journal of Obesity and Related Metabolic Disorders, 1996. **20**(1): p. 47-55.

12. French, S.A., et al., *Predictors of weight change over two years among a population of working adults: The Healthy Worker Project.* International Journal of Obesity, 1994. **18**: p. 145-154.

13. Korkeila, M., et al., *Weight-loss attempts and risk of major weight gain.* American Journal of Clinical Nutrition, 1999. **70**: p. 965-973.

14. Shunk, J.A. and L.L. Birch, *Girls at risk for overweight at age 5 are at risk for dietary restraint, disinhibited overeating, weight concerns, and greater weight gain from 5 to 9 years.* Journal of the American Dietetic Association, 2004. **104**(7): p. 1120-6.

15. Williamson, D.F., et al., *Prospective study of intentional weight loss and mortality in never-smoking overweight U.S. white women aged 40-64 years.* American Journal of Epidemiology, 1995. **141**: p. 1128-1141.

16. Williamson, D.F., et al., *Prospective study of intentional weight loss and mortality in overweight white men aged 40-64 years.* American Journal of Epidemiology, 1999. **149**(6): p. 491-503.

17. Andres, R., D.C. Muller, and J.D. Sorkin, *Long-term effects of change in body weight on all-cause mortality. A review.* Annals of Internal Medicine, 1993. **119**: p. 737-743.

18. Yaari, S. and U. Goldbourt, *Voluntary and involuntary weight loss: associations with long term mortality in 9,228 middle-aged and elderly men.* American Journal of Epidemiology, 1998. **148**: p. 546-55.

19. Gaesser, G., *Thinness and weight loss: Beneficial or detrimental to longevity.* Medicine and Science in Sports and Exercise, 1999. **31**(8): p. 1118-1128.

20. Sørensen, T., et al., *Intention to lose weight, weight changes, and 18-y mortality in overweight individuals without co-morbidities.* PLoS Med, 2005. **2**: p. E171.

21. Fagard, R.H., *Physical activity in the prevention and treatment of hypertension in the obese.* Med Sci Sports Exerc, 1999. **31**(11 Suppl): p. S624-30.

22. Appel, L.J., et al., *A clinical trial of the effects of dietary patterns on blood pressure.* New England Journal of Medicine, 1997. **33**: p. 1117-1124.

23. Kraus, W.E., et al., *Effects of the amount and intensity of exercise on plasma lipoproteins.* N Engl J Med, 2002. **347**(19): p. 1483-92.

24. Lamarche, B., et al., *Is body fat loss a determinant factor in the improvement of carbohydrate and lipid metabolism following aerobic exercise training in obese women?* Metabolism, 1992. **41**: p. 1249-1256.

25. Bjorntorp, P., et al., *The effect of physical training on insulin production in obesity.* Metabolism, 1970. **19**: p. 631-638.

26. National Center for Health Statistics, *Health, United States, 2007. With Chartbook on Trends in the Health of Americans.* 2007, Hyattsville, MD.

27. Rosamond, W., et al., *Heart Disease and Stroke Statistics 2008 Update. A Report From the American Heart Association Statistics Committee and Stroke Statistics Subcommittee.* Circulation, 2007.

28. Mathers, C. and D. Loncar, *Projections of Global Mortality and Burden of Disease from 2002 to 2030.* PLoS Med, 2006. **3**(11): p. 2011-2029.

29. Social Security Administration, *Periodic Life Table.* 2007 (updated 7/9/07).

FRIENDS AND FAMILY: HOW YOU CAN BEST SUPPORT ME IN GOOD HEALTH

To My Friends and Family:

I understand that you care about me and that you are concerned about my health and well-being. I've learned a lot about issues related to weight, and I've come to believe that I can be healthy and happy at my current weight. I have also learned, both from personal experience and studying the physiology of weight regulation, that dieting and trying to lose weight typically cause more problems than they solve and are usually unsuccessful, despite strong determination and willpower.

As a result, I've switched my focus to feeling better about the body I currently have and improving my lifestyle habits for health and well-being, rather than weight change. I am not giving up—I am moving on.

I'd like your support. What I need from you is to accept and appreciate me as I am and to stop commenting on my weight, weight loss, or the food I eat. Being nagged about what I weigh or how I eat has never been helpful and has only made me feel worse.

If you are interested, I'd be happy to share what I am learning.

Thanks for your love and concern.

Signature: _____

HEALTH CARE PROVIDERS:
PROVIDING SENSITIVE CARE
FOR PEOPLE OF ALL SIZES

To _____:

Your patient is providing you with this fact sheet because he or she would like your support in incorporating sustainable health habits as opposed to focusing on weight loss or restrictive eating.

Many people assume that weight loss is a prerequisite for good health. It's not. Believing that it is leads many people to feel helpless about their health.

Despite admonitions to lose weight and a proliferation of weight-loss attempts, Americans aren't getting thinner. Many people will continue to live out their lives in larger bodies. You can accept this and support them in being as healthy as possible.

Abundant research demonstrates that health habits prove to be more important than weight. Please partner with your patient in celebrating his or her body and making choices that honor it.

Here's the easy prescription:

- Supply your patient with the same treatment you would provide to a thinner patient with a similar concern. Focus on treating the condition rather than the weight.
- Show compassion for how difficult it is to live in a culturally stigmatized body. Support your larger clients in handling the unique challenges of their bodies.

Educate yourself about Health at Every Size. Attached is the Health at Every Size Manifesto, a short synopsis of the underlying issues. Join increasing numbers of professionals in this exciting new paradigm shift, making a difference in their patients' lives.

Patient Name _____

MOVING ON:
FROM WEIGHT TO WHAT MATTERS

Weight.

Few topics are as complicated and consuming. That's because most of us view the world through a weight lens, whether considering if we can afford the calories in a dessert, calculating the exercise price we should pay for indulging, judging ourselves when we look in a mirror, or making assumptions about someone's character based on their body size.

Weight is an easy scapegoat. We blame it for health problems or problems getting a date. We use it as an excuse not to buy clothes we want, not to approach people who interest us, and not to take chances, whether socially, recreationally, or professionally. After all, we think, "Why would they want to hire me? I'm too fat." "Those pants just won't look good until I lose weight." We also use weight to discriminate against others: "We can't have her in the reception area—we want to project competence." We consider thinness a virtue and weight loss a requirement for heavier people to achieve good health and get respect.

Then there are the ideas about how to lose weight. As in: A virtuous person monitors and controls his or her calorie intake, just says "no" to dessert, and spends two hours a day at the gym to work off last night's cheesecake. Drugs, surgery, a worthy person should do anything to help win the weight-loss game.

It may come as a surprise to learn that these common assumptions are not supported by science or reason. Buying into them is the true source of our collective discontent. Conversely, understanding the reality behind these weight myths can be your journey to salvation.

So let's do some debunking.

- Fat is not the killer we've been led to believe.
- Fat's role in poor health has been greatly exaggerated.
- Dieting and exercise are not effective techniques for long-term weight loss.

We can choose to appreciate the body we are living in . . . and move on. We can adopt good health habits and let our weight fall where it will naturally.

There's a revolution happening. It's called "Health at Every Size." Participation is simple: Honor the body you live in. Take good care of it. Develop and nurture connections with others. Eat well. Find pleasurable ways of moving. Live fully.

The road to health and happiness is wide enough to include **you**—and everyone who crosses over that arbitrary boundary we call "fat."

Want the data, rationale, and a strategy that supports this way of living? Check out *Health at Every Size: The Surprising Truth About Your Weight* (www.HAESbook.com).

A MESSAGE FOR PEOPLE WHO HAVE DISEASES BLAMED ON THEIR WEIGHT

Maybe you think that if you'd done a better job of controlling your food intake and weight, you wouldn't have diabetes or heart disease or hypertension—or whatever your diagnosis is. But chances are you've tried to diet and manage your weight. Perhaps you shed some pounds that later returned. You wonder why you can't just take better care of yourself.

Stop blaming yourself!

The scientific reality is that genes play a greater role than weight in the development of all diseases associated with weight, including diabetes, atherosclerosis, hypertension, and cancer. We're all born with challenges written into our genetic code; this just happens to be your challenge. Your body is genetically vulnerable to a particular disease(s) and environmental components triggered that genetic propensity. While other people may be able to live a lifestyle that allows them to not pay much attention to how they eat and how active they are, this lifestyle doesn't work as well for you. It's just the way it is, and learning to accept it will bring unexpected benefits into your life.

Your diagnosis woke you up to the fact that your body is having trouble. Now you can rise to the challenge. You can learn how to better manage your health and nourish yourself.

The first step to healing is to let go of those assumptions that stop you from moving on, starting with the idea that you need to lose weight. The value of achieving and maintaining weight loss has long been an unchallenged assumption for so many diseases and you may be surprised to learn that there is very little evidence as to its veracity. In fact, an abundance of evidence suggests the pursuit of weight loss is actually harmful, setting us up for physical and emotional difficulties and distracting us from what really matters.

While it is true that some diseases are *associated* with weight, that just means these diseases are more likely to be found in heavier people—not that that the weight itself causes the disease. The research that determines these associations rarely considers such factors as fitness, activity, history of dieting, stress, nutrient intake, weight cycling, or socioeconomic status. Yet all play a role.

When studies *do* control for these factors, the increased risk of disease disappears or is significantly reduced. What's likely going on is that some or all of these other factors increase disease risk as well as the risk of weight gain. In other words, there's much more involved in the relationship between weight and disease than weight itself. The role of weight has been misrepresented and exaggerated.

All health indicators, such as blood pressure, cholesterol levels, or blood sugar control, can be improved through lifestyle changes, even without weight loss.

The new paradigm in health care is called Health at Every Size (HAES). HAES encourages you to focus on wellness rather than body size, making changes that more directly affect your health and well-being. HAES helps you focus on what truly matters and allows your body to determine the weight that's best for you.

Can HAES really help me improve my health?

The answer is a resounding YES! HAES has been evaluated in several studies and the results published in well-respected scientific journals. The studies find that HAES is much more effective in improving health than the pursuit of weight loss is. They also show that people enjoy HAES and are much more likely to make it a part of their lives on an ongoing basis than dieting. This enjoyment leads to ongoing changes in eating and exercise behaviors—changes that can last a lifetime.

Is it really okay to stop trying to lose weight?

It's not only okay—it's the basis of positive change. Living a *Health at Every Size* lifestyle isn't about giving up, it's about moving on.

This commentary was abridged and adapted from the article, "Reclaiming Pleasure in Eating," by Linda Bacon and Judith Matz, *Diabetes Management* magazine, (2010, in press).

For more information, check out *Health at Every Size: The Surprising Truth About Your Weight* (www.HAESbook.com).

A MESSAGE FOR PEOPLE
CONSIDERING THEIR NEXT DIET

This is for you if you are contemplating your next weight loss attempt. Maybe you're making a list of the foods you plan to give up, the food journal you plan to keep, the calorie-counting you'll do. You're picturing the deprivation and the forced exercise, resenting it but feeling that there's no other way to get the body you want, the *smaller* body you crave. You're also thinking about all the wonderful rewards that come with a thinner you, such as attention, admiration, and respect. The possibility of thinness is stronger than any concern about how hard and uncomfortable it will be to get there. You're motivated and ready!

Before you jump on the diet bandwagon yet again, however, I'd like to encourage you to think farther into the future—*after* you lose weight. Think two years from now, when it's quite likely that you'll have returned to your starting weight, maybe even higher. I understand that you don't want to consider this. You're probably tempted to stop reading now and are angry at the spoilsport "friend" who slipped you this paper.

Indulge me for just a few more paragraphs. I don't intend to take away your hope, but, instead, to help you reframe your thoughts so you can actually achieve what you're looking for.

It's way too easy to believe that a thin body will right everything wrong in your world. That your life will automatically improve once you're thin enough to take the steps you feel your weight prevents you from taking today. But it won't. The reality is that this fantasy of weight loss is what's stopping you from achieving your dreams—not your weight itself. The pursuit of weight loss rarely produces the thin, happy life many people dream of.

It's also way too easy to believe that you can control your weight through disciplined diet and exercise. The science just doesn't support that myth. The reality is that biologic safeguards underlie your body's resistance to maintaining weight loss. Research demonstrates that most people, regardless of willpower or diet or exercise, regain the weight they lose. In fact, research shows that dieting is a strong predictor of weight gain! *It's not your fault* that you are among the majority who hasn't been able to keep off the weight thus far.

I'm not asking you to give up on your dreams. What I am suggesting is that you move on. When you stop trying to control your weight, you allow your body to do the job for you—naturally and much more effectively. If you stop fighting yourself, achieving and maintaining a weight that is healthy for your body becomes effortless.

Just think how much fun it would be if you didn't have to worry about your weight!

Curious about the science that supports this? Want strategies and support for getting in tune with your body? Check out *Health at Every Size: The Surprising Truth About Your Weight* (www.HAESbook.com).

Health at Every Size has been evaluated in several research studies, the results published in top scientific journals. Adopting a Health at Every Size lifestyle can give you what you want much more effectively than a diet ever will. You have nothing to lose by trying.

And be nice to the friend who gave you this! He or she is trying to support you in achieving *your* goals.

A MESSAGE FOR PEOPLE CONSIDERING · BARIATRIC SURGERY

Bariatric surgery is among the highest-paying surgical specialties, which may partially explain why accuracy and integrity in reporting the results of these operations tend to go by the wayside. Combine that with the vulnerability of patients (desperation to lose weight is not conducive to good judgment) and bariatric surgery is a setup for disaster.

We are misled about the extent and severity of the health risks associated with weight. We are also told that bariatric surgery is a solution for those health risks. It's not.

Bariatric surgery is better described as a high-risk, disease-inducing, cosmetic surgery - not a health-enhancing procedure. Unlike a diet, however, you usually can't abandon it when you realize you made a mistake, despite claims otherwise.

Bottom line: Bariatric surgery is a big decision with life-altering results. Make yours an informed decision. Consider the facts and stories not being told.

To learn the other side of the story:

- Read *Health at Every Size: The Surprising Truth About Your Weight*, by Linda Bacon. An excerpt from the book that discusses bariatric surgery is available at www.HAESbook.com.
- Read the bariatric surgery series at the JunkFood Science blog: http://junkfoodscience.blogspot.com.
- Check out the Obesity Surgery Information Center: http://obesitysurgery-info.com. Be sure to read the personal testimonials.
- Surf over to http://suethsayings.blogspot.com and read about "The reality of obesity, weight loss surgery and other things."

■ Read the personal story: *I Want To Live: Gastric Bypass Reversal*, by Dani Hart.

There is an evidence-based compassionate alternative to bariatric surgery: Health at Every Size. To learn more, visit www.HAES book.com.

A MESSAGE FOR HEALTH CARE PROVIDERS AND ADMINISTRATORS AND STAFF OF OBESITY PREVENTION OR TREATMENT PROGRAMS

Obesity is said to have reached epidemic proportions, posing drastic threats to public health, increasing morbidity, mortality and health care costs, and lowering quality of life. These concerns have spawned obesity prevention and treatment efforts by many well-intentioned and caring people.

However, scientific research shows that these common assumptions just don't hold up to the evidence. For example, dozens of studies indicate that weight doesn't adversely affect longevity for the vast majority of people—and less than a handful of studies suggest otherwise. And when factors such as activity, nutrition, dieting and weight cycling history, and socioeconomic status are considered, the relationship between weight and disease disappears or is significantly reduced. Studies also show that biologic safeguards prevent most people from maintaining weight loss, despite vigilant dieting and exercise.

Trumpeting obesity concerns and admonishing people to lose weight is not just misguided, but downright damaging. It leads to repeated cycles of weight loss and regain, to food and body preoccupation, self-hatred, eating disorders, weight discrimination, and poor health. Few of us are at peace with our bodies, whether because we're fat or because we fear becoming fat. Every time you make fat the problem, these are side effects, however unintended they may be.

This is an important turning point in history. The weight of the evidence clearly trumps the assumptions of the current paradigm. I urge you: Be part of the solution, not the problem. The price society pays when you do not challenge yourself is too high.

There is an evidence-based, compassionate alternative to the war on obesity. It's called *Health at Every Size*. It involves switching your focus from weight to health and supporting your patients in doing the same. Everyone can benefit from good health behaviors.

For more information:

- Check out the book, *Health at Every Size: The Surprising Truth About Your Weight* (www.HAEbook.com); the website includes many free downloads.
- The (free) HAES Community Resources (www.HAES Community.Org) helps you find resources and individuals supporting HAES and allows you to register your voice.
- Consider joining the Association for Size Diversity and Health (www.sizediversityandhealth.org), an organization for professionals committed to HAES values.

A MESSAGE FOR LEGISLATORS/ POLITICIANS ON OBESITY TREATMENT AND PREVENTION POLICIES

Obesity is a hot topic in health care reform. It is said to have reached epidemic proportions, posing drastic threats to public health, increasing morbidity, mortality and health care costs, and lowering quality of life. These concerns have spawned a variety of obesity prevention and treatment efforts.

Despite good intentions, these obesity policies have backfired, causing more problems than they solve. Americans *are* trying to lose weight, but efforts at weight management generally result in repeated cycles of damaging weight loss and regain, food and weight preoccupation, reduced self-esteem, feelings of failure, and increased risk for life-threatening eating disorders. As Americans strive to shed pounds, they move further away from the original intent of improved health.

The focused attention on weight has also led to an increase in stigmatization and weight discrimination, to the extent that discrimination based on weight now equals or exceeds that based on race or gender. Weight-based discrimination reduces quality of life and worsens health.

Every time you make fat the problem, these are side effects, however unintended they may be.

We've got some tough decisions looming in health care policy. As we consider various health reform policies, whether they're about nutrition labeling in restaurants, taxing beverages and snack foods, incentivizing health behaviors, or building school gardens, let's direct them towards health promotion instead of obesity prevention. When we consider health insurance, let's ensure that people of all sizes have equal access to compassionate and unbiased health care.

We need to remove the obstacles that get in the way of people of all sizes making healthy choices. Health policies that are promoted for their own sake, rather than as obesity prevention measures, are more likely to bring about desired results—and without the damaging consequences that come when done in the name of obesity prevention. All people deserve access to good food, useful nutrition information, and exercise opportunities. Everyone should feel welcome in the White House garden—which just won't happen when it is promoted for the prevention of obesity.

There is an evidence-based, compassionate alternative to the war on obesity. It's called Health at Every Size. It involves switching our focus from weight to the behaviors that make people healthy. Everyone can benefit from good health behaviors.

More information can be found in *Health at Every Size: The Surprising Truth About Your Weight* (www.HAESbook.com) and at the HAES Community Resources (www.HAESCommunity.org).

A MESSAGE FOR SCHOOL
ADMINISTRATORS AND TEACHERS

Much concern has been expressed about children's weight, spurring a variety of school-based interventions such as body mass index (BMI) screening, weight-related "report cards," and campaigns emphasizing the dangers of carrying excess weight.

These anti-obesity campaigns are damaging and ineffective. Think about the impact of BMI report cards: the heavier kids get pathologized, bullied, and teased by their peers, and are put on diets and exercise programs that set them up for a lifetime of struggle, feelings of failure, and a greater risk for developing a life-threatening eating disorder. The thinner kids—who may have similar health habits or be maintaining their low weights through damaging diets or obsessive exercise—get ignored. Meanwhile, every child across the weight spectrum is saddled with a fear of fat and a bias against fat people.

It's tough enough for kids to enjoy their bodies. Few are at peace in their bodies, whether they're fat or fear becoming fat. Every time we make fat the problem, these are side effects, however unintended they may be.

Eating well and being regularly active are valuable for kids of all sizes. Good health habits can be promoted for their own sake, rather than as obesity prevention measures.

Here are a few ideas you can implement in your school:

- Take the focus off weight and put it on health and self-esteem. Dump weight-based programs like BMI screening.
- Teach children that their bodies deserve love and respect no matter how much they weigh.
- Implement media literacy programs that challenge the current thin ideal in the media. Discuss body size as a diversity issue as you would race or gender.

- Avoid words like "overweight" and "obese," which promote judgment and stigma.
- Create an environment that supports enjoyable physical activity, honoring that different body types are suited to different types of movement. A fat child may have more difficulty running than a thin child, for example, but may excel at swimming.
- Encourage kids to honor their body signals of hunger, fullness, and appetite. Discourage dieting; all diets undermine the dieters' ability to trust their own capacity to meet their own needs. It also sets the dieter up for feelings of failure and inadequacy.
- Display artwork and images in your classroom that celebrate children of varying sizes.
- Enforce zero-tolerance policies regarding weight-based victimization and bullying. Be available and approachable to students who are victims of such bullying.
- You are a role model for students. Challenge your own size bias and incorporate healthy habits and attitudes into your own life.

It's hard to challenge the common dogma that stigmatizes weight and promotes dieting as a virtue. But there is substantial evidence that these ideas have backfired, causing more problems than they solve. Educate yourself about the new paradigm in health promotion, which has proven to be much more successful than fighting obesity. It's called Health at Every Size.

More details can be found in the book, *Health at Every Size: The Surprising Truth about Your Weight* (www.HAESbook.com). Visit the HAES Community Resources (www.HAESCommunity.Org) to get connected with the community and discover school-based programs that incorporate Health at Every Size.

A MESSAGE FOR FITNESS PROFESSIONALS

No doubt you got into the fitness field because you're enthusiastic about good health and want to support and inspire others. However, you may be surprised to learn that some of the most basic assumptions you hold about weight and health aren't supported by scientific evidence. Despite your best intentions, the work you are doing may actually *harm* your clients.

Consider the calorie balance equation. You and your clients likely believe that if they just increase the amount of calories expended relative to the amount taken in, they should lose weight, right? Exercise should be the ultimate panacea in the weight war since it burns calories in the moment while also building muscle, an ongoing calorie-burning furnace.

Unfortunately, it doesn't work that way. We can't control the calorie balance equation to the extent we've long believed. It's easy in the short term, which is why short-term weight loss typically occurs. But over the long-term the body has compensatory mechanisms that undermine its ability to maintain weight loss. Long-term studies show that few people maintain significant weight or fat loss by increasing their physical activity, *even when exercise habits are maintained*.

Another common misconception is that thin=fit. But did you know that it's possible to be both fat and fit? And that research consistently shows that fitness is a much better indicator of health than weight? Not only are there are plenty of metabolically healthy fat people, but when you take fitness into account, many of the health risks associated with weight disappear or, at the very least, are significantly reduced.

I know it may be hard to believe these contentions given the current bias in the field. But when you consider that supporting people in their weight-loss goals is not just misguided, it's downright damaging, it becomes critical that you consider these challenges seriously. After all, you want to help people, not hurt them, right?

The reality is that few of us are at peace with our bodies, whether because we're fat or because we fear becoming fat. Repeated cycles of weight loss and regain, unhealthy weight loss behaviors, poor body image, eating disorders, stress, stigmatization, and discrimination are all collateral damage in the war against fat. Every time you make fat the problem, these are the side effects, however unintended they may be.

It doesn't have to be that way. Here's an easy prescription to do good:

- Support your clients in focusing on health and well-being, not weight. Help them understand that the problem is in cultural attitudes about weight, not their body.
- Support your clients in handling the unique challenges they may have with their bodies. Show compassion for the difficulties that arise from living in a culturally stigmatized body.
- Provide a friendly, non-judgmental environment that acknowledges and celebrates body diversity.
- Help your clients develop *sustainable* behavioral changes that easily fit into their busy lives.

For more information, check out *Health at Every Size: The Surprising Truth About Your Weight* (www.HAESbook.com).

A MESSAGE FOR PEOPLE COMMITTED TO FOOD JUSTICE AND SUSTAINABLE AGRICULTURE

You care about sustainability and you're committed to making a difference. Obesity, viewed as a visible result of a food system gone wrong, is an easy rallying call.

But here's the rub. No matter how often and authoritatively you trumpet fears about obesity, scientific research shows that common assumptions just don't hold up to the evidence. Despite assumptions to the contrary, research shows that the fat and thin are not eating remarkably differently. The fact that some people are heavier is largely a reflection of their particular biological response to current lifestyle habits and environmental conditions. Research also shows that lifestyle changes are much more effective at health improvement than weight loss, even in those rare cases where weight loss is maintained. What we do is much more important than what we weigh.

Trumpeting obesity concerns is not just misguided, but downright damaging. It leads to repeated cycles of weight loss and regain, to food and body preoccupation, self-hatred, eating disorders, weight discrimination, and poor health. Few of us are at peace with our bodies, whether because we're fat or because we fear becoming fat. Every time you make fat the problem, these are side effects, however unintended they may be.

By encouraging good food policy on its own merits, you can address real health concerns, giving both fat and thin people the support they deserve, and avoiding stigmatizing people and worsening the problem.

There is relatively little size diversity among people participating in the food justice movement. This has less to do with the idea that heavier people don't share a commitment to good food, and more to do with the community stigmatization. Given that the majority of the U.S. population now fits into the stigmatized categories, anti-obesity campaigns alienate a huge pool of potential supporters and sabotage the cause.

Foodies, I plead with you: Lay off the fat people. Science and reason do not support the value of a weight focus. Switch the emphasis to advocating for good food directly. Stop the demonization and instead invite fat people to join you at the table, celebrating the diversity they bring. Help people of all sizes feel welcome in the White House organic garden. You can make a powerful argument for good food based on social justice, environmental stewardship, animal welfare, or a host of other reasons—you don't need to do it on the backs of fat people.

If you examine the data with an open mind, you can also find some other facts that may surprise you. Did you know that the obesity epidemic—if there ever was such a thing—is long over: child, teen, and adult obesity rates leveled off years ago? That dozens of studies indicate that weight doesn't adversely affect longevity for the vast majority of people—and less than a handful of studies suggest otherwise? And when factors such as activity, nutrition, dieting and weight cycling history, and socioeconomic status are considered, the relationship between weight and disease disappears or is significantly reduced? Studies also show that biologic safeguards prevent most people from maintaining weight loss, despite vigilant dieting and exercise.

Get on board with the new paradigm that shifts the emphasis from weight to health. It's called Health at Every Size. More information can be found in *Health at Every Size: The Surprising Truth About Your Weight* (www.HAESbook.com).

A MESSAGE FOR JOURNALISTS/ WRITERS/PEOPLE IN THE MEDIA ON COVERING WEIGHT CONCERNS

A growing number of scientists, health professionals, civil rights advocates, educators, and other concerned people are challenging conventional ideas about weight. We argue that many currently accepted ideas are unsupported by scientific evidence and have resulted in significant damage to people of all body sizes.

Assumptions that support the current weight paradigm are so strongly part of our cultural landscape that they are not even recognized, with the result that fairness and accuracy in reporting get compromised. For example, did you know that the "obesity epidemic"—if there ever was one—is long over: child, teen and adult obesity rates leveled off years ago? That dozens of studies indicate that weight doesn't adversely affect longevity for the vast majority of people—and less than a handful of studies suggest otherwise? And when factors such as activity, nutrition, dieting and weight cycling history, and socioeconomic status are considered, the relationship between weight and disease disappears or is greatly lessened? Studies also show that biologic safeguards prevent most people from maintaining weight loss, despite vigilant dieting and exercise.

Despite ample evidence published in top scientific journals, these contentions are rarely given credence or fair exposure in the media. If we are to truly provide accurate information and improve the health of the American people, it is time to challenge status quo belief systems about weight and health.

To be fair-minded, consider the following points when reporting stories on weight:

- Recognize that just because something is conventionally accepted doesn't mean it's true. Journalists have an obligation to remain open-minded and give air time to perspectives that aren't typically heard.

■ Listen to and report on what fat people have to say—and keep an open mind. Don't make assumptions about their health practices and don't limit your story to "experts" describing the experiences of fat people. "Nothing about us without us" is a rallying call of many stigmatized groups.

■ Stage fair fights. If you interview a health expert talking about the dangers of obesity, pair her or him with a health expert who can dispute the conventional view of weight and health. Paring a conventional obesity "expert" with a fat person talking about their experience is an unfair setup.

■ Show images of fat people being physically active, eating nutritious foods, and participating in their lives, rather than the usual photos that reinforce the stereotypes. Depict fat people as complete human beings. The typical stock photo of the "headless fatty" is dehumanizing. It sends a message that this body is so shameful that it doesn't deserve a face.

■ Language has meaning. Think about terms like "obesity," "overweight" and "fat" and what they convey. Discover why a growing number of health professionals don't use the terms "overweight" or "obesity."

■ When you report on weight loss, be sure to consider long-term evidence. Many techniques deliver short-term, but those results can be deceptive when the long term is considered.

■ Cover stories about people doing work to help people of all sizes improve their health without a focus on weight or weight loss.

■ Remember that the proliferation of stories about the evils of fat and other misinformation can contribute to an increase in unhealthy weight loss behaviors, painful food and weight preoccupation, damaging cycles of weight loss and regain, poor body image, life-threatening eating disorders, stress, stigmatization, and discrimination. Don't be part of the problem.

The media hold considerable power. Use yours respectfully.

To learn more about these issues, check out *Health at Every Size: The Surprising Truth About Your Weight* (www.HAESbook.com) or contact Dr. Linda Bacon at linda@lindabacon.org. Other helpful resources include The Association for Size Diversity and Health (www.sizediversityandhealth.org) and the National Association to Advance Fat Acceptance (www.NAAFA.org).

A MESSAGE FOR THERAPISTS
ON COMPASSIONATE THERAPY
FOR WEIGHT CONCERNS

We are all raised with assumptions that fat is bad, that the pursuit of weight loss is positive self-care, and that body weight can be controlled through dietary change and exercise. These assumptions are so strongly a part of our cultural landscape that they are regarded as self-evident. As a result, many well-intentioned, caring people unknowingly collude and transmit these and other cultural biases regarding weight. A review of the science shows, however, that these ideas are social constructs that stand in the way of healthy development.

As therapists, it is important for us to look deeply at our biases and the ways they may show up in our work with clients. Taking the steps to identify your own implicit assumptions about body size, eating behaviors, and health will minimize the potential of your beliefs negatively influencing the way you work with those who come to you for help. The Health at Every Size (HAES) movement can help you develop a framework for conceptualizing weight and working with weight concerns. I encourage you to educate yourself about HAES.

Here are some suggestions on how to conceptualize and work with three common scenarios from a HAES perspective.

1. Clients on diets.
When clients announce they have just started a diet, you may feel tempted to view this as positive self-care and want to support their plan. Diets are seductive in their ability to make people believe that following a prescribed structure can bring about a feeling of "doing something." However, following the rules of an outside authority

undermines dieters' ability to trust their own capacity to meet their own needs. It also sets them up for feelings of failure and inadequacy. Sound science shows that biology often underlies the inability to sustain weight loss, even when that weight loss results from positive behavior change.

People who say they want to lose weight are speaking in code. It is up to you to help your clients identify what they are really looking for. Is it happiness, respect, health, feeling attractive? You can help your clients refocus their awareness on what they are really looking for and affirm their right to live in the world no matter what their size or shape.

If a client believes weight is the problem, then weight loss becomes the only solution. But if you reassure your client that his or her body is acceptable just as it is, your client can begin to pull their energy away from weight loss towards self-care behaviors that honor who they really are.

2. Clients who lose weight.

When clients share their success at weight loss, it is natural to want to celebrate with them. Doing so, however, affirms that thinner is "better." It also reinforces bad feelings if (when) the weight returns. Instead, help your clients re-frame their achievement as a positive behavior change and self-nurturance. They can hold on to that regardless of their weight outcome.

3. Fat vs. Thin Clients.

Behaviors such as counting calories (or carbs or fat grams), using exercise to burn calories, exercising several times a day, etc., are suspicious when they come from an "underweight" client, raising a red flag for eating disorders. But larger clients who talk about these same behaviors are often applauded. Help your clients see that it's not how big or small they are, but how they nourish themselves that is important.

For more information about Health at Every Size:

■ Check out *Health at Every Size: The Surprising Truth About Your Weight* (www.HAESbook.com).

■ Consider joining the Association for Size Diversity and Health (www.sizediversityandhealth.org), an organization for HAES-sensitive professionals.

■ Visit the (free) HAES Community Resources (www.HAES Community.org) to register your voice, inform others about your work, and learn about other HAES-sensitive individuals and resources.

A MESSAGE FOR PEOPLE WHO HAVE LOST WEIGHT

So you've lost some weight and kept it off for a while. Perhaps you worked hard for your weight loss, enduring a restrictive diet or challenging exercise program. Or maybe you lost your weight by skipping one dessert at a time. Regardless, you must be feeling quite proud of yourself and enjoying the attention and praise from others.

Often, when people lose weight they want to tell everyone about their accomplishment. Maybe you feel like you've found the secret—and you want to share it with others. Plus, many of your friends and coworkers may be asking you for advice on how to do what you've done.

The problem with doing this is that there are many factors that influence weight and they are highly individual. While your strategy worked for you, it is unlikely it will work for someone else. Someone could eat exactly what you ate, exercise the same way and in the same amounts, and still end up with completely different results. In fact, odds are they will. After all, you are the statistical anomaly. Research shows that the vast majority of people who lose weight regain it—often with additional pounds.

Think about it this way. Suppose you won the lottery by choosing numbers based on your children's birth years. Would you tell others that if they did the same they, too, could win the lottery? Of course not. You recognize that you beat the odds—the lottery was about chance, not skill.

Weight loss is exactly the same. Oh sure, you may *think* it's different. After all, *everyone knows* that if people just ate less and exercised more they could lose weight. Right?

Wrong!

While it is commonly believed that losing weight is a simple matter of taking in fewer calories than you burn off in exercise, research shows this just isn't true. It may work on a short-term basis, but the vast majority of people have built in biological compensatory mechanisms that prevent diet and exercise from working in the long-term.

So when you share your weight-loss success with others, you may actually be setting them up to fail, rendering serious physical and emotional harm in the process.

Am I advising you to tell others to give up? Absolutely not. But instead of focusing on the weight, focus on the healthy things you did to get where you are such as taking good care of yourself, eating well, and engaging in regular physical activity. When you support these behaviors, disentangle them from the weight loss. Because the majority of people won't lose weight or, even if they *do* lose weight, it will be temporary. You don't want their feelings of failure on your conscience, do you?

Talking about your weight loss could backfire on you, too. If you happen to gain some weight back, you might feel like you've failed and be tempted to stop your health-promoting behaviors. So it is important that you make life-enhancing choices for yourself regardless of the impact it may have on your weight. Eating healthfully and moving joyfully have health benefits regardless of weight loss.

Please don't promote the belief that if someone is disciplined enough, they can *choose* to be thin. This is not true for the vast majority of people. Many fat people face a great deal of discrimination and stereotyping because of the false belief that weight loss just takes discipline.

If you want to encourage people to exercise without shaming them, say something like: "I feel really good when I run. Want to try it?", rather than saying, "I've lost weight running; maybe you should try it."

We live in a culture that stigmatizes fatness. Focusing on weight loss continues this misperception and mistreatment of people who are simply a bigger size than this culture says they should be. Please don't be a part of the fat hatred that consumes our society and causes countless eating disorders, body hatred, despair, discrimination, suffering, and misery. Think about the impact of what you say on other people. Everyone deserves to feel good about themself and enjoy their life, regardless of their size.

You have the opportunity to help people pursue healthy lifestyle choices for the sake of their health and general well being. You also have the opportunity to do a lot of damage. Which route will you choose?

For more information, check out *Health at Every Size: The Surprising Truth About Your Weight* (www.HAESbook.com).

REFLECTIONS ON THIN PRIVILEGE
AND RESPONSIBILITY

The word "privilege" is used to describe receiving unjust advantages at the expense of others. These advantages are often largely invisible—especially to those who enjoy them. For instance, I have what is called "thin privilege," a consequence of weight discrimination.

Because I'm relatively thin, it's been easier for me to meet and get approval from other people. This has helped me make friends, find a life partner, develop professional contacts, and secure jobs. It also means I am treated with greater respect when I shop or eat in a restaurant. It means I have a larger choice of fashions at less expensive prices and never have to pay for more than one airline seat, making travel and its accompanying opportunities more accessible. I could go on for days listing the ways in which I have benefited from others' perception of my weight, but I believe these simple examples make the point. I can think of very little in my life that is untainted by "thin privilege."

Thin privilege is as strong as it is because weight bias is so pervasive. Research documents that fatter people face discrimination in employment (including lower wages), barriers in education, biased attitudes and lower quality of care from health professionals, stereotypes in the media, stigma in interpersonal relationships, and, overall, are judged negatively and treated with less respect. Weight discrimination has reached such great proportions that it now equals or exceeds discrimination based on race and gender.

In addition to the advantages thinner people receive from thin privilege, however, there are also costs. For instance, since I know that fat people are expected to meet greater demands for achievement, I can't have a full sense of legitimacy in *my* achievements. I know that I landed my nutrition professorship in part because many potential competitors were eliminated before they even reached the rigors of academia while other were weeded out along the way due to others' biased assumptions about their nutritional habits. We do not live in a meritocracy.

Another cost we pay is not being able to feel truly valued for who we are. This is commonly noticed by people who lose weight and suddenly get more attention. They also feel enormous pressure, worried that if they regain the weight they will lose their new-found admirers. This wreaks havoc with their self-esteem.

All of us regularly judge and react to others. Sadly, we have all perpetuated weight bias ourselves. When we are subjected repeatedly to images of fat people as lazy gluttons, to images of thin people as attractive, desirable, and healthy, to notions that weight is completely controllable by diet and exercise or that fat causes people to get sick and die early, it should come as no surprise that these ideas have become ingrained in our psyches. Yet these "beliefs" are nothing more than cultural constructs of dubious scientific and social merit.[1]

Weight bias harms everyone across the size spectrum. To understand how it might harm thinner people, consider these examples:

■ As long as it is more difficult to live in a fat body, everyone fears becoming fat. The internalization of the belief that thinner is better drives the body anxiety that most people—fat *or* thin—experience. It fuels our preoccupation with obtaining or maintaining that "ideal" weight and conjures up the feelings of shame if we don't. It also supports the development of eating disorders.

---

[1] This is a short essay on thin privilege and it's beyond space constraints to bust those myths here. For easy reading on those topics, download the "Health at Every Size (HAES) Manifesto" at www.HAESbook.com, or, for more detail, check out my book, *Health at Every Size: The Surprising Truth About Your Weight.*

■ An enormous amount of time, money, and energy is wasted trying to maintain or achieve a thinner body. Many of us put many aspects of our lives on hold until we achieve those elusive results. We avoid certain clothes, skip out on parties or other social ventures, postpone job searches, or hide in the background, not wanting to draw attention to ourselves until we lose the weight and feel more presentable.

■ The oppressive values we absorb limit our world. When prejudice rears its ugly head, we become blinded by our preconceptions, unable to see people for who they really are. We are cheated out of seeing people in all their wonderful uniqueness because we've formed ideas about who they are long before we can really know someone. How many friendships and networking opportunities do we miss out on due to this prejudice?

Until our society fundamentally changes, we can't completely escape or renounce the various privileges we have, whether it's based on our size, skin color, socioeconomic status, education, or other attributes. We're taught to recognize oppression as individual acts of meanness, not as a system (often invisible) conferring advantages. It may be painful to own our role as unfairly advantaged individuals, reaping benefits that at the same time limit and hurt others and ourselves. But whether or not you have actively chosen your privilege, if you are committed to fairness and social justice, I challenge you to be accountable for it; unearned privilege comes with responsibility.

Tips on Living Responsibly with Thin Privilege

Reflect on your privilege. How would your life be different if you were heavier? Think about your daily activities, whether it's meeting a new person, buying a candy bar, ordering fried chicken, shopping for clothes, or speaking out on weight bias. Would others view or treat you differently? Would *you* feel more or less self-conscious about others' judgments? More or less entitled in whatever you're doing?

If you think weight bias doesn't affect you, if you're not outraged by what you learn from this exercise, keep repeating it until you understand. It may be hard to see yourself as a person of privilege; after all, you probably sincerely want to do the right thing and be a good person. Give yourself a break. You can accept your privilege without blaming yourself. No one expects you to carry the weight of our culture's sins on your shoulders alone. You can use your privilege to make this a fairer, more compassionate world.

Challenge your assumptions about weight. No doubt you have absorbed some of the assumptions of our culture without critical thought. It's not too late to do that critical thinking. Listen to what fat people say about their own lives and read the exposés that have been written about weight. Commit to fighting oppression. Explore the movements for Health at Every Size and Fat Acceptance.

Use your privilege responsibly.
What are you going to do to lessen or end it?

This is an abridged version of a longer article that can be accessed through the Resources link at www.LindaBacon.org.

More information can be found in *Health at Every Size: The Surprising Truth About Your Weight* (www.HAESbook.com).

FINAL WORDS:
FOR HEALTH PROFESSIONALS RESISTANT TO HEALTH AT EVERY SIZE

So you've been exposed to the **Health at Every Size** concept and still you don't agree with it. Resistance is understandable. Beliefs such as "Fat poses substantial risk to health and longevity," "Dieting is a helpful strategy for improving health," and "Anyone can achieve permanent weight loss if only they try hard enough" are firmly embedded in our medical ideology and culture. Why should you challenge these ideas when they appear so well-established and well-supported?

Because we're losing the war on obesity. No matter how authoritatively we repeat the "lose weight" mantra, America's average weight is not declining. Instead of helping people get healthier, we've inadvertently supported rampant food and body preoccupation, damaging cycles of weight loss and regain, eating disorders, reduced self-esteem, weight discrimination, and poor health. We are violating the basic tenet of medical practice: "First, do no harm." Rather than take responsibility for our failed paradigm, we blame our patients for failed weight loss attempts and don't consider the well-documented biological resistance to weight loss or other challenges.

Health at Every Size (HAES) is the new paradigm, providing a compassionate alternative to the war on obesity. No harm comes from supporting people of all sizes in adopting good health behaviors.

It may be particularly difficult for educated health professionals to consider HAES seriously. Ironically, our education gets in the way of our ability to learn. The more experienced and "expert" we are in a particular field, the more likely we are to apply our "knowledge."

This can prevent us from giving serious consideration to innovative ideas.

The lens of conventional assumptions taints nearly every weight-related paper published in scientific journals. When we see the well-established association between weight and certain diseases, for example, we extrapolate that weight is the problem. It is only when we let go of conventional assumptions that other possibilities emerge. For instance, how much of the association between weight and health risk can be explained by damage caused by the weight cycling resulting from repeated diet attempts? How much is caused by the stress response resulting from weight bias? In actuality, some of the health risk may be iatrogenic, caused by the assumptions of the currently accepted weight paradigm rather than adiposity itself. Some of the risk can also be explained by lifestyle habits that are common across the weight spectrum, not physically obvious in people with a lesser biologic propensity to store fat. We ignore this at-risk "normal weight" population because of our weight focus.

It can be threatening to consider the ramifications that may come if you adopt HAES: Would it jeopardize your career if you stopped promoting weight loss? Would you lose the respect of colleagues if you adopted such a contrarian view? What would it feel like to assume a position that provokes considerable resistance? It takes a lot of courage to open your mind to a challenge when the stakes are so high.

Indeed, it may not be a conscious choice to avoid fully engaging with the HAES challenge. Many of us have strong defense mechanisms that keep us rooted to the safe and familiar. Defense mechanisms frequently operate below the level of conscious thought, allowing us to dismiss information before it threatens our worldview.

But you owe it to yourself and others to take on this challenge. Too much damage has already occurred as a result of misguided quests to support good health.

———

I'd like to end with some words of support for those of you who do rise to the HAES challenge. In the past, you may have recommended weight loss, thinking it was a responsible and kind thing to do. It can be very painful to reflect back on your history and consider that the advice you gave was actually quite destructive. It's not uncommon for people to feel considerable grief when they first embrace HAES.

Don't be too hard on yourself. You were well intentioned and did the best you could given the information you had at the time. You didn't invent the problem. But you can seize the opportunity to undo that damage now. You will not be alone. There is a large community of health care professionals committed to HAES. Join us! Consider joining the Association for Size Diversity and Health (ASDAH) at www.sizediversityandhealth.org, an association for HAES professionals.

For more information, read *Health at Every Size: The Surprising Truth About Your Weight* (www.HAESbook.com). Visit the HAES Community Resources (www.HAESCommunity.org) to learn more about your colleagues and to register your voice.

FOR PEOPLE WHO CONSIDER SIZE
ACCEPTANCE DANGEROUS

We've all heard the weight fears: obesity is said to have reached epidemic proportions, posing drastic threats to public health, increasing morbidity, mortality and health care costs, and lowering quality of life. Many well-intentioned people strongly believe that we need to fight obesity and that people who promote size acceptance are dangerous.

But here's the rub. History shows that admonishing people to lose weight is just plain ineffective. The weight loss literature has been consistent for decades: while many weight loss methods are successful for short-term weight loss, only a tiny minority of people actually maintain that weight loss over the long term. Whether you blame willpower or accept the more scientific argument that biologic mechanisms underlie the resistance to weight loss, the simple fact remains: admonishments to lose weight don't result in maintained weight loss for the vast majority of people. You can choose to adopt a self-righteous attitude and blame the individual, or, you can take responsibility and acknowledge that for whatever reason, your advice is not achieving the desired outcome.

Trumpeting obesity fears and hounding people to lose weight is not just ineffective, but downright damaging. They lead to repeated cycles of weight loss and regain, to food and body preoccupation, self-hatred, eating disorders, weight discrimination, and poor health. Few of us are at peace with our bodies, whether because we're fat or because we fear becoming fat. Every time you make fat the problem, these are side effects, however unintended they may be.

Those of us who advocate for size acceptance care deeply about people's health. A large scientific literature demonstrates that improved health behaviors can improve health directly, regardless of whether weight changes. The psychological literature additionally indicates that people make better health choices when they feel better about themselves.

The argument for size acceptance doesn't need to depend on whether you accept the considerable challenges to the current assumptions about weight and health. It's really very simple: Your strategy has not only failed, but backfired. Shame doesn't help people make better health choices—though it does contribute to considerable "dis-ease." I urge you: Lay off the fat people. Science and reason do not support the value of a weight focus.

There is a compassionate alternative to the war on obesity. It's called Health at Every Size and it involves shifting focus from weight to health.

For more information, check out *Health at Every Size: The Surprising Truth About Your Weight* (www.HAESbook.com).

JOIN THE HAES REVOLUTION

Interest in Health at Every Size (HAES) is growing fast. People are tired of diets, tired of feeling like failures, and tired of being scared of food. They are excited to find a paradigm that respects the diversity of human bodies and starts from the very basic premise that they can trust themselves—a paradigm that respects pleasure rather than denial.

We're at a transition point. Many people are ready to move on from feeling shame about their bodies and being preoccupied with their weight, yet our institutions are still mired in damaging old-school thought. Large publishers hesitate to publish HAES books, worried that only books promising weight loss will sell. Many health professionals and organizations cling to the belief that fearmongering about weight and promising weight loss motivate people to improve their health practices. The mainstream media are reluctant to give Health at Every Size sufficient air time, apparently convinced that reinforcing people's weight insecurities generates more attention.

I hope this book helps you to envision a different, more compassionate, and more respectful world, and that it gives you ideas and tools to help you make that vision reality.

I invite you to also consider some other simple, important things you can do.

The HAES Pledge: Making our Presence Known

Sign the online HAES pledge to show your commitment to HAES. As word spreads, this will show others our strength in numbers. We'll hasten institutional change by demonstrating that there is a large audience for HAES-affirming practices.

The HAES Registry and Resource List

So many of us incorporate HAES values into our work and activities: psychotherapists, dieticians, artists, academics, bloggers. . . . The

HAES Registry and Resource List have been established to foster community, educate people, and nurture the development of HAES values. Become a part of the HAES Registry. Or search the Registry to find who or what you're looking for. Check out the Resource List to learn more about HAES-affirming books, Web sites, videos, and more—or add your resource to the list. You can even find listings for job, volunteer, research, or activism opportunities.

The HAES Pledge, Registry, and Resource List: The Fine Print

The HAES Registry and Resource List are located at www.HAESCommunity.org. Participation is free. You will be asked to sign the HAES Pledge, reproduced below. The Registry and Resource List are intended to facilitate dialogue and connections between those interested in HAES and to support a diversity of HAES vantage points, not just the limited perspective presented in this book.

The Health at Every Size Pledge

Health at Every Size is based on the simple premise that the best way to improve health is to honor your body. It supports people in adopting health habits for the sake of health and well-being (rather than weight control). Health at Every Size encourages:

- Accepting and respecting the natural diversity of body sizes and shapes.
- Eating in a flexible manner that values pleasure and honors internal cues of hunger, satiety, and appetite.
- Finding the joy in moving one's body and becoming more physically vital.

I pledge my support for Health at Every Size.

Signature _____

RESOURCE GUIDE

Visit www.HAESCommunity.org to find more extensive resource listings and a searchable database.

HAES Professional Organization

The Association for Size Diversity and Health (ASDAH) is an international professional organization composed of individuals and organizations committed to the principles of Health at Every Size. ASDAH's mission "is to promote education, research, and the provision of services which enhance health and well-being, and which are free from weight-based assumptions and weight discrimination."

ASDAH can be reached in the following ways:

Web Site: www. sizediversityandhealth.org
E-mail: contact@sizediversityandhealth.org
Phone: 877-576-1102 (toll free)

Not all of the below-listed resources are entirely consistent with HAES though they all have valuable aspects. Please use your judgment.

Books

HAES for Professionals (also accessible for the general public)

Kratina, Karin, Nancy L. King, and Dale Hayes. *Moving Away From Diets*. Lake Dallas, TX: Helm Seminars Publishing, 1996.

Matz, Judith and Ellen Frankel. *Beyond a Shadow of a Diet: The Therapist's Guide to Treating Compulsive Eating*. New York: Brunner-Routledge, 2004.

Robison, Jon and Karen Carrier. *The Spirit and Science of Holistic Health: More than Broccoli, Jogging, and Bottled Water . . . More than Yoga, Herbs, and Meditation.* Bloomington, IN: AuthorHouse, 2004.

Weight-Related Exposés

Basham, Patrick, Gio Gori, and John Luik. *Diet Nation: Exposing the Obesity Crusade.* United Kingdom: Social Affairs Unit, 2006.

Campos, Paul. *The Diet Myth: Why America's Obsession with Weight is Hazardous to Your Health.* New York: Gotham Books, 2004.

Fraser, Laura. *Losing It: False Hopes and Fat Profits in the Diet Industry.* New York: Penguin Group, 1998.

Gaesser, Glenn. *Big Fat Lies: The Truth about Your Weight and Your Health.* Carlsbad: Gurze Books, 2002.

Gard, Michael and Jan Wright. *The Obesity Epidemic: Science, Morality and Ideology.* Oxon, UK: Routledge, 2005.

Kolata, Gina B. *Rethinking Thin: The New Science of Weight Loss—and the Myths and Realities of Dieting.* 1st ed. New York: Farrar, Straus, and Giroux, 2007.

Oliver, J. Eric. *Fat Politics: The Real Story Behind America's Obesity Epidemic.* New York: Oxford University Press, 2006.

Intuitive Eating

Hirschmann, Jane R. and Carol H. Munter. *Overcoming Overeating: Living Free in a World of Food.* Reading, MA: Addison-Wesley Publishing Co., 1988.

Kano, Susan. *Making Peace with Food: Freeing Yourself from the Diet/Weight Obsession.* Rev. ed. New York: Perennial Library, 1989.

Koenig, Karen R. *The Rules of "Normal" Eating: A Commonsense Approach for Dieters, Overeaters, Undereaters, Emotional Eaters, and Everyone in Between!* 1st ed. Carlsbad, CA: Gurze Books, 2005.

————. *The Food & Feelings Workbook: A Full Course Meal on Emotional Health.* Carlsbad, CA: Gurze Books, 2007.

Matz, Judith and Ellen Frankel. *Diet Survivor Handbook: 60 Lessons in Eating, Acceptance and Self-Care.* Naperville, IL: Sourcebooks, Inc., 2006.

May, Michelle. *Eat What You Love, Love What You Eat: How to Break Your Eat-Repent-Repeat Cycle.* Greenleaf Book Group Press, 2009.

Normandi, Carol Emery and Laurelee Roark. *It's Not About Food.* New York: Grosset/Putnam, 1998.

Omichinski, Linda. *You Count, Calories Don't.* Hugs International Inc. (www.hugs.com), 1999.

————. *Staying Off the Diet Rollercoaster.* Washington, D.C.: Advice-Zone (www.hugs.com) 2000.

Roth, Geneen. *When Food is Love: Exploring the Relationship Between Eating and Intimacy.* New York: Dutton, 1991.

————. *Breaking Free from Compulsive Eating.* New York: Plume, 1993.

————. *Feeding the Hungry Heart: The Experience of Compulsive Eating.* New York: Plume, 1993.

————. *Appetites: On the Search for True Nourishment.* New York: Dutton, 1996.

————. *When You Eat at the Refrigerator, Pull Up a Chair: 50 Ways to be Thin, Gorgeous, and Happy (When You Feel Anything But).* 1st ed. New York: Hyperion, 1998.

————. *The Craggy Hole in My Heart and the Cat Who Fixed It: Over the Edge and Back with My Cat, My Dad, and Me.* 1st ed. New York: Harmony Books, 2004.

Tribole, Evelyn and Elyse Resch. *Intuitive Eating: A Revolutionary Program That Works.* Newly revised and updated ed. New York: St. Martin's Griffin, 2003.

Size Acceptance and Empowerment/Body Image/Self-Esteem

Ballard, Pat. *10 Steps to Loving Your Body (No Matter What Size You Are)*. Pearlsong Press, 2008.

Bernell, Bonnie. *Bountiful Women: Large Women's Secrets for Living the Life They Desire*. Berkeley, CA: Wildcat Canyon Press, 2000.

Bliss, Kelly. *Don't Weight: Eat Healthy and Get Moving Now!* Haverford, PA: Infinity Publishing, 2002.

Bruno, Barbara Altman. *Worth Your Weight: What You Can Do About a Weight Problem*. Bethel, CT: Rutledge Books, Inc., 1996.

Erdman, Cheri K. *Nothing to Lose: A Guide to Sane Living in a Larger Body*. 1st ed. San Francisco: HarperSanFrancisco, 1995.

———. *Live Large!: Ideas, Affirmations, and Actions for Sane Living in a Larger Body*. 1st ed. San Francisco: HarperCollinsPublishers, 1997.

———. *Live Large!: Affirmations for Living the Life You Want in the Body You Already Have*. Carlsbad, CA: Gurze Books, 2003.

Frater, Lara. *Fat Chicks Rule!: How to Survive in a Thin-Centric World*. Brooklyn, NY: IG Publishing, 2005.

Harding, Kate and Marianne Kirby. *Lessons from the Fat-o-sphere: Quit Dieting and Declare a Truce with Your Body*. New York: Perigee Books, 2009.

Hirschmann, Jane R. and Carol Munter. *When Women Stop Hating Their Bodies*. New York City: Fawcett Columbine, 1995.

Hutchinson, Marcia G. *Transforming Body Image: Learning to Love the Body You Have*. Trumansburg, NY: Crossing Press, 1985.

———. *200 Ways to Love the Body You Have*. Freedom, CA: Crossing Press, 1999.

Johnson, Carol. *Self-esteem Comes in All Sizes: How to be Happy and Healthy at Your Natural Weight*. Rev. ed. Carlsbad, CA: Gurze Books, 2001.

Maine, Margo. *Body Wars: Making Peace with Women's Bodies: An Activist's Guide*. 1st ed. Carlsbad, CA: Gurze Books, 2000.

Martin, Courtney E. *Perfect Girls, Starving Daughters: The Frightening New Normalcy of Hating Your Body*. New York: Free Press, 2007.

Orbach, Suzy. *Fat is a Feminist Issue*. New York: Galahad Books, 1997.

Rothblum, Esther and Sondra Solovay (eds). *The Fat Studies Reader*. NYU Press, 2009.

Sarasohn, Lisa. *The Woman's Belly Book: Finding Your True Center for More Energy, Confidence, and Pleasure*. Novato, CA: New World Library, 2006.

Solovay, Sondra. *Tipping the Scales of Justice*. Amherst, NY: Prometheus Books, 2000.

Thomas, Pattie and Carl Wilkerson. *Taking Up Space: How Eating Well & Exercising Regularly Changed My Life*. Nashville: Pearlsong Press, 2005.

Wann, Marilyn. *Fat!So?: For People Who Don't Apologize for their Size*. Berkeley: Ten Speed Press, 1999.

Wolf, Naomi. *The Beauty Myth: How Images of Beauty Are Used Against Women*. New York: Perennial, 2002.

Size-Accepting Fitness

Lyons, Pat and Debby Burgard. *Great Shape: The First Fitness Guide for Large Women*. iUniverse, 2000.

General Weight or HAES-Related Titles

Berg, Francie. *Women Afraid to Eat: Breaking Free in Today's Weight-Obsessed World*. Hettinger: Healthy Weight Network, 2000.

Brown, Harriet (ed). *Feed Me!: Writers Dish About Food, Eating, Weight, and Body Image*. Ballantine Books, 2009.

Holmes, Betty, Suzy Pelican, and Fred Heede. *Let Their Voices Be Heard*. Chicago: Discovery Association Publishing House, 2005.

Plus-Size Resources

Bliss, Kelly. *Kelly Bliss' Yellow Pages*. Philadelphia, PA: Infinity Publishing, 2007.

Kids

Berg, Francie M. *Children and Teens Afraid to Eat: Helping Youth in Today's Weight-Obsessed World*. Hettinger, ND: Healthy Weight Network, 2001.

————. *Underage and Overweight: America's Childhood Obesity Crisis—What Every Family Needs to Know*. Long Island City, NY: Hatherleigh Press, 2004.

Kater, Kathy. *Real Kids Come in All Sizes: Ten Essential Lessons to Build Your Child's Body Esteem*. New York: Broadway Books, 2004.

Satter, Ellyn. *How to Get Your Kid to Eat—But Not Too Much*. Palo Alto, CA: Bull Publising Co., 1987.

————. *Secrets of Feeding a Healthy Family: How to Eat, How to Raise Good Eaters and How to Cook*. Madison, WI: Kelcy Press, 2008.

————. *Child of Mine: Feeding with Love and Good Sense*. Palo Alto, CA: Bull Publishing, 2000.

Nutrition/Food Politics

Bacon, Linda. *Eat Well: For Your Self, For the World* (manuscript in progress). http://www.LindaBacon.org

Campbell, T. Colin and Thomas M. Campbell. *The China Study: The Most Comprehensive Study of Nutrition Ever Conducted and the Startling Implications for Diet, Weight Loss and Long-term Health*. 1st BenBella Books ed. Dallas: BenBella Books, 2005.

Edell, Dean and Melissa Houtte. *Life, Liberty, and the Pursuit of Healthiness: Dr. Dean's Commonsense Guide for Anything That Ails You*. 1st ed. New York: Harper Collins, 2004.

Edell, Dean and David Schrieberg. *Eat, Drink, and Be Merry: America's Doctor Tells You Why the Health Experts are Wrong.* 1st ed. New York: HarperCollins Publishers, 1999.

Glassner, Barry. *The Gospel of Food: Everything You Think You Know About Food is Wrong.* 1st ed. New York: Ecco, 2007.

Omichinski, Linda and Heather Wiebe Hildebrand, *Tailoring Your Tastes.* Winnipeg, Canada: TAMOS Books, Inc., 1995. (Available at www.hugs.com)

Pollan, Michael. *The Omnivore's Dilemma: A Natural History of Four Meals.* New York: Penguin Press, 2006.

———. *In Defense of Food: An Eater's Manifesto.* New York: Penguin Group, 2008.

Simon, Michele. *Appetite for Profit: How the Food Industry Undermines our Health and How to Fight Back.* New York: Nation Books, 2006.

Weil, Andrew. *Eating Well for Optimum Health: The Essential Guide to Food, Diet, and Nutrition.* 1st ed. New York: Knopf: Distributed by Random House, Inc., 2000.

Web Sites

Web Sites and Organizations That Promote Size Acceptance Advocacy/Activism

Association for Size Diversity and Health (ASDAH): http://www.sizediversityandhealth.org/

Big Fat Blog: http://www.bigfatblog.com/

Council on Size and Weight Discrimination (CSWD): http://www.cswd.org/

Fat!So?: http://www.fatso.com

Healthy Weight Network: http://www.healthyweight.net/

Largesse: http://www.largesse.net/

National Association to Advance Fat Acceptance (NAAFA): http://www.naafa.org

Web Sites and Organizations That Provide Body Image Education/Support, from a Health at Every Size Perspective

Body Image Health: http://www.bodyimagehealth.org/
Body Positive: http://www.bodypositive.com/
The Body Positive: http://www.thebodypositive.org/
HUGS International Inc: http://www.hugs.com/

Plus-Size Health Resources

Fat Friendly Health Professionals List: http://cat-and-dragon
.com/stef/fat/ffp.html
Fat-Acceptance Diabetes Support List: http://ww3.telerama.com/
~moose/fa-diab.html
Plus-Size Pregnancy Web site: http://www.plus-size-pregnancy.org/

Plus-Size Exercise Clothing

A Big Attitude.com: http://www.abigattitude.com
Always for Me: http://store.alwaysforme.com
Bodysuit.com: http://www.bodysuit.com/plussizes.html
Danskin: http://www.danskin.com/plus.html
Junonia: http://www.junonia.com
Living XL: http://www.livingxl.com
NetSweat.com: http://www.netsweat.com/A_Big_Attid/index.html
Swimsuitsforall.com: http://www.swimsuitsforall.com

Additional Plus-Size Resources, including apparel, accessories, art
and other categories, can be found at the Plus Size Yellow Pages:
http://www.plussizeyellowpages.com/

ACKNOWLEDGMENTS

Thanks to the women who participated in the Health at Every Size research study, originally known as the Healthy Living Project, for their courage in considering new ideas and challenging their values, and their generosity in sharing their journeys. I feel incredibly fortunate to have shared in the research groups.

I could not have a more supportive and loving family. Special appreciation goes to my life partner, Anne Coyle, for providing the safe haven that makes everything possible. Anne was instrumental in every aspect of this volume; her insight, editing skill, and compassion, in particular, helped make this a much better book. She endured my stress, distraction, and endless discussions about the book while patiently helping me envision new strategies for achieving better balance between work and play. Thanks also to our son, Isaac Bacon Coyle, who is living proof that inhabiting one's body and eating in a way that is health-enhancing and environmentally friendly can be a natural and joyful experience, and to my parents, Janet and Bob Bacon, for their ongoing support, love, and confidence in me. Additional thanks to my mother-in-law Herta Coyle and to Pam Tyson, also loving and supportive presences in my life.

I am also grateful to my friends and colleagues in the Health at Every Size community, who have been incredibly generous in helping to shape these ideas. Our ongoing "Show Me the Data" mailing list dialogue, in particular, helped to inform my views and provided much-needed support. I cannot imagine a more insightful, stimulating, or encouraging online community. I have also been nurtured by participation in the Bay Area "HAES Think Tank," the "Fat Studies" electronic list, the Association for Size Diversity and Health, and the size-acceptance community.

Many reviewers helped along the way, providing commentary on parts or all of the text. Anne Coyle, Barbara Altman Bruno, and Judith Matz read and commented on the manuscript more times than anyone should have to. I am also grateful to the others who gave it a full read, including Roki Abakoui, Keith Bachman, Christian Bachmann, Bonnie Bernell, Brenda Buck, Lisa Carvalho, Sigrun Danielsdottir, Peggy Elam, Paul Ernsberger, Ellen Frankel, Glenn Gaesser, Julie Hanna, Ellyn Herb, Nancy Keim, Dave Mager, Tamara Mucha, Lily O'Hara, Lisa Sarasohn, Judy Stern, Pattie Thomas, Pam Tyson, and Marilyn Wann. Michele Simon and Sue Widemark also critiqued aspects, and Lara Frater, Lynn McAfee, and Jon Robison were always available for help. A brief mention clearly doesn't do justice to the extraordinary amount of time, energy, and support many people put into their review. I'd like to particularly acknowledge Keith Bachman, Kathy Barron, Deb Burgard, Carmen Cool, Sigrun Danielsdottir, Peggy Elam, Paul Ernsberger, Judith Matz, Lisa Sarasohn, Elizabeth Scott, Connie Sobczak, and Marilyn Wann for always being available to challenge me and delve into aspects on a deeper level. And thanks to all those friends who called me on some difficulties and helped ensure the integrity of the message. Thanks also to Daniel Jackson and Doris and Tom Smeltzer for their support and insight.

Writing a book proposal and sorting through publisher contracts was made much easier with advice from Paul Campos, Peggy Elam, Glenn Gaesser, and Marilyn Wann. Coleen O'Shea initially served as my agent, helping to pitch the book to publishers in its early stages, and I am grateful for her support. Thanks also to Deb Gordon for smoothing out aspects of the writing and for her general support and great ideas, and to Lisa Sarasohn for pulling through in the final hour.

I also owe a debt to the institutions that employed me while writing this book: City College of San Francisco and University of

California, Davis (thank you to my mentor, Judy Stern); and to the other institutions that helped support the research or my education: the National Institutes of Health, the National Science Foundation, and the Western Human Nutrition Research Center, a division of the United States Department of Agriculture (thanks in particular to Nancy Keim and Marta Van Loan). I'd like to also acknowledge Joe Reyes, a beacon of support and friendship at City College.

I am particularly grateful to have found a press with heart, passion, and integrity. (It wasn't easy to find a publishing company worthy of this accolade!) Thanks to Glenn Yeffeth for his vision and kindness, and to Jennifer Canzoneri, Leah Wilson, Laura Watkins, Yara Abuata, and everyone who worked behind the scenes at Ben-Bella for their friendliness and skill.

REFERENCES

1. Bacon, L., *Tales of mice and leptin: False promises and new hope in weight control*. Healthy Weight Journal, 2003. 17(2): p. 24-7.
2. Bacon, L., et al., *Evaluating a "Non-diet" Wellness Intervention for Improvement of Metabolic Fitness, Psychological Well-Being and Eating and Activity Behaviors*. International Journal of Obesity, 2002. 26(6): p. 854-865.
3. Bacon, L., et al., *Size Acceptance and Intuitive Eating Improve Health for Obese, Female Chronic Dieters*. Journal of the American Dietetic Association, 2005. 105: p. 929-36.
4. Wood, Marcia, "Health at Every Size: New Hope for Obese Americans?" *Agricultural Research* (2006).
5. Friedman, Jeffrey M., "Modern Science Versus the Stigma of Obesity," *Nature Medicine* 10, no. 6 (2004): 563–9.
6. Centers for Disease Control and Prevention. *Ten-State Nutrition Survey 1968–1970*. U.S. DHEW Publication No. (HSM) 72-8131.
7. Schwartz, W., Michael, "Brain Pathways Controlling Food Intake and Body Weight," *Experimental Biology and Medicine* 226, no. 11 (2001): 978–81.
8. Anand, B. K. and John R. Brobeck, "Localization of A 'Feeding Center' in the Hypothalamus of the Rat," *Proceedings of the Society of Experimental Biology and Medicine* 77 (1951): 323–4.
9. Hess, Walter Rudolf, *Diencephalon: Autonomic and Extrapyramidal Functions*. New York: Grune & Stratton, 1954.
10. Kessey, R., the Psychiatric Clinics of North America. "Set-Points and Body Weight Regulation." Symposium on Obesity: Basic Mechanisms and Treatment. 1978.

11. Mitchel, J. S. and Richard E. Keesey, "Defense of a Lowered Weight Maintenance Level by Lateral Hypothalamically Lesioned Rats: Evidence from a Restriction-Refeeding Regimen," *Physiology and Behavior* 18 (1977): 1121–5.
12. Corbett, S. W., E. J. Wilterdink, and R. E. Keesey, "Resting Oxygen Consumption in Over- and Underfed Rats with Lateral Hypothalamic Lesions," *Physiology and Behavior* 35 (1985): 971–7.
13. Hetherington, A. W. and S. W. Ranson, "Hypothalamic Lesions and Adiposity in the Rat," *Anatomical Record* 78 (1940): 149.
14. Olds, James, "Effects of Hunger and Male Sex Hormone on Self-Stimulation of the Brain," *Journal of Comparative and Physiological Psychology* 51 (1958): 320–24.
15. Bennett, William and Joel Gurin, *The Dieter's Dilemma: Eating More and Weighing Less*. New York: Basic Books, Inc., 1982.
16. Sclafani, A., D. Springer, and L. Kluge, "Effects of Quinine Adulterated Diets on the Food Intake and Body Weight of Obese and Non-Obese Hypopthalamic Hyperphagic Rats," *Physiology and Behavior* 16 (1976): 631–40.
17. Leibel, Rudolph L., Michael Rosenbaum, and Jules Hirsch, "Changes in Energy Expenditure Resulting from Altered Body Weight," *New England Journal of Medicine* 332 (1995): 621–28.
18. Zhang, Yiying, et al., "Positional Cloning of the Mouse Obese Gene and Its Human Homologue," *Nature* 372.6505 (1994): 425–32.
19. Heymsfield, Steven B., et al., "Recombinant Leptin for Weight Loss in Obese and Lean Adults," *Journal of the American Medical Association* 282 (1999): 1568–75.
20. Montague, Carl T., et al., "Congenital Leptin Deficiency Is Associated with Severe Early-Onset Obesity in Humans," *Nature* 387.6636 (1997): 903–8.
21. Wadden, Thomas A., et al., "Short- and Long-Term Changes in Serum Leptin in Dieting Obese Women: Effects of Calorie Restriction and Weight Loss," *Journal of Clinical Endocrinology and Metabolism* 83 (1998): 214–18.
22. Laessle, R. G., H. Wurmser, and K. M. Pirke, "Restrained Eating and Leptin Levels in Overweight Preadolescent Girls," *Physiology and Behavior* 70, no. 1–2 (2000): 45–47.
23. Macaulay, Vincent, et al., "The Emerging Tree of West Eurasian Mtdnas: A Synthesis of Control-Region Sequences and Rflps," *American Journal of Human Genetics* 64, no. 1 (1999): 232–49.
24. Rozin, P., et al., "Attitudes to Food and the Role of Food in Life in the U.S.A., Japan, Flemish Belgium and France: Possible Implications for the Diet-Health Debate," *Appetite* 33, no. 2 (1999): 163–80.

25. Wansink, Brian, *Mindless Eating: Why We Eat More Than We Think.* New York: Bantam Books, 2006.

26. Corstorphine, Emma, et al., "Changes in Internal States across the Binge-Vomit Cycle in Bulimia Nervosa," *Journal of Nervous and Mental Disorders* 194, no. 6 (2006): 446–49.

27. Redlin, J. A., et al., "Functional Assessment of Binge Eating in a Clinical Sample of Obese Binge Eaters," *Eating and Weight Disorders* 7, no. 2 (2002): 106–15.

28. Herman, C. Peter and Janet Polivy, "A Boundary Model for the Regulation of Eating." *Eating and Its Disorders.* Eds. Albert J. Stunkard and Eliot Stellar. New York: Raven Press, 1984.

29. Hawks, Steven, R. M. Merrill, and H. N. Madanat, "The Intuitive Eating Scale: Development and Preliminary Evaluation," *American Journal of Health Education* 35, no. 2 (2004): 90–99.

30. Gallo, Anthony E., "Food Advertising in the United States." *America's Eating Habits: Changes and Consequences.* Ed. E. Frazao. Washington, DC: USDA, 1999.

31. Herman, C. Peter, M. P. Olmsted, and Janet Polivy, "Obesity, Externality, and Susceptibility to Social Influence: An Integrated Analysis," *Journal of Personality and Social Psychology* 45 (1983): 926–34.

32. Herman, C. Peter, Janet Polivy, and V. M. Esses, "The Illusion of Counterregulation," *Appetite* 9 (1987): 161–69.

33. Herman, C. Peter and Janet Polivy, "Studies of Eating in Normal Dieters." *Eating Behavior in Eating Disorders.* Ed. B. T. Walsh. Washington, DC: American Psychiatric Association Press, 1988.

34. Raben, A., et al., "Evidence for an Abnormal Postprandial Response to a High-Fat Meal in Women Predisposed to Obesity," *American Journal of Physiology* 267 (1994): E549–59.

35. Platte, P., et al., "Resting Metabolic Rate and Diet-Induced Thermogenesis in Restrained and Unrestrained Eaters," *International Journal of Eating Disorders* 20 (1996): 33–41.

36. Keim, Nancy L. and William F. Horn, "Restrained Eating Behavior and the Metabolic Response to Dietary Energy Restriction in Women," *Obesity Research* 12, no. 1 (2004): 141–49.

37. Tuschl, R. J., et al., "Energy Expenditure and Everyday Eating Behavior in Healthy Young Women," *American Journal of Clinical Nutrition* 52 (1990): 81–86.

38. Poehlman, Eric T., H. F. Viers, and M. Detzer, "Influence of Physical Activity and Dietary Restraint on Resting Energy Expenditure in Young, Non-Obese Females," *Canadian Journal of Physiological Pharmacology* 69 (1991): 320–26.

39. Westerterp-Plantenga, Margriet S., et al., "Diet-Induced Thermogenesis and Cumulative Food Intake Curves as a Function of Familiarity with Food and Dietary Restraint in Humans," *Physiology and Behavior* 51 (1992): 457–65.

40. Keys, Ancel, et al. *The Biology of Human Starvation*. Minneapolis: University of Minnesota Press, 1950.

41. Howard, Barbara V., et al., "Low-Fat Dietary Pattern and Weight Change over 7 Years: The Women's Health Initiative Dietary Modification Trial," *Journal of the American Medical Association* 295, no. 1 (2006): 39–49.

42. Gardner, Christopher D., et al., "Comparison of the Atkins, Zone, Ornish, and Learn Diets for Change in Weight and Related Risk Factors among Overweight Premenopausal Women: The A to Z Weight Loss Study: A Randomized Trial," *Journal of the American Medical Association* 297, no. 9 (2007): 969–77.

43. Coakley, E. H., et al., "Predictors of Weight Change in Men: Results from the Health Professionals Follow-Up Study," *International Journal of Obesity and Related Metabolic Disorders* 22 (1998): 89–96.

44. Bild, Diane E., et al., "Correlates and Predictors of Weight Loss in Young Adults: The CARDIA study," *International Journal of Obesity and Related Metabolic Disorders* 20, no. 1 (1996): 47–55.

45. French, S. A., et al., "Predictors of weight change over two years among a population of working adults: The Healthy Worker Project," *International Journal of Obesity and Related Metabolic Disorders* 18 (1994): 145–54.

46. Korkeila, Maarit, et al., "Weight-loss attempts and risk of major weight gain," *American Journal of Clinical Nutrition* 70 (1999): 965–73.

47. Stice, Eric, et al., "Naturalistic weight-reduction efforts prospectively predict growth in relative weight and onset of obesity among female adolescents," *Journal of Consulting and Clinical Psychology* 67 (1999): 967–74.

48. Shunk, Jennifer A. and Leann L. Birch, "Girls at risk for overweight at age 5 are at risk for dietary restraint, disinhibited overeating, weight concerns, and greater weight gain from 5 to 9 years," *Journal of the American Dietetic Association* 104, no. 7 (2004): 1120–26.

49. Stice, Eric, Katherine Presnell, and Heather Shaw, "Psychological and Behavioral Risk Factors for Obesity Onset in Adolescent Girls: A Prospective Study," *Journal of Consulting and Clinical Psychology* 73, no. 2 (2005): 195–202.

50. Cella, F., et al., "Effects of Dietary Restriction on Serum Leptin Concentration in Obese Women," *International Journal of Obesity* 23 (1999): 494–97.

51. Keim, Nancy L., Judith S. Stern, and Peter J. Havel, "Relation between Circulating Leptin Concentrations and Appetite During a Prolonged, Moderate Energy Deficit in Women," *American Journal of Clinical Nutrition* 68 (1998): 794–801.

52. Kern, P. A., et al., "The Effects of Weight Loss on the Activity and Expression of Adipose Tissue Lipoprotein Lipase in Very Obese Humans," *New England Journal of Medicine* 322 (1990): 1053–59.

53. Gerardo-Gettens, G., et al., "Exercise Decreases Fat Selection in Female Rats During Weight Cycling," *American Journal of Physiology* 260 (1991): R518–24.

54. Reed, Danielle R., et al., "Weight Cycling in Female Rats Increases Dietary Fat Selection and Adiposity," *Physiology and Behavior* 42 (1988): 389–95.

55. Blundell, John E., et al., "Cross Talk between Physical Activity and Appetite Control: Does Physical Activity Stimulate Appetite?" *Proceedings of the Nutrition Society* 62. no. 3 (2003): 651–61.

56. Tsofliou, F., et al., "Moderate Physical Activity Permits Acute Coupling between Serum Leptin and Appetite-Satiety Measures in Obese Women," *International Journal of Obesity and Related Metabolic Disorders* 27, no. 11 (2003): 1332–39.

57. Chu, N. F., et al., "Dietary and Lifestyle Factors in Relation to Plasma Leptin Concentrations among Normal Weight and Overweight Men," *International Journal of Obesity and Related Metabolic Disorders* 25, no. 1 (2001): 106–14.

58. van Aggel-Leijssen, D. P., et al., "Regulation of Average 24h Human Plasma Leptin Level; the Influence of Exercise and Physiological Changes in Energy Balance," *International Journal of Obesity and Related Metabolic Disorders* 23, no. 2 (1999): 151–58.

59. Lee, I-Min, et al., "Physical Activity and Coronary Heart Disease in Women: Is 'No Pain, No Gain' Passé?" *Journal of the American Medical Association* 285 (2001): 1447–54.

60. Sesso, Howard D., Ralph S. Paffenbarger, Jr., and I-Min Lee, "Physical Activity and Coronary Heart Disease in Men: The Harvard Alumni Health Study," *Circulation* 102, no. 9 (2000): 975–80.

61. Miller, Wayne C., D. M. Koceja, and E. J. Hamilton, "A Meta-Analysis of the Past 25 Years of Weight Loss Research Using Diet, Exercise or Diet Plus Exercise Intervention," *International Journal of Obesity and Related Metabolic Disorders* 21. no. 10 (1997): 941–47.

62. Wilmore, Jack H., et al., "Alterations in Body Weight and Composition Consequent to 20 Wk of Endurance Training: The Heritage Family Study," *American Journal of Clinical Nutrition* 70, no. 3 (1999): 346–52.

63. Ballor, D. L. and Richard E. Keesey, "A Meta-Analysis of the Factors Affecting Exercise-Induced Changes in Body Mass, Fat Mass and Fat-Free Mass in Males and Females," *International Journal of Obesity and Related Metabolic Disorders* 15, no. 11 (1991): 717–26.

64. Donnelly, Joseph E., et al., "Effects of a 16-Month Randomized Controlled Exercise Trial on Body Weight and Composition in Young, Overweight Men and Women: The Midwest Exercise Trial," *Archives of Internal Medicine* 163, no. 11 (2003): 1343–50.

65. Lamarche, Benoit, et al., "Is body fat loss a determinant factor in the improvement of carbohydrate and lipid metabolism following aerobic exercise training in obese women?" *Metabolism* 41 (1992): 1249–56.

66. Blundell, John E. and Neil A. King, "Physical Activity and Regulation of Food Intake: Current Evidence," *Medicine and Science in Sports and Exercise* 31, no. 11 (Supplement) (1999): S573–83.

67. Blair, Steven N., et al., "Body Weight Change, All-Cause Mortality, and Cause-Specific Mortality in the Multiple Risk Factor Intervention Trial," *Annals of Internal Medicine* 119 (1993): 749–57.

68. Vickers, Mark H., et al., "Sedentary Behavior During Postnatal Life Is Determined by the Prenatal Environment and Exacerbated by Postnatal Hypercaloric Nutrition," *American Journal of Physiology—Regulatory, Integrative, and Comparative Physiology* 285, no. 1 (2003): R271–73.

69. Nishitani, N. and H. Sakakibara, "Relationship of Obesity to Job Stress and Eating Behavior in Male Japanese Workers," *International Journal of Obesity (London)* 30, no. 3 (2006): 528–33.

70. Brunner, Eric J., Tarani Chandola, and Michael G. Marmot, "Prospective Effect of Job Strain on General and Central Obesity in the Whitehall II Study," *American Journal of Epidemiology* 165, no. 7 (2007): 828–37.

71. Kuo, Lydia E., et al., "Neuropeptide Y Acts Directly in the Periphery on Fat Tissue and Mediates Stress-Induced Obesity and Metabolic Syndrome," *Nature Medicine* (2007).

72. DeFalco, Jeff, et al., "Virus-Assisted Mapping of Neural Inputs to a Feeding Center in the Hypothalamus," *Science* 291 (2001): 2608–13.

73. Locard, E., et al., "Risk Factors of Obesity in a Five Year Old Population. Parental Versus Environmental Factors," *International Journal of Obesity and Related Metabolic Disorders* 16, no. 10 (1992): 721–29.

74. Vioque, J., A. Torres, and J. Quiles, "Time Spent Watching Television, Sleep Duration and Obesity in Adults Living in Valencia, Spain,"

International Journal of Obesity and Related Metabolic Disorders 24, no. 12 (2000): 1683–88.

75. von Kries, R., et al., "Reduced Risk for Overweight and Obesity in 5- and 6-Y-Old Children by Duration of Sleep—a Cross-Sectional Study," *International Journal of Obesity and Related Metabolic Disorders* 26, no. 5 (2002): 710–16.

76. Hasler, Gregor, et al., "The Association between Short Sleep Duration and Obesity in Young Adults: A 13-Year Prospective Study," *Sleep* 27, no. 4 (2004): 661–66.

77. Gupta, Neeraj K., et al., "Is Obesity Associated with Poor Sleep Quality in Adolescents?" *American Journal of Human Biology* 14 (2002): 762–68.

78. Taheri, Shahrad, et al., "Short Sleep Duration Is Associated with Reduced Leptin, Elevated Ghrelin, and Increased Body Mass Index," *PLoS Med* 1, no. 3 (2004): e62.

79. Spiegel, Karine, et al., "Brief Communication: Sleep Curtailment in Healthy Young Men Is Associated with Decreased Leptin Levels, Elevated Ghrelin Levels, and Increased Hunger and Appetite," *Annals of Internal Medicine* 141, no. 11 (2004): 846–50.

80. Pasarica, Magdalena, et al., "Human Adenovirus 36 Induces Adiposity, Increases Insulin Sensitivity, and Alters Hypothalamic Monoamines in Rats," *Obesity (Silver Spring)* 14, no. 11 (2006): 1905–13.

81. Dhurandhar, Nikhil V., et al., "Human Adenovirus Ad-36 Promotes Weight Gain in Male Rhesus and Marmoset Monkeys," *Journal of Nutrition* 132, no. 10 (2002): 3155–60.

82. Dhurandhar, Nikhil V., *234th National Meeting of the American Chemical Society*. Boston, 2007.

83. Renvert, Stefan, et al., "Bacterial Profile and Burden of Periodontal Infection in Subjects with a Diagnosis of Acute Coronary Syndrome," *Journal of Periodontology* 77, no. 7 (2006): 1110–19.

84. Vasilakopoulou, A. and C. W. le Roux, "Could a Virus Contribute to Weight Gain?" *International Journal of Obesity (London)* 31, no. 9 (2007): 1350–56.

85. Wolf, George, "Gut Microbiota: A Factor in Energy Regulation," *Nutrition Reviews* 64, no. 1 (2006): 47–50.

86. Turnbaugh, Peter J., et al., "An Obesity-Associated Gut Microbiome with Increased Capacity for Energy Harvest Microbial Ecology: Human Gut Microbes Associated with Obesity," *Nature* 444.7122 (2006): 1027–31.

87. Ley, Ruth E., et al., "Microbial Ecology: Human Gut Microbes Associated with Obesity," *Nature* 444.7122 (2006): 1022–23.

88. Sears, Cynthia L., "A Dynamic Partnership: Celebrating Our Gut Flora," *Anaerobe* 11, no. 5 (2005): 247–51.

89. Bhatnagar, Aruni, "Environmental Cardiology: Studying Mechanistic Links between Pollution and Heart Disease," *Circulation Research* 99, no. 7 (2006): 692–705.

90. Tabb, Michelle M. and Bruce Blumberg, "New Modes of Action for Endocrine-Disrupting Chemicals," *Molecular Endocrinology* 20, no. 3 (2006): 475–82.

91. Grun, Felix and Bruce Blumberg, "Environmental Obesogens: Organotins and Endocrine Disruption Via Nuclear Receptor Signaling," *Endocrinology* 147, no. 6 (Supplement) (2006): S50–55.

92. Grun, Felix and Bruce Blumberg, "Perturbed Nuclear Receptor Signaling by Environmental Obesogens as Emerging Factors in the Obesity Crisis," *Reviews in Endocrine & Metabolic Disorders* 8, no. 2 (2007): 161–71.

93. Grun, Felix, et al., "Endocrine-Disrupting Organotin Compounds Are Potent Inducers of Adipogenesis in Vertebrates," *Molecular Endocrinology* 20, no. 9 (2006): 2141–55.

94. Blumberg, Bruce, "Do These Genes Make Me Look Fat? Genetics, Environment, and Obesity." *The Genetics and Public Policy Center's Genetic Perspectives on Policy Seminar.* December 5, 2006.

95. Chevrier, J., et al., "Body Weight Loss Increases Plasma and Adipose Tissue Concentrations of Potentially Toxic Pollutants in Obese Individuals," *International Journal of Obesity and Related Metabolic Disorders* 24, no. 10 (2000): 1272–78.

96. Sundl, Isabella, et al., "Effects of Orlistat Therapy on Plasma Concentrations of Oxygenated and Hydrocarbon Carotenoids," *Lipids* 41, no. 2 (2006): 113–18.

97. Lucas, Kristy H. and Barbara Kaplan-Machlis, "Orlistat—a Novel Weight Loss Therapy," *Annals of Pharmacotherapy* 35, no. 3 (2001): 314–28.

98. Rucker, Diana, et al., "Long Term Pharmacotherapy for Obesity and Overweight: Updated Meta-Analysis," *British Medical Journal* 15 (2007): 15.

99. GlaxoSmithKline. "Alli: Treatment Effects." November 7, 2007. http://www.myalli.com/howdoesitwork/treatmenteffects.aspx

100. Pajecki, Denis, et al., "Follow-up of Roux-En-Y Gastric Bypass Patients at 5 or More Years Postoperatively," *Obesity Surgery* 17, no. 5 (2007): 601–7.

101. American College of Gastroenterology. "Gastric Bypass Surgery May Cause Post-Op Nutrient Deficiencies." *ScienceDaily.* November 10, 2007.

102. Folope, V., M. Coeffier, and P. Dechelotte, "[Nutritional Deficiencies Associated with Bariatric Surgery]," *Gastroenterologie Clinique et Biologique* 31.4 (2007): 369–77.

103. Bernert, C. Poitou, et al., "Nutritional Deficiency after Gastric Bypass: Diagnosis, Prevention and Treatment," *Diabetes Metabolism Review* 33, no. 1 (2007): 13–24.

104. Shah, Meena, Vinaya Simha, and Abhimanyu Garg, "Review: Long-Term Impact of Bariatric Surgery on Body Weight, Comorbidities, and Nutritional Status," *Journal of Clinical Endocrinology and Metabolism* 91, no. 11 (2006): 4223–31.

105. Malinowski, Scott S., "Nutritional and Metabolic Complications of Bariatric Surgery," *American Journal of Medical Science* 331, no. 4 (2006): 219–25.

106. Flum, David R., et al., "Early Mortality among Medicare Beneficiaries Undergoing Bariatric Surgical Procedures," *Journal of the American Medical Association* 294 (2005): 1903–8.

107. American Society for Metabolic and Bariatric Surgery. "Gastric Bypass and Laparoscopic Gastric Bypass." Chap. 3 in *The Story of Surgery for Obesity: A Brief History and Summary of Bariatric Surgery*, 2005.

108. Correa, T., "Dying to Lose Weight." *Fresno Bee*, December 30, 2001.

109 Omalu, B.I., et al., *Death rates and causes of death after bariatric surgery for Pennsylvania residents, 1995 to 2004*. Arch Surg, 2007. **142**(10): p. 923-8; discussion 929.]

110. Swarzc, S., *The other side of the story — Part Two, Junkfood Science (blog)*. April 27, 2008.

111. Ernsberger, Paul and S. Swarzc, Personal Communication (2007).

112. Mitka, Mike, "Demand Soars Amid Scientific, Ethical Questions," *Journal of the American Medical Association* 289 (2003): 1761–62.

113. Edward E. Mason, "Surgery for Obesity," *International Bariatric Surgery Registry (ISBR) Newsletter* (Fall 1999).

114. Emergency Care Research Institute. *Bariatric Surgery for Obesity*. 2004.

115. Mitchell, James E., et al., "Long-Term Follow-up of Patients' Status after Gastric Bypass," *Obesity Surgery* 11, no. 4 (2001): 464–68.

116. Avinoah, E., et al., "[Long-Term Weight Changes after Roux-En-Y Gastric Bypass for Morbid Obesity]," *Harefuah* 124, no. 4 (1993): 185–87, 248.

117. Sjostrom, Lars, et al., "Lifestyle, Diabetes, and Cardiovascular Risk Factors 10 Years after Bariatric Surgery," *New England Journal of Medicine* 351.26 (2004): 2683–93.

118. American Society for Metabolic and Bariatric Surgery. "Bariatric Surgery: Post-Operative Concerns." <www.asbs.org/html/pdf/asbs_bspc .pdf>

119. Pajecki, Denis P., et al., "Follow-up of Rygbp Cases 5 to 9 Years after Operation," *Obesity Surgery* 15 (2005).

120. Adams, Ted D., et al., "Long-Term Mortality after Gastric Bypass Surgery," *New England Journal of Medicine* 357, no. 8 (2007): 753–61.

121. Rea, J. D., et al., "Influence of Complications and Extent of Weight Loss on Quality of Life after Laparoscopic Roux-En-Y Gastric Bypass," *Surgical Endoscopy* 21, no. 7 (2007): 1095–1100.

122. United States Department of Agriculture. The Agriculture Fact Book 2001-2002: Agriculture Dept., Office of Communications; 2002.

123. Wooley, Susan and O. W. Wooley, "Should Obesity Be Treated at All?" *Eating and Its Disorders*, Eds. A. J. Stunkard and E. J. Stellar. New York: Raven, 1984.

124. Garrow, J. S., *Energy Balance and Obesity in Man*. New York: Elsevier, 1974.

125. Braitman, L. E., E. V. Adlin, and J. L. Stanton, Jr., "Obesity and Caloric Intake: The National Health and Nutrition Examination Survey of 1971–1975 (HANES I)," *Journal of Chronic Disease* 38, no. 9 (1985): 727–32.

126. National Resource Council (National Academy of Sciences). "Diet and Health: Implications for Reducing Chronic Disease." Ed. Committee on Diet and Health (Food and Nutrition Board/Commission on Life Sciences): National Academy Press, 1999.

127. Wooley, Susan, O. W. Wooley, and S. Dyrenforth, "Theoretical, Practical and Social Issues in Behavioral Treatments of Obesity," *Journal of Applied Behavior Analysis* 12 (1979): 3–25.

128. Schoonover, Heather and Mark Muller, *Food without Thought: How U.S. Farm Policy Contributes to Obesity*. Minneapolis: Institute for Agriculture and Trade Policy, 2006.

129. Appleby, P. N., et al., "Low Body Mass Index in Non-Meat Eaters: The Possible Roles of Animal Fat, Dietary Fibre and Alcohol," *International Journal of Obesity and Related Metabolic Disorders* 22, no. 5 (1998): 454–60.

130. Levin, N., J. Rattan, and T. Gilat, "Energy Intake and Body Weight in Ovo-Lacto Vegetarians," *Journal of Clinical Gastroenterology* 8 (1986): 451–53.

131. Campbell, Colin T., "Energy Balance: Interpretation of Data from Rural China," *Toxicological Sciences* 52 (1999): 87–94.

132. Fang, Jing, et al., "Exercise, Body Mass Index, Caloric Intake, and Cardiovascular Mortality," *American Journal of Preventive Medicine* 25, no. 4 (2003): 283–89.

133. Raynor, Holly A. and Leonard H. Epstein, "Dietary Variety, Energy Regulation, and Obesity," *Psychological Bulletin* 127, no. 3 (2001): 325–41.

134. McCrory, Megan A., et al., "Dietary Variety within Food Groups: Association with Energy Intake and Body Fatness in Men and Women," *American Journal of Clinical Nutrition* 69, no. 3 (1999): 440–47.

135. Peck, J. W., "Rats Defend Different Body Weights Depending on Palatability and Accessibility of Their Food," *Journal of Comparative and Physiological Psychology* 92 (1978): 555–70.

136. Putnam, Judy, Jane Allshouse, and Linda Scott Kantor, "U.S. Per Capita Food Supply Trends: More Calories, Refined Carbohydrates, and Fats," *Food Review* 25.3 (2002): 1–14.

137. Reavan, Gerald, Terry Strom, and Barry Fox, *Syndrome X the Silent Killer*. New York: Fireside, 2000.

138. Newby, P. Kirstin, et al., "Dietary Patterns and Changes in Body Mass Index and Waist Circumference in Adults," *American Journal of Clinical Nutrition* 77, no. 6 (2003): 1417–25.

139. Gaesser, Glenn, "Carbohydrate Quantity and Quality in Relation to Body Mass Index," *Journal of the American Dietetic Association* 107 (2007): 1768–80.

140. Holt, Susanne H., et al., "A Satiety Index of Common Foods," *European Journal of Clinical Nutrition* 49, no. 9 (1995): 675–90.

141. Cordain, Loren, "The Nutritional Characteristics of a Contemporary Diet Based Upon Paleolithic Food Groups," *Journal of the American Neutraceutical Association* 5 (2002): 15–24.

142. Meyer, Katie A., et al., "Carbohydrates, Dietary Fiber, and Incident Type 2 Diabetes in Older Women," *American Journal of Clinical Nutrition* 71, no. 4 (2000): 921–30.

143. Lairon, Denis, et al., "Dietary Fiber Intake and Risk Factors for Cardiovascular Disease in French Adults," *American Journal of Clinical Nutrition* 82, no. 6 (2005): 1185–94.

144. Cho, Sungsoo, et al., "The Effect of Breakfast Type on Total Daily Energy Intake and Body Mass Index: Results from the Third National Health and Nutrition Examination Survey (NHANES III)," *Journal of American College of Nutrition* 22, no. 4 (2003): 296–302.

145. Barton, Bruce A., et al., "The Relationship of Breakfast and Cereal Consumption to Nutrient Intake and Body Mass Index: The National

Heart, Lung, and Blood Institute Growth and Health Study," *Journal of the American Dietetic Association* 105, no. 9 (2005): 1383–89.

146. Prewitt, T. E., et al., "Changes in Body Weight, Body Composition, and Energy Intake in Women Fed High- and Low-Fat Diets," *American Journal of Clinical Nutrition* 54, no. 2 (1991): 304–10.

147. de Oliveira, Maria Conceição, Rosely Sichieri, and Anibal Sanchez Moura, "Weight Loss Associated with a Daily Intake of Three Apples or Three Pears among Overweight Women," *Nutrition* 19 (2003): 253–56.

148. Liu, Simin, et al., "Whole Grain Consumption and Risk of Coronary Heart Disease: Results from the Nurses' Health Study," *American Journal of Clinical Nutrition* 70, no. 3 (1999): 412–19.

149. Kahn, H. S., et al., "Stable Behaviors Associated with Adults' 10-Year Change in Body Mass Index and Likelihood of Gain at the Waist," *American Journal of Public Health* 87, no. 5 (1997): 747–54.

150. Rolls, Barbara J., Julia A. Ello-Martin, and Beth Carlton Tohill, "What Can Intervention Studies Tell Us about the Relationship between Fruit and Vegetable Consumption and Weight Management?" *Nutrition Reviews* 62, no. 1 (2004): 1–17.

151. Bray, George A., Samara Joy Nielsen, and Barry M. Popkin, "Consumption of High-Fructose Corn Syrup in Beverages May Play a Role in the Epidemic of Obesity," *American Journal of Clinical Nutrition* 79, no. 4 (2004): 537–43.

152. Tordoff, Michael G. and Annette M. Alleva, "Oral Stimulation with Aspartame Increases Hunger," *Physiology and Behavior* 47, no. 3 (1990): 555–59.

153. Anderson, J. W., et al., "Metabolic Effects of Fructose Supplementation in Diabetic Individuals," *Diabetes Care* 12, no. 5 (1989): 337–44.

154. Raben, Anne, et al., "Sucrose Compared with Artificial Sweeteners: Different Effects on Ad Libitum Food Intake and Body Weight after 10 Wk of Supplementation in Overweight Subjects," *American Journal of Clinical Nutrition* 76, no. 4 (2002): 721–29.

155. Bray, George A., Samara Joy Nielsen, and Barry M. Popkin, "Consumption of High-Fructose Corn Syrup in Beverages May Play a Role in the Epidemic of Obesity," *American Journal of Clinical Nutrition* 79, no. 4 (2004): 537–43.

156. Davidson, Terry L. and Susan E. Swithers, "A Pavlovian Approach to the Problem of Obesity," *International Journal of Obesity* 28, no. 7 (2004): 933–35.

157. USDA Economic Research Service. "The ERS Food Consumption (Per Capita) Data System."

158. Enns, Cecilia Wilkinson, Joseph D. Goldman, and Annetta Cook, "Trends in Food and Nutrient Intakes by Adults: Nfcs 1977–78, Csfii

1989–91, and Csfii 1994–95," *Family Economics and Nutrition Review* 10, no. 4 (1997): 2–15.

159. United States Department of Agriculture, "Major Trends in the U.S. Food Supply, 1909–99," *FoodReview* 23, no. 1 (2000): 8–15.

160. Havel, Peter J., et al., "High-Fat Meals Reduce 24-H Circulating Leptin Concentrations in Women," *Diabetes* 48 (1999): 334–41.

161. Lawton, C., et al., *Dietary fat and appetite control in obese subjects: weak effects on satiation and satiety.* International Journal of Obesity, 1993. 17(7): p. 409-16.

162. Cummings, D.E., *Ghrelin and the short- and long-term regulation of appetite and body weight.* Physiol Behav, 2006. 89(1): p. 71-84.

163. Hill, James O., et al., "Development of Dietary Obesity in Rats: Influence of Amount and Composition of Dietary Fat," *International Journal of Obesity and Related Metabolic Disorders* 16, no. 5 (1992): 321–33.

164. Horton, Tracy J., et al., "Fat and Carbohydrate Overfeeding in Humans: Different Effects on Energy Storage," *American Journal of Clinical Nutrition* 62, no. 1 (1995): 19–29.

165. Tataranni, Pietro Antonio and Eric Ravussin, "Effect of Fat Intake on Energy Balance," *Annals of New York Academy Sciences* 819 (1997): 37–43.

166. Tremblay, Angelo, et al., "Impact of Dietary Fat Content and Fat Oxidation on Energy Intake in Humans," *American Journal of Clinical Nutrition* 49, no. 5 (1989): 799–805.

167. Bray, George A. and Barry M. Popkin, "Dietary Fat Intake Does Affect Obesity!" *American Journal of Clinical Nutrition* 68, no. 6 (1998): 1157–73.

168. Lovejoy, Jennifer C., "The Influence of Dietary Fat on Insulin Resistance," *Current Diabetes Report* 2, no. 5 (2002): 435–40.

169. Harris, Ruth B. and Helen Kor, "Insulin Insensitivity Is Rapidly Reversed in Rats by Reducing Dietary Fat from 40 to 30% of Energy," *Journal of Nutrition* 122, no. 9 (1992): 1811–22.

170. Flatt, J. P., "Energetics of Intermediary Metabolism." *Substrate and Energy Metabolism in Man.* Eds. J. S. Gatrow and D. Halliday. London: John Libbey and Co., 1985.

171. Shell, Ellen Ruppel, *The Hungry Gene: The Science of Fat and the Future of Thin.* New York: Atlantic Monthly Press, 2002.

172. Widdowson, Peter S., et al., "Inhibition of Food Response to Intracerebroventricular Injection of Leptin Is Attenuated in Rats with Diet-Induced Obesity," *Diabetes* 46 (1997): 1782–85.

173. Havel, Peter J., et al., "Relationship of Plasma Leptin to Plasma Insulin and Adiposity in Normal Weight and Overweight Women:

Effects of Dietary Fat Content and Sustained Weight Loss," *Journal of Clinical Endocrinology and Metabolism* 81, no. 12 (1996): 4406–13.

174. Gregersen, Søren, et al., "Impact of Dietary FA and Energy Restriction on Plasma Leptin and Ob Gene Expression in Mice," *Lipids* 38, no. 5 (2003): 513–17.

175. Steerenberg, P. A., et al., "Long-Term Effect of Fish Oil Diet on Basal and Stimulated Plasma Glucose and Insulin Levels in Ob/Ob Mice," *Diabetes, Nutrition and Metabolism* 15, no. 4 (2002): 205–14.

176. Wang, Hongqin, Len H. Storlien, and Xu-Feng Huang, "Effects of Dietary Fat Types on Body Fatness, Leptin, and Arc Leptin Receptor, Npy, and Agrp Mrna Expression," *American Journal of Physiology, Endocrinology and Metabolism* 282, no. 6 (2002): E1352–59.

177. Cha, Ming C. and Peter J. H. Jones, "Tissue Fatty Acid Deposition Is Influenced by an Interaction of Dietary Oil Source and Energy Intake Level in Rats," *Journal of Nutritional Biochemistry* 7 (1996): 650–58.

178. Cha, Ming C. and Peter J. H. Jones, "Dietary Fat Type and Energy Restriction Interactively Influence Plasma Leptin Concentration in Rats," *Journal of Lipid Research* 39, no. 8 (1998): 1655–60.

179. Eaton, S. Boyd, et al., "Dietary Intake of Long-Chain Polyunsaturated Fatty Acids During the Paleolithic," *World Review of Nutrition and Diet* 83 (1998): 12–23.

180. Porrini, M., et al., "Weight, Protein, Fat, and Timing of Preloads Affect Food Intake," *Physiology and Behavior* 62, no. 3 (1997): 563–70.

181. Gerstein, Dana E., et al., "Clarifying Concepts About Macronutrients' Effects on Satiation and Satiety," *Journal of the American Dietetic Association* 104, no. 7 (2004): 1151–53.

182. Spencer, Elizabeth A., et al., "Diet and Body Mass Index in 38,000 Epic-Oxford Meat-Eaters, Fish-Eaters, Vegetarians and Vegans," *International Journal of Obesity and Related Metabolic Disorders* 27, no. 6 (2003): 728–34.

183. Wurtman, Judith J., et al., "Carbohydrate Craving in Obese People: Suppression by Treatments Affecting Serotoninergic Transmission," *International Journal of Eating Disorders* (1981).

184. United States Department of Agriculture. "USDA National Nutrient Database for Standard Reference, Release 20." (2007).

185. Halton, Thomas L., et al., "Low-Carbohydrate-Diet Score and the Risk of Coronary Heart Disease in Women," *New England Journal of Medicine* 355, no. 19 (2006): 1991–2002.

186. Lutsey, Pamela L., Lyn M. Steffen, and June Stevens, "Dietary Intake and the Development of the Metabolic Syndrome," *Circulation* (2008).

187. Greger, Michael, *Carbophobia: The Scary Truth About America's Low Carb Craze*. Lantern Books, 2005.

188. Lesser, Lenard I., et al., "Relationship between Funding Source and Conclusion among Nutrition-Related Scientific Articles," *PLoS Med* 4, no. 1 (2007): e5.

189. Schlosser, Eric, *Fast Food Nation*. New York: Houghton Mifflin Company, 2001.

190. Thompson, Olivia M., et al., "Food Purchased Away from Home as a Predictor of Change in BMI Z-Score among Girls," *International Journal of Obesity* 28 (2004): 282–89.

191. Ma, Yunsheng, et al., "Association between Eating Patterns and Obesity in a Free-Living Us Adult Population," *American Journal of Epidemiology* 158, no. 1 (2003): 85–92.

192. Smith, A. P., "Stress, Breakfast Cereal Consumption and Cortisol," *Nutritional Neuroscience* 5, no. 2 (2002): 141–44.

193. Cook's Illustrated.com. "Tasting Lab: The Scoop on Vanilla Ice Cream—Updated." May 2006.

194. Simon, Michele, *Appetite for Profit: How the Food Industry Undermines Our Health and How to Fight Back*. New York: Nation Books, 2006.

195. Tillotson, James E., "America's Obesity: Conflicting Public Policies, Industrial Economic Development, and Unintended Human Consequences," *Annual Review of Nutrition* 24 (2004): 617–43.

196. Lambert, Craig, "The Way We Eat Now: Ancient Bodies Collide with Modern Technology to Produce a Flabby, Disease-Ridden Populace," *Harvard Magazine* (2004).

197. Bovard, James, *Archer Daniels Midland: A Case Study in Corporate Welfare*. Cato Institute, 1995.

198. Imhoff, Dan, *The Citizen's Guide to a Food and Farm Bill*. Watershed Media, 2007.

199. Diliberti, Nicole, et al., "Increased Portion Size Leads to Increased Energy Intake in a Restaurant Meal," *Obesity Research* 12, no. 3 (2004): 562–68.

200. Levine, Allen S., Catherine M. Kotz, and Blake A. Gosnell, "Sugars and Fats: The Neurobiology of Preference," *Journal of Nutrition* 133, no. 3 (2003): 831S–34S.

201. Levine, A.S., C.M. Kotz, and B.A. Gosnell, Sugars and fats: the neurobiology of preference. *Journal of Nutrition*, 2003. 133(3): p. 831S–834S.

202. Drewnowski, Adam and Allen S. Levine, "Sugar and Fat—from Genes to Culture," *Journal of Nutrition* 133, no. 3 (2003): 829S–30S.

203. Nestle, Marion, *Food Politics. How the Food Industry Influences Nutrition and Health*. Berkeley: University of California Press, Ltd., 2002.

204. Center for Science in the Public Interest. *Lifting the Veil of Secrecy. Corporate Support for Health and Environmental Professional Associations, Charities and Industry Front Groups.* Washington, DC, 2003.

205. American Academy of Family Physicians News Staff. *Coca-Cola Grant Launches AAFP Consumer Alliance Program Program Focused on Helping Consumers Make Better Choices.* 2009 [cited 2009 November 21]; Available from: http://www.aafp.org/online/en/home/publications/news/news-now/inside-aafp/20091006cons-alli-coke.html

206. American Dietetic Association. "Fact Sheet on Straight Facts on Beverage Choices." June 25, 2004. http://www.nsda.org/softdrinks/CSD Health/Nutrition/901percent20Softpercent20drink percent20sheet.pdf

207. Lesser, Lenard I., et al., "Relationship between Funding Source and Conclusion among Nutrition-Related Scientific Articles," *PLoS Med* 4, no. 1 (2007): 1–6.

208. Mello, Michelle M., Brian R. Clarridge, and David M. Studdert, "Academic Medical Centers' Standards for Clinical-Trial Agreements with Industry," *New England Journal of Medicine* 352. no. 21 (2005): 2202–10.

209. Committee on Nutrition in Medical Education. *Nutrition Education in U.S. Medical Schools.* Washington, DC: National Academy of Sciences, 1985.

210. Zeisel, Steven H. and Claudia S. Plaisted, "CD-Roms for Nutrition Education," *Journal of American College of Nutrition* 18 (1999): 287.

211. Fairfield, Kathleen M., et al., "A Prospective Study of Dietary Lactose and Ovarian Cancer," *International Journal of Cancer* 110 (2004): 271–77.

212. Genkinger, Jeanine M., et al., "Dairy Products and Ovarian Cancer: A Pooled Analysis of 12 Cohort Studies," *Cancer Epidemiology, Biomarkers and Prevention* 15 (2006): 364–72.

213. Larsson, Susanna C., Nicola Orsini, and Alicja Wolk, "Milk, Milk Products and Lactose Intake and Ovarian Cancer Risk: A Meta-Analysis of Epidemiological Studies," *International Journal of Cancer* 118, no. 2 (2006): 431–41.

214. Virtanen, Suvi M., et al., "Cow's Milk Consumption, Hla-Dqb1 Genotype, and Type 1 Diabetes: A Nested Case-Control Study of Siblings of Children with Diabetes. Childhood Diabetes in Finland Study Group," *Diabetes* 49, no. 6 (2000): 912–17.

215. Akerblom, Hans K. and Mikael Knip, "Putative Environmental Factors in Type 1 Diabetes," *Diabetes Metabolism Review* 14, no. 1 (1998): 31–67.

216. Karjalainen, J., et al., "A Bovine Albumin Peptide as a Possible Trigger of Insulin-Dependent Diabetes Mellitus," *New England Journal of Medicine* 327, no. 5 (1992): 302–7.

217. Scott, Fraser W., "Cow Milk and Insulin-Dependent Diabetes Mellitus: Is There a Relationship?" *American Journal of Clinical Nutrition* 51, no. 3 (1990): 489–91.

218. Hankinson, Susan E., et al., "Circulating Concentrations of Insulin-Like Growth Factor 1 and Risk of Breast Cancer," *Lancet* 351.9113 (1998): 1393–96.

219. Cardogan J., et al., "Milk Intake and Bone Mineral Acquisition in Adolescent Girls: Randomised, Controlled Intervention Trial," *British Medical Journal* 315, no. 7118 (1997): 1255–60.

220. Chan, June M., et al., "Plasma Insulin-Like Growth Factor-1 [Igf-1] and Prostate Cancer Risk: A Prospective Study," *Science* 279 (1998): 563–66.

221. Heaney, R. P., et al., "Dietary Changes Favorably Affect Bone Remodeling in Older Adults," *Journal of the American Dietetic Association* 99, no. 10 (1999): 1228–33.

222. Scrimshaw, Nevin S. and Edwina B. Murray, "The Acceptability of Milk and Milk Products in Populations with a High Prevalence of Lactose Intolerance," *American Journal of Clinical Nutrition* 48 (1988): 1083–85.

223. Kirk, Andrea B., et al., "Perchlorate in Milk," *Environmental Science and Technology* 37, no. 21 (2003): 4979–81.

224. Environmental Protection Agency (EPA), "Perchlorate Environmental Contamination," *NCEA-1-0503* (2002).

225. *New York Times Magazine*, February 1, 1998.

226. Lanou, Amy Joy, Susan E. Berkow, and Neal D. Barnard, "Calcium, Dairy Products, and Bone Health in Children and Young Adults: A Reevaluation of the Evidence," *Pediatrics* 115, no. 3 (2005): 736–43.

227. Weinsier, Roland L. and Carlos L. Krumdieck, "Dairy Foods and Bone Health: Examination of the Evidence," *American Journal of Clinical Nutrition* 72 (2000): 681–89.

228. Feskanich, Diane, et al., "Milk, Dietary Calcium, and Bone Fractures in Women: A 12-Year Prospective Study," *American Journal of Public Health* 87, no. 6 (1997): 992–97.

229. Midkiff, Ken, *The Meat You Eat. How Corporate Farming Has Endangered America's Food Supply*. New York: St. Martin's Press, 2004.

230. Mulkern, Anne C. "When Advocates Become Regulators." *Denver Post*, May 24, 2004.

231. Drewnowski, Adam, "The Real Contribution of Added Sugars and Fats to Obesity," *Epidemiology Reviews* 29 (2007): 160–71.

232. Popkin, Barry M., "The Nutrition Transition and Obesity in the Developing World," *Journal of Nutrition* 131, no. 3 (2001): 871S–73S.
233. CNN.com. "Surgeon General to Cops: Put Down the Donuts." August 18, 2004. http://www.cnn.com/2003/HEALTH/02/28/obesity.police/index.html
234. Mokdad, Ali H., et al., "Actual Causes of Death in the United States, 2000," *Journal of the American Medical Association* 291 (2004): 1238–45.
235. Flegal, Katherine M., et al., "Excess Deaths Associated with Underweight, Overweight, and Obesity," *Journal of the American Medical Association* 293, no. 15 (2005): 1861–67.
236. Gibbs, W., "Obesity: An Overblown Epidemic?" *Scientific American.* Vol June; 2005.
237. Flegal, Katherine M., et al., "Supplement: Response To 'Can Fat Be Fit,'" *Scientific American* January 2008.
238. Al Snih, Soham, et al., "The Effect of Obesity on Disability vs Mortality in Older Americans," *Archives of Internal Medicine* 167.8 (2007): 774–80.
239. Dolan, Chantal M., et al., "Associations between Body Composition, Anthropometry, and Mortality in Women Aged 65 Years and Older," *American Journal of Public Health* 97, no. 5 (2007): 913–18.
240. Janssen, Ian, "Morbidity and Mortality Risk Associated with an Overweight BMI in Older Men and Women," *Obesity (Silver Spring)* 15, no. 7 (2007): 1827–40.
241. McTigue, Kathleen, et al., "Mortality and Cardiac and Vascular Outcomes in Extremely Obese Women," *Journal of the American Medical Association* 296, no. 1 (2006): 79–86.
242. Gu, Dongfeng, et al., "Body Weight and Mortality among Men and Women in China," *Journal of the American Medical Association* 295, no. 7 (2006): 776–83.
243. Arndt, Volker, et al., "Body Mass Index and Premature Mortality in Physically Heavily Working Men-a Ten-Year Follow-up of 20,000 Construction Workers," *Journal of Occupational and Environmental Medicine* 49, no. 8 (2007): 913–21.
244. Laara, Esa and Paula Rantakallio, "Body Size and Mortality in Women: A 29 Year Follow up of 12,000 Pregnant Women in Northern Finland," *Journal of Epidemiology and Community Health* 50, no. 4 (1996): 408–14.
245. Waaler, Hans T., "Height and Weight and Mortality: The Norwegian Experience," *Acta Medica Scandinavica Supplementum* 679 (1984): 1–56.
246. McGee, Daniel L., "Body Mass Index and Mortality: A Meta-Analysis Based on Person-Level Data from Twenty-Six Observational Studies," *Annals of Epidemiology* 15, no. 2 (2005): 87–97.

248. Olshansky, S. Jay, et al., "A Potential Decline in Life Expectancy in the United States in the 21st Century," *New England Journal of Medicine* 352, no. 11 (2005): 1138–45.

249. National Center for Health Statistics. *Health, United States, 2007. With Chartbook on Trends in the Health of Americans.* Hyattsville, MD, 2007.

250. Rosamond, W., et al., "Heart Disease and Stroke Statistics 2008 Update. A Report from the American Heart Association Statistics Committee and Stroke Statistics Subcommittee," *Circulation* (2007).

251. Mathers, Colin D. and Dejan Loncar, "Projections of Global Mortality and Burden of Disease from 2002 to 2030," *PLoS Med* 3, no. 11 (2006): 2011–29.

252. Social Security Administration. "Periodic Life Table." 2007 (updated 7/9/07).

253. Wildman, R. P., P. Muntner, K. Reynolds, et al., The obese without cardiometabolic risk factor clustering and the normal weight with cardiometabolic risk factor clustering: prevalence and correlates of 2 phenotypes among the US population (NHANES 1999-2004). *Arch. Intern. Med.* Aug 11 2008;168(15):1617-1624.

254. Iacobellis, G., M. C. Ribaudo, A. Zappaterreno, C. V. Iannucci, and F. Leonetti, Prevalence of uncomplicated obesity in an Italian obese population. *Obes. Res.* Jun 2005;13(6):1116-1122.

255. Lotutu, P. A., et al., "Male Pattern Baldness and Coronary Heart Disease," *Archives of Internal Medicine* 160 (2000): 165–71.

256. Barlow, Carolyn E., et al., "Physical Fitness, Mortality and Obesity," *International Journal of Obesity* 19 (Supplement 4) (1995): S41–S44.

257. Lee, Chong Do, Steven N. Blair, and Andrew S. Jackson, "Cardiorespiratory Fitness, Body Composition, and All-Cause and Cardiovascular Disease Mortality in Men," *American Journal of Clinical Nutrition* 69, no. 3 (1999): 373–80.

258. Farrell, Stephen W., et al., "The Relation of Body Mass Index, Cardiorespiratory Fitness, and All-Cause Mortality in Women," *Obesity Research* 10 (2002): 417–23.

259. Church, Timothy S., et al., "Exercise Capacity and Body Composition as Predictors of Mortality among Men with Diabetes," *Diabetes Care* 27, no. 1 (2004): 83–8.

260. Blair, Steven N. and Suzanne Brodney, "Effects of Physical Inactivity and Obesity on Morbidity and Mortality: Current Evidence and Research Issues," *Medicine and Science in Sports and Exercise* 31, no. 11 (Supplement) (1999): S646–62.

261. Gulati, Martha, et al., "Exercise Capacity and the Risk of Death in Women: The St James Women Take Heart Project," *Circulation* 108, no. 13 (2003): 1554–59.

262. Sui, Xuemei, et al., "Cardiorespiratory Fitness and Adiposity as Mortality Predictors in Older Adults," *Journal of the American Medical Association* 298, no. 21 (2007): 2507–16.
263. Fraser, Laura, *Losing It. False Hopes and Fat Profits in the Diet Industry.* New York: Plume, 1998.
264. Frishman, William H., et al., "Cardiovascular Manifestations of Substance Abuse: Part 2: Alcohol, Amphetamines, Heroin, Cannabis, and Caffeine," *Heart Disease* 5, no. 4 (2003): 253–71.
265. Olson, Marian B., et al., "Weight Cycling and High-Density Lipoprotein Cholesterol in Women: Evidence of an Adverse Effect," *Journal of the American College of Cardiology* 36 (2000): 1565–71.
266. Fontaine, Kevin R., et al., "Body Weight and Health Care among Women in the General Population," *Archives of Family Medicine* 7, no. 4 (1998): 381–84.
267. Olson, C. L., H. D. Schumaker, and B. P. Yawn, "Overweight Women Delay Medical Care," *Archives of Family Medicine* 3, no. 10 (1994): 888–92.
268. Amy, N., A. Aalborg, P. Lyons, and L. Keranen, Barriers to routine gynecological cancer screening for White and African-American obese women. *Int. J. Obes. Relat. Metab. Disord.* 2006;30(1):147-155.
269. Puhl, R., and K. Brownell Bias, discrimination and obesity. *Obes. Res.* 2001;9(12):788-805.
270. Puhl, R. M., and C. A. Heuer, The stigma of obesity: a review and update. *Obesity (Silver Spring).* May 2009;17(5):941-964.
271. Griggs, J. J., M. E. Sorbero, and G. H. Lyman, Undertreatment of obese women receiving breast cancer chemotherapy. *Arch. Intern. Med.* Jun 13 2005;165(11):1267-1273.
272. Flegal, Katherine M., et al., "Overweight and Obesity in the United States: Prevalence and Trends, 1960–1994," *International Journal of Obesity* 22 (1998): 39–47.
273. Brook, Robert D., "Is Air Pollution a Cause of Cardiovascular Disease? Updated Review and Controversies," *Review of Environmental Health* 22, no. 2 (2007): 115–37.
274. Ranjit, Nalini, et al., "Psychosocial Factors and Inflammation in the Multi-Ethnic Study of Atherosclerosis," *Archives of Internal Medicine* 167, no. 2 (2007): 174–81.
275. Chandola, T., E. Brunner, and M. Marmot, Chronic stress at work and the metabolic syndrome: prospective study. *BMJ.* Mar 4 2006;332(7540):521-525.
276. McEwen, B. S., Protective and damaging effects of stress mediators. *N. Engl. J. Med.* Jan 15 1998;338(3):171-179.

277. Vitaliano, P. P., J. M. Scanlan, J. Zhang, M. V. Savage, I. B. Hirsch, and I. C. Siegler, A path model of chronic stress, the metabolic syndrome, and coronary heart disease. *Psychosom. Med.* May-Jun 2002;64(3):418–435.

278. Muennig, Peter, et al., "Gender and the Burden of Disease Attributable to Obesity," *American Journal of Public Health* 96, no. 9 (2006): 1662–68.

279. Fontaine, Kevin R., et al., "Years of Life Lost Due to Obesity," *Journal of the American Medical Association* 289, no. 2 (2003): 187–93.

280. Paeratakul, Sahasporn, et al., "Sex, Race/Ethnicity, Socioeconomic Status, and BMI in Relation to Self-Perception of Overweight," *Obesity Research* 10, no. 5 (2002): 345–50.

281. Cash, Thomas F., et al., "Measuring 'Negative Body Image': Validation of the Body Image Disturbance Questionnaire in a Nonclinical Population," *Body Image* 1, no. 4 (2004): 363–72.

282. Muennig, Peter, et al., "I Think Therefore I Am: Perceived Ideal Weight as a Determinant of Health," *American Journal of Public Health* March (2008).

283. Puhl, R. M., T. Andreyeva, and K. D. Brownell, Perceptions of weight discrimination: prevalence and comparison to race and gender discrimination in America. *Int J Obes* (Lond). Mar 4 2008.

284. Akram, D. S., et al. *Obesity: Preventing and Managing the Global Epidemic. Report of a WHO Consultation on Obesity.* Geneva, Switzerland: World Health Organization, 1997.

285. Ernsberger, Paul and Richard J. Koletsky, "Biomedical Rationale for a Wellness Approach to Obesity: An Alternative to a Focus on Weight Loss," *Journal of Social Issues* 55, no. 2 (1999): 221–60.

286. Ernsberger, Paul and D. O. Nelson, "Effects of Fasting and Refeeding on Blood Pressure Are Determined by Nutritional State, Not by Body Weight Change," *American Journal of Hypertension* (1988): 153S–57S.

287. Guagnano, M. T., et al., "Weight Fluctuations Could Increase Blood Pressure in Android Obese Women," *Clinical Sciences (London)* 96, no. 6 (1999): 677–80.

288. Ernsberger, Paul, et al., "Consequences of Weight Cycling in Obese Spontaneously Hypertensive Rats," *American Journal of Physiology: Regulatory, Integrative and Comparative Physiology* 270 (1996): R864–R72.

289. Ernsberger, Paul, et al., "Refeeding Hypertension in Obese Spontaneously Hypertensive Rats," *Hypertension* 24 (1994): 699–705.

290. Chernin, K., *The Obsession: Reflections on the Tyranny of Slenderness.* New York: Harper & Row, 1981.

291. Barrett-Connor, Elizabeth and K. T. Khaw, "Is Hypertension More Benign When Associated with Obesity?" *Circulation* 72 (1985): 53–60.

292. Cambien, Francois, et al., "Is the Relationship between Blood Pressure and Cardiovascular Risk Dependent on Body Mass Index?" *American Journal of Epidemiology* 122 (1985): 434–42.

293. Weinsier, Roland L., et al., "Body Fat: Its Relationship to Coronary Heart Disease, Blood Pressure, Lipids, and Other Risk Factors Measured in a Large Male Population," *American Journal of Medicine* 61 (1976): 815–24.

294. Uretsky, Seth, et al., "Obesity Paradox in Patients with Hypertension and Coronary Artery Disease," *American Journal of Medicine* 120, no. 10 (2007): 863–70.

295. Kang, Xingping, et al., "Impact of Body Mass Index on Cardiac Mortality in Patients with Known or Suspected Coronary Artery Disease Undergoing Myocardial Perfusion Single-Photon Emission Computed Tomography," *Journal of the American College of Cardiology* 47, no. 7 (2006): 1418–26.

296. Nowson, Caryl A., et al., "Blood Pressure Change with Weight Loss Is Affected by Diet Type in Men," *American Journal of Clinical Nutrition* 81, no. 5 (2005): 983–89.

297. McDonald, K. Colleen, Jean C. Blackwell, and Linda N. Meurer, "Clinical Inquiries. What Lifestyle Changes Should We Recommend for the Patient with Newly Diagnosed Hypertension?" *Journal of Family Practice* 55, no. 11 (2006): 991–93.

298. Delichatsios, Helen K. and Francine K. Welty, "Influence of the Dash Diet and Other Low-Fat, High-Carbohydrate Diets on Blood Pressure," *Current Atherosclerosis Reports* 7, no. 6 (2005): 446–54.

299. Gregg, Edward W., et al., "Secular Trends in Cardiovascular Disease Risk Factors According to Body Mass Index in Us Adults," *Journal of the American Medical Association* 293, no. 15 (2005): 1868–74.

300. McGill, Henry C., Jr., *The Geographic Pathology of Atherosclerosis.* Baltimore: Williams and Wilkins, 1986.

301. Montenegro, M. R. and L. A. Solberg, "Obesity, Body Weight, Body Length, and Atherosclerosis," *Laboratory Investigations* 18 (1968): 134–43.

302. Gaesser, Glenn, *Big Fat Lies: The Truth About Your Weight and Your Health.* Carlsbad: Gurze Books, 2002.

303. Patel, Y. C., D. A. Eggen, and Jack P. Strong, "Obesity, Smoking and Atherosclerosis. A Study of Interassociations," *Atherosclerosis* 36, no. 4 (1980): 481–90.

304. Warnes, C. A. and W. C. Roberts, "The Heart in Massive (More Than 300 Pounds or 136 Kilograms) Obesity: Analysis of 12 Patients Studied at Necropsy," *American Journal of Cardiology* 54, no. 8 (1984): 1087–91.

305. Chambless, Lloyd E., et al., "Risk Factors for Progression of Common Carotid Atherosclerosis: The Atherosclerosis Risk in Communities Study, 1987–1998," *American Journal of Epidemiology* 155, no. 1 (2002): 38–47.

306. Salonen, Riitta and Jukka T. Salonen, "Progression of Carotid Atherosclerosis and Its Determinants: A Population-Based Ultrasonography Study," *Atherosclerosis* 81, no. 1 (1990): 33–40.

307. Applegate, William B., J. P. Hughes, and R. Vander Zwaag, "Case-Control Study of Coronary Heart Disease Risk Factors in the Elderly," *Journal of Clinical Epidemiology* 44, no. 4–5 (1991): 409–15.

308. Lissner, Lauren, et al., "Variability of Body Weight and Health Outcomes in the Framingham Population," *New England Journal of Medicine* 324, no. 26 (1991): 1839–44.

309. Bray, George A., "Health Hazards of Obesity," *Endocrinology and Metabolism. Clinics of North America* 25, no. 4 (1996): 907–19.

310. Pi-Sunyer, F. Xavier, "Medical Hazards of Obesity," *Annals of Internal Medicine* 119 (1993): 655–60.

311. Neel, James V., Alan B. Weder, and Stevo Julius, "Type 2 Diabetes, Essential Hypertension, and Obesity As "Syndromes of Impaired Genetic Homeostasis": The 'Thrifty Genotype' Hypothesis Enters the 21st Century," *Perspectives in Biology and Medicine* 42, no. 1 (1998): 44–74.

312. Bennett, Peter H., "More About Obesity and Diabetes," *Diabetologia* 29. no. 10 (1986): 753–54.

313. Ciliska, Donna, et al., "A Review of Weight Loss Interventions for Obese People with Non-Insulin Dependent Diabetes Mellitus," *Canadian Journal of Diabetes Care* 19 (1995): 10–15.

314. Klein, Samuel, et al., "Absence of an Effect of Liposuction on Insulin Action and Risk Factors for Coronary Heart Disease," *New England Journal of Medicine* 350, no. 25 (2004): 2549–57.

315. Barnard, R. James, T. Jung, and S. B. Inkeles, "Diet and Exercise in the Treatment of Niddm," *Diabetes Care* 17 (1994): 1469–72.

316. Barnard, R. James, et al., "Role of Diet and Exercise in the Management of Hyperinsulinemia and Associated Atherosclerotic Risk Factors," *American Journal of Cardiology* 69 (1992): 440–44.

317. Boule, Normand G., et al., "Effects of Exercise on Glycemic Control and Body Mass in Type 2 Diabetes Mellitus: A Meta-Analysis of Controlled Clinical Trials," *Journal of the American Medical Association* 286, no. 10 (2001): 1218–27.

318. Gaesser, Glenn A., "Weight Loss for the Obese: Panacea or Pound-Foolish?" *Quest* 56 (2004): 12–27.

319. Ross, C., Robert D. Langer, and Elizabeth Barrett-Connor, "Given Diabetes, Is Fat Better Than Thin?" *Diabetes Care* 20, no. 4 (1997): 650–2.

320. American Institute for Cancer Research. *Food, Nutrition, Physical Activity, and the Prevention of Cancer: A Global Perspective. The Second Expert Report.* Washington, DC, 2007.

321. BBC World Report Radio. Is Obesity-Cancer Link Fear-Mongering?November 5, 2009.

322. Flegal, Katherine M., et al., "Cause-Specific Excess Deaths Associated with Underweight, Overweight, and Obesity," *Journal of the American Medical Association* 298, no. 17 (2007): 2028–37.

323. Wolf, Anne M. and Graham A. Colditz, "Current Estimates of the Economic Cost of Obesity in the United States," *Obesity Research* 6, no. 2 (1998): 97–106.

324. Barrett-Connor, Elizabeth L., "Obesity, Atherosclerosis and Coronary Artery Disease," *Annals of Internal Medicine* 103 (1985): 1010–19.

325. Srinivasan Beddhu, "The Body Mass Index Paradox and an Obesity, Inflammation, and Atherosclerosis Syndrome in Chronic Kidney Disease," *Seminars in Dialysis* 17, no. 3 (2004): 229–32.

326. Ernsberger, Paul and Paul Haskew, "Health Implications of Obesity: An Alternative View," *Journal of Obesity and Weight Regulation* 9, no. 2 (1987): 39–40.

327. Lavie, Carl J., Richard V. Milani, and Hector O. Ventura, "Obesity, Heart Disease, and Favorable Prognosis—Truth or Paradox?" *American Journal of Medicine* 120, no. 10 (2007): 825–26.

328. Gruberg, Luis, et al., "Impact of Body Mass Index on the Outcome of Patients with Multivessel Disease Randomized to Either Coronary Artery Bypass Grafting or Stenting in the Arts Trial: The Obesity Paradox II?" *American Journal of Cardiology* 95, no. 4 (2005): 439–44.

329. Lavie, Carl J., et al., "Body Composition and Prognosis in Chronic Systolic Heart Failure: The Obesity Paradox," *American Journal of Cardiology* 91, no. 7 (2003): 891–94.

330. Schmidt, Darren S. and Abdulla K. Salahudeen, "Obesity-Survival Paradox—Still a Controversy?" *Seminars in Dialysis* 20, no. 6 (2007): 486–92.

331. Kulminski, Alexander M., et al., "Body Mass Index and 9-Year Mortality in Disabled and Nondisabled Older U.S. Individuals," *Journal of the American Geriatrics Society* (2007).

332. Ogden, C., M. Carroll, M. McDowell, and K. Flegal, *Obesity Among Adults in the United States - No Statistically Significant Change Since*

2003-2004. Hyattsville, MD: National Center for Health Statistics; November 2007.

333. National Center for Health Statistics. http://www.cdc.gov/nchs/about/major/nhanes/datalink.htm. Accessed January 3, 2008.

334. Flegal, Katherine M., et al., "Prevalence and Trends in Obesity among US Adults, 1999–2000," *Journal of the American Medical Association* 288 (2002): 1723–27.

335. Ogden, C. L., M. D. Carroll, L. R. Curtin, M. M. Lamb, and K. M. Flegal, Prevalence of High Body Mass Index in US Children and Adolescents, 2007-2008. *JAMA.* 2010:242–249.

336. Ogden, Cynthia L., et al., "Mean Body Weight, Height, and Body Mass Index, United States 1960–2002," *Advance Data* 347 (2004): 1–17.

337. Gaesser, G., *Big Fat Lies.* New York: Fawcett Columbine; 1996.

338. Williamson, David F., et al., "Prospective Study of Intentional Weight Loss and Mortality in Never-Smoking Overweight U.S. White Women Aged 40–64 Years," *American Journal of Epidemiology* 141 (1995): 1128–41.

339. Yaari, Shlomit and Uri Goldbourt, "Voluntary and Involuntary Weight Loss: Associations with Long Term Mortality in 9,228 Middle-Aged and Elderly Men," *American Journal of Epidemiology* 148 (1998): 546–55.

340. Diehr, Paula, et al., "Body Mass Index and Mortality in Nonsmoking Older Adults: The Cardiovascular Health Study," *American Journal of Public Health* 88 (1998): 623–29.

341. French, S. A., et al., "Prospective Study of Intentionality of Weight Loss and Mortality in Older Women: The Iowa Women's Health Study," *American Journal of Epidemiology* 149 (1999): 504–15.

342. Williamson, David F., et al., "Prospective Study of Intentional Weight Loss and Mortality in Overweight White Men Aged 40–64 Years," *American Journal of Epidemiology* 149, no. 6 (1999): 491–503.

343. Williamson, David F., et al., "Intentional Weight Loss and Mortality in Overweight Individuals with Diabetes," *Diabetes Care* 23 (2000): 1499–504.

344. National Institutes of Health (NIH), "Methods for Voluntary Weight Loss and Control (Technology Assessment Conference Panel)," *Annals of Internal Medicine* 116, no. 11 (1992): 942–49.

345. Gaesser, Glenn, "Thinness and Weight Loss: Beneficial or Detrimental to Longevity," *Medicine and Science in Sports and Exercise* 31, no. 8 (1999): 1118–28.

346. Dulloo, Abdul G., Jean Jacquet, and Jean-Pierre Montani, "Pathways from Weight Fluctuations to Metabolic Diseases: Focus on Maladap-

tive Thermogenesis During Catch-up Fat," *International Journal of Obesity and Related Metabolic Disorders* 26 (Supplement 2) (2002): S46–57.

347. Miller, Wayne C., "How Effective Are Traditional Dietary and Exercise Interventions for Weight Loss?" *Medicine and Science in Sports and Exercise* 31, no. 8 (1999): 1129–34.

348. Wayne C. Miller, "Fitness and Fatness in Relation to Health: Implications for a Paradigm Shift," *Journal of Social Issues* 55, no. 2 (1999): 207–19.

349. Dengel, J. L., Leslie I. Katzel, and Andrew P. Goldberg, "Effect of an American Heart Association Diet, with or without Weight Loss, on Lipids in Obese Middle-Aged and Older Men," *American Journal of Clinical Nutrition* 62 (1995): 715–21.

350. Stunkard, Albert J., et al., "An Adoption Study of Human Obesity," *New England Journal of Medicine* 314, no. 4 (1986): 193–98.

351. Stunkard, Albert J., T. T. Foch, and Zdenek Hrubec, "A Twin Study of Human Obesity," *Journal of the American Medical Association* 256, no. 1 (1986): 51–54.

352. Stunkard, Albert J., et al., "The Body-Mass Index of Twins Who Have Been Reared Apart," *New England Journal of Medicine* 322 (1990): 1483–87.

353. Allison, David B., et al., "The Heritability of Body Mass Index among an International Sample of Monozygotic Twins Reared Apart," *International Journal of Obesity and Related Metabolic Disorders* 20, no. 6 (1996): 501–6.

354. Douglas, K., "Supersize This: Some More Susceptible to Obesity Than Others," *New Scientist* (2007).

355. Nystrom, Fredrik. *Gut*. Accepted for publication January 2008.

356. Williams, Paul T., et al., "Concordant Lipoprotein and Weight Responses to Dietary Fat Change in Identical Twins with Divergent Exercise Levels," *American Journal of Clinical Nutrition* 82 (2005): 181–87.

357. Poehlman, Eric T., et al., "Heredity and Changes in Body Composition and Adipose Tissue Metabolism after Short-Term Exercise-Training," *European Journal of Applied Physiology* 56, no. 4 (1987): 398–402.

358. Bouchard, C., *The Journal of the Federation of American Societies for Experimental Biology* (1992): 1647 (Abstract).

359. Mann, Traci, et al., "Medicare's Search for Effective Obesity Treatments: Diets Are Not the Answer," *American Psychologist* 62, no. 3 (2007): 220–33.

360. Garner, David and Susan Wooley, "Confronting the Failure of Behavioral and Dietary Treatments for Obesity," *Clinical Psychology Review* 11 (1991): 748–54.

361. Wing, Rena R. and James O. Hill, "Successful Weight Loss Maintenance," *Annual Review of Nutrition* 21 (2001): 323–41.
362. Ikeda, Joanne, et al., "The National Weight Control Registry: A Critique," *Journal of Nutrition Education and Behavior* 37, no. 4 (2005): 203–5.
363. Shick, S. M., et al., "Persons Successful at Long-Term Weight Loss and Maintenance Continue to Consume a Low-Energy, Low-Fat Diet," *Journal of the American Dietetic Association* 98, no. 4 (1998): 408–13.
364. Neighbors, Lori A. and Jeffery Sobal, "Prevalence and Magnitude of Body Weight and Shape Dissatisfaction among University Students," *Eating Behavior* 8, no. 4 (2007): 429–39.
365. Marketdata Enterprises. *The U.S. Weight Loss and Diet Control Market (Ninth Edition)*. Lynbrook, N.Y., 2009.
366. Oliver, J. Eric, *Fat Politics: The Real Story Behind America's Obesity Epidemic*. New York: Oxford University Press, 2006.
367. Marsh, P., *An epidemic of confusion:* Social Issues Research Centre;2005.
368. Ernsberger, Paul and Richard J. Koletsky, "Weight Cycling," *Journal of the American Medical Association* 273, no. 13 (1995): 998–99.
369. National Institutes of Health National Task Force on the Prevention and Treatment of Obesity, "Long-Term Pharmacotherapy in the Management of Obesity," *Journal of the American Medical Association* 276, no. 23 (1996): 1907–15.
370. National Institutes of Health. *Clinical Guidelines on the Identification, Evaluation, and Treatment of Overweight and Obesity in Adults: The Evidence Report*, 1998.
371. Andres, Reubin, "Beautiful Hypotheses and Ugly Facts: The BMI-Mortality Association," *Obesity Research* 7, no. 4 (1999): 417–19.
372. Troiano, R. P., et al., "The Relationship between Body Weight and Mortality: A Quantitative Analysis of Combined Information," *International Journal of Obesity and Related Metabolic Disorders* 20 (1996): 63–75.
373. Stern, Judith S., Comment originally made in 1999. Verified in personal communication August 2007.
374. James, Philip, "The Worldwide Obesity Epidemic," *Obesity Research* 4 (2001).
375. Mundy, Alicia, *Dispensing with the Truth*. New York: St. Martin's Press, 2001.
376. Campos, Paul, *The Diet Myth: Why America's Obsession with Weight Is Hazardous to Your Health*. New York: Gotham Books, 2004.
377. Basham, Patrick, Gio Gori, and John Luik, *Diet Nation: Exposing the Obesity Crusade*. United Kingdom: Social Affairs Unit, 2006.

378. Moore, Thomas, *Lifespan: New Perspectives on Extending Human Longevity*. New York: Touchstone, 1993.
379. Phrasing coined by fat activist Marilyn Wann.
380. Provencher, V., C. Begin, and A. Tremblay, et al. Health-at-every-size and eating behaviors: 1-year follow-up results of a size acceptance intervention. *J. Am. Diet. Assoc.* Nov 2009;109(11):1854-1861.
381. Suggestions provided by Lesleigh Owen, Personal Communication, May 22, 2008.
382. Schwartz, Marlene B., et al., "Weight Bias among Health Professionals Specializing in Obesity," *Obesity Research* 11, no. 9 (2003): 1033–39.
383. Adolfsson, Birgitta, et al., "Are Sexual Dissatisfaction and Sexual Abuse Associated with Obesity? A Population-Based Study," *Obesity Research* 12, no. 10 (2004): 1702–9.
384. Polivy, Janet, Julie Coleman, and C. Peter Herman, "The Effect of Deprivation on Food Cravings and Eating Behavior in Restrained and Unrestrained Eaters," *International Journal of Eating Disorders* 38, no. 4 (2005): 301–9.
385. Baldaro, B., et al., "Effects of an Emotional Negative Stimulus on Cardiac, Electrogastrographic, and Respiratory Responses," *Perceptual and Motor Skills* 71, no. 2 (1990): 647–55.
386. Giduck, Sharon A., et al., "Cephalic Reflexes: Their Role in Digestion and Possible Roles in Absorption and Metabolism," *Journal of Nutrition* 117, no. 7 (1987): 1191–96.
387. Barclay, G. R., "Effect of Psychosocial Stress on Salt and Water Transport in the Human Jejunum," *Gastroenterology* 93, no. 1 (1987).
388. Zverev, Yuriy P., "Effects of Caloric Deprivation and Satiety on Sensitivity of the Gustatory System," *BMC Neuroscience* 5 no. 1 (2004): 5.
389. Hetherington, Marion, Barbara J. Rolls, and Victoria J. Burley, "The Time Course of Sensory-Specific Satiety," *Appetite* 12, no. 1 (1989): 57–68.
390. Wansink, Brian, "Can Package Size Accelerate Usage Volume?" *Journal of Marketing* 60, no. 3 (1996): 1–14.
391. Wansink, Brian and Matthew M. Cheney, "Super Bowls: Serving Bowl Size and Food Consumption," *Journal of the American Medical Association* 293, no. 14 (2005): 1727–28.
392. Wansink, Brian and Junyong Kim, "Bad Popcorn in Big Buckets: Portion Size Can Influence Intake as Much as Taste," *Journal of Nutrition Education and Behavior* 37, no. 5 (2005): 242–45.
393. Wansink, Brian, Koert van Ittersum, and James E. Painter, "Ice Cream Illusions: Bowls, Spoons, and Self-Served Portion Sizes," *American Journal of Preventive Medicine* 31, no. 3 (2006): 240–43.

394. Rolls, Barbara and Robert A. Barnett, *The Volumetrics Weight Control Plan*. 2002.

395. Kral, Tanja V. and Barbara J. Rolls, "Energy Density and Portion Size: Their Independent and Combined Effects on Energy Intake," *Physiology and Behavior* 82, no. 1 (2004): 131–38.

396. Jakicic, John M., et al., "Effects of Intermittent Exercise and Use of Home Exercise Equipment on Adherence, Weight Loss, and Fitness in Overweight Women," *Journal of the American Medical Association* 282 (1999): 1554–60.

397. Murphy, Marie H. and Adrianne Hardman, "Training Effects of Short and Long Term Bouts of Brisk Walking in Sedentary Women," *Medicine and Science in Sports and Exercise* 30 (1998): 152–57.

398. Boreham, Colin A. G., William F. M. Wallace, and Alan Nevill, "Training Effects of Accumulated Daily Stair-Climbing Exercise in Previously Sedentary Young Women," *Preventive Medicine* 30 (2000): 277–81.

399. Coleman, Karen J., et al., "Providing Sedentary Adults with Choices of Meeting Their Walking Goals," *Preventive Medicine* 28 (1999): 510–19.

400. Dunn, Andrea L., Ross E. Andersen, and John M. Jakicic, "Lifestyle Physical Activity Interventions. History, Short- and Long-Term Effects, and Recommendations," *American Journal of Preventive Medicine* 15, no. 4 (1998): 398–412.

401. Andersen, Ross E., et al., "Effects of Lifestyle Activity vs. Structured Aerobic Exercise in Obese Women," *Journal of the American Medical Association* 281 (1999): 335–40.

402. Jakicic, John M., et al., "Prescribing Exercise in Multiple Short Bouts Versus One Continuous Bout: Effects on Adherence, Cardiorespiratory Fitness, and Weight Loss in Overweight Women," *International Journal of Obesity* 19 (1995): 893–901.

403. Jakicic, John M. and Rena R. Wing, "Strategies to Improve Exercise Adherence: Effect of Short-Bouts Versus Long-Bouts of Exercise," *Medicine and Science in Sports and Exercise* 1997, no. 29 (Supplement) (1997): S42 (abstract).

404. Elmer, Patricia J., et al., "Lifestyle Intervention: Results of the Treatment of Mild Hypertension Study (Tomhs)," *Preventive Medicine* 24 (1995): 378–88.

405. Satter, Ellyn, "Eating Competence: Nutrition Education with the Satter Eating Competence Model," *Journal of Nutrition Education and Behavior* 39 (2007): S189–S94.

406. Fisher, Jennifer O. and Leann L. Birch, "Restricting Access to Palatable Foods Affects Children's Behavioral Response, Food Selection, and Intake," *American Journal of Clinical Nutrition* 69, no. 6 (1999): 1264–72.

407. Spruijt-Metz, Donna, et al., "Relation between Mothers' Child-Feeding Practices and Children's Adiposity," *American Journal of Clinical Nutrition* 75.3 (2002): 581–86.

408. Birch, Leann L., et al., "'Clean up Your Plate': Effects of Child Feeding Practices on the Conditioning of Meal Size," *Learning and Motivation* 18 (1987): 301–17.

409. Birch, Leann L. and Jennifer O. Fisher, "Development of Eating Behaviors among Children and Adolescents," *Pediatrics* 101.3 Pt 2 (1998): 539–49.

410. Birch, Leann L., "Development of Food Acceptance Patterns," *Developmental Psychology* 26, no. 4 (1990): 515–9.

411. Gillman, Matthew W., et al., "Family Dinner and Diet Quality among Older Children and Adolescents," *Archives of Family Medicine* 9, no. 3 (2000): 235–40.

412. Eisenberg, Marla E., et al., "Correlations between Family Meals and Psychosocial Well-Being among Adolescents," *Archives of Pediatric and Adolescent Medicine* 158, no. 8 (2004): 792–96.

413. Center on Addiction and Substance Abuse. *The Importance of Family Dinners IV*. National Center on Addiction and Substance Abuse at Columbia University, 2007.

414. Center for Ecoliteracy. *Education for Sustainability. Findings from the Evaluation Study of the Edible Schoolyard*, 2003.

415. Morley, John E. and Allen S. Levine, "The Role of the Endogenous Opiates as Regulators of Appetite," *American Journal of Clinical Nutrition* 35, no. 4 (1982): 757–61.

416. Hallberg, Leif, et al., "Iron Absorption from Southeast Asian Diets. II. Role of Various Factors That Might Explain Low Absorption," *American Journal of Clinical Nutrition* 30, no .4 (1977): 539–48.

417. *Human Senses* TV Programmes, Programme 3: "Taste." BBC One. July 14, 2003.

418. Birch, Leann L., C. Johnson, and Jennifer O. Fisher, "Children's Eating: The Development of Food-Acceptance Patterns," *Young Child* 50 (1995): 71–8.

419. Pliner, Patricia, "The Effects of Mere Exposure on Liking for Edible Substances," *Appetite* 3 (1982): 283–90.

420. Unlu, Nuray Z., et al., "Carotenoid Absorption from Salad and Salsa by Humans Is Enhanced by the Addition of Avocado or Avocado Oil," *Journal of Nutrition* 135 (2005): 431–36.

421. Brown, Melody J., et al., "Carotenoid Bioavailability Is Higher from Salads Ingested with Full-Fat Than with Fat-Reduced Salad Dressings as Measured with Electrochemical Detection," *American Journal of Clinical Nutrition* 80, no. 2 (2004): 396–403.

422. Hu, Frank B., JoAnn E. Manson, and Walter C. Willett, "Types of Dietary Fat and Risk of Coronary Heart Disease: A Critical Review," *Journal of the American College of Nutrition* 20, no. 1 (2001): 5–19.

423. Hetherington, Marion M., "Pleasure and Excess: Liking for and Over-consumption of Chocolate," *Physiology and Behavior* 57, no. 1 (1995).

424. Drewnowski, Adam, "Taste Preferences and Food Intake," *Annual Review of Nutrition* 17 (1997): 237–53.

425. Rozin, Paul, E. Levine, and C. Stoess, "Chocolate Craving and Liking," *Appetite* 17, no. 3 (1991): 199–212.

426. Barnard, Neal D., et al., "Diet and Sex-Hormone Binding Globulin, Dysmenorrhea, and Premenstrual Symptoms," *Obstetrics and Gynecology* 95, no. 2 (2000): 245–50.

427. Hoegg, JoAndrea and Joseph W. Alba, "Taste Perception: More Than Meets the Tongue," *Journal of Consumer Research* 33 (2006): 490–98.

428. Robinson, Thomas N., et al., "Effects of Fast Food Branding on Young Children's Taste Preferences," *Archives of Pediatric and Adolescent Medicine* 161, no. 8 (2007): 792–97.

429. Bertino, Mary, Gary K. Beauchamp, and Karl Engelman, "Increasing Dietary Salt Alters Salt Taste Preference," *Physiology and Behavior* 38, no. 2 (1986): 203–13.

430. Beauchamp, Gary K., Mary Bertino, and Karl Engelman, "Modification of Salt Taste," *Annals of Internal Medicine* 98.5 Pt 2 (1983): 763–69.

431. Bertino, Mary, Gary K. Beauchamp, and Karl Engelman, "Long-Term Reduction in Dietary Sodium Alters the Taste of Salt," *American Journal of Clinical Nutrition* 36, no. 6 (1982): 1134–44.

432. Mattes, Richard D., "Fat Preference and Adherence to a Reduced-Fat Diet," *American Journal of Clinical Nutrition* 57, no. 3 (1993): 373–81.

433. Rada, Pedro, Nicole M. Avena, and Bartley G. Hoebel, "Daily Bingeing on Sugar Repeatedly Releases Dopamine in the Accumbens Shell," *Neuroscience* (2005).

434. Spangler, Rudolph, et al., "Opiate-Like Effects of Sugar on Gene Expression in Reward Areas of the Rat Brain," *Brain Research. Molecular Brain Research* 124, no. 2 (2004): 134–42.

435. Erlanson-Albertsson, Charlotte, "[Sugar Triggers Our Reward-System. Sweets Release Opiates Which Stimulates the Appetite for Sucrose—Insulin Can Depress It]," *Lakartidningen* 102.21 (2005): 1620–22, 1625, 1627.

436. Cottone, P., V. Sabino, M. Roberto, et al. CRF system recruitment mediates dark side of compulsive eating. *Proc. Natl. Acad. Sci. U. S. A.* Nov 24 2009;106(47):20016-20020.

437. Wang, Gene-Jack, et al., "Brain Dopamine and Obesity," *Lancet* 357.9253 (2001): 354–57.

INDEX

6-n-propylthiouracil (PROP), 237–240

A

Abbott Laboratories, 154
addictive nature of food, 247–250
adenovirus-36, 57
advertising affecting food choices, 113–120
Alli, 60–61
American Institute for Cancer Research, 136
American Medical Association, 62
American Obesity Association, 154
American Society for Metabolic and Bariatric Surgery, 62, 64–65
Amgen, 40
amino acids, 117, 247
amphetamines, 130
analyzing your eating journal, 202–208
Association for Size Diversity and Health (ASDAH), 294, 305–308, 318, 323, 329
atherosclerosis, 133–134. see also cholesterol, high
Atkins diet, 48, 89
author's HAES journey, 268–69
autonomic nervous system, 14

B

bacteroidetes, 58
bariatric surgery, 62–65, 132, 151–152
beauty as related to weight, 146–149
beets, balsamic braised, 226–227
beverages, effect on hunger, 89–90
blood pressure, high. see hypertension
body, respecting your, 173–191
Body Mass Index (BMI)
    and body image, 131
    obesity range, 124

as related to mortality, 153
relationship to cancer, 137
"report cards", 267
standards changing, 153
of twins, 142

C

calories, putting into perspective, 44–45
cancer, 54, 136–137
carbohydrates, 76–81, 241–242
Carmona, Richard, 123
celebrating your hunger, 269–270
Centers for Disease Control, 124–125, 137, 151, 152
children, establishing healthy habits for, 229–233
cholecystokinin, 237
cholesterol, high, 54. see also atherosclerosis
Community Supported Agriculture (CSA), 253
consumer's HAES journey, 264–266
context of food relating to taste, 237–240
control, internal of ideal weight. see setpoint weight
cooking, learning to enjoy, 254
corn syrup, high-fructose, 81–83, 84, 91, 105–106
cortisol, 55, 221
couch potatoes, 50–51, 55
cravings, sugar, 241–242
culture, changing weight attitudes of, 190–192
cynarin, 265

D

DASH diet, 132

■ 367 ■

ABOUT LINDA BACON, PHD

Like many men and women, Linda Bacon used to be preoccupied with her own weight. Bacon's pain and obsession about her weight fueled her determination to understand everything about weight regulation.

Bacon earned a master's degree in psychotherapy, with a specialty in eating disorders and body image, and began work as a psychotherapist. Her career led her to a greater understanding about herself and her relationship with food and weight. With questions still unanswered, Bacon went back to school to pursue a master's degree in exercise science, specializing in metabolism. Bacon continued to broaden her education and went on to complete a doctoral program in physiology with a focus in nutrition and weight regulation from the University of California, Davis.

Through all of her studies and research, Bacon continually stumbled across the same disconnect. The science of weight regulation directly contradicts cultural assumptions as well as those promoted by the "experts." Bacon's experiences and academic training led her to an entirely different paradigm in weight regulation, where she finally found relief from her painful preoccupation and developed a healthy and pleasurable relationship with her body and with food.

Bacon feels fortunate to have conquered her food and weight obsession, and empathizes with the many others engaged in their own personal battle with food and weight. She has dedicated her career towards helping others on that journey, designing the Health at Every Size program, which she tested meticulously in a clinical research study funded by the National Institutes of Health and co-sponsored by the U.S. Department of Agriculture. *Health at Every Size: The Surprising Truth About Your Weight* chronicles the remarkable findings of that study: that people can indeed overcome their weight problems and improve their health—without dieting, deprivation, or a focus on weight loss.

Bacon is currently a nutrition professor in the biology department at City College of San Francisco. She also serves as an associate nutritionist at the University of California, Davis and maintains a private consulting practice. A popular and compelling public speaker, she consistently draws large and enthusiastic crowds.

Bacon is well published in the scientific literature. She has also been a guest on national television and radio and has been cited as an expert in numerous print publications. Her credits include *Good Morning America*, ABC, ABC Nightline News, ABC 7 News, *Allure Magazine*, AOL Health, the *Atlantic*, BBC World News Radio, the *Economist*, Fox TV News, *Health Magazine*, the *Los Angeles Times*, MSNBC TV, MSN Life & Style, National Public Radio, the *New York Times*, *Newsweek*, *Prevention*, *Reuters*, *Self*, *Shape*, *U.S. News & World Report*, *The Washington Post*, WebMD, and *Women's Health*.